Clinical Immunology

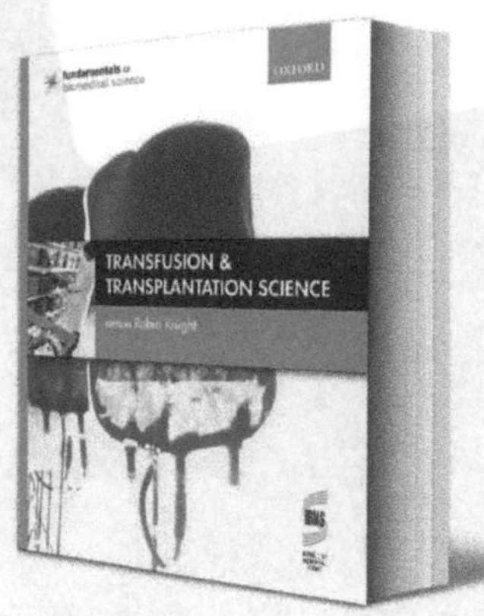
OXFORD
TRANSFUSION &
TRANSPLANTATION SCIENCE

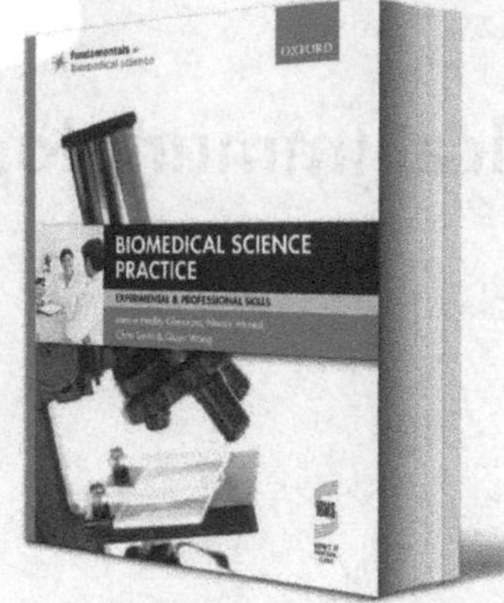
OXFORD
BIOMEDICAL SCIENCE
PRACTICE

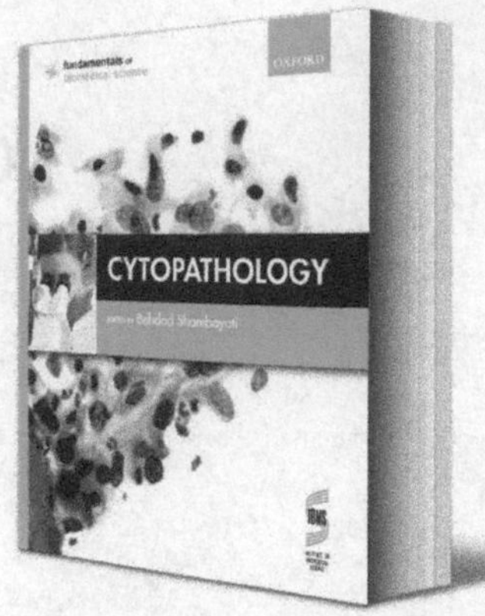
OXFORD
CYTOPATHOLOGY

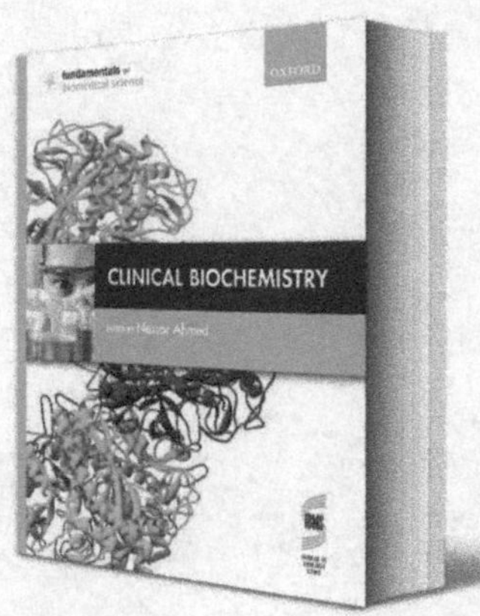
OXFORD
CLINICAL BIOCHEMISTRY

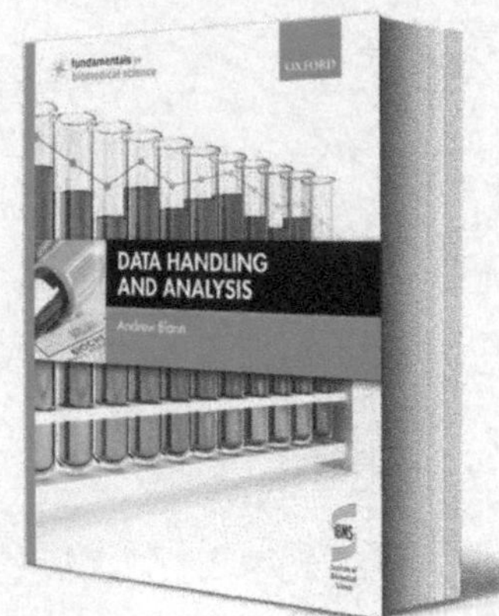
OXFORD
DATA HANDLING
AND ANALYSIS
Andrew Blann

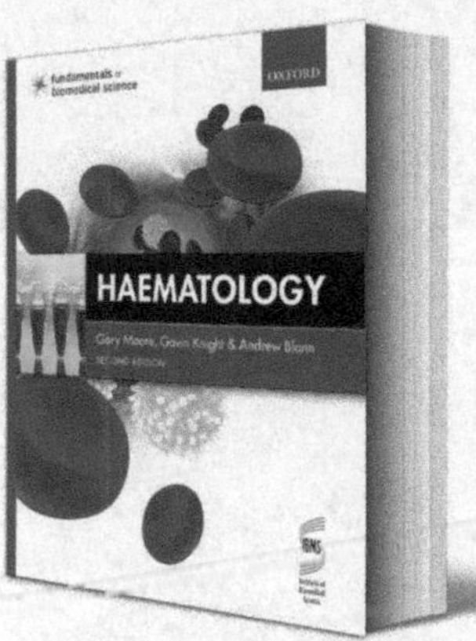
OXFORD
HAEMATOLOGY
Gary Moore, Gavin Knight & Andrew Blann

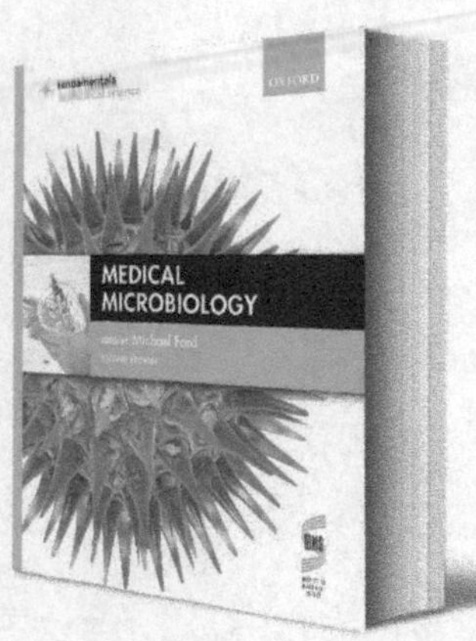
OXFORD
MEDICAL
MICROBIOLOGY

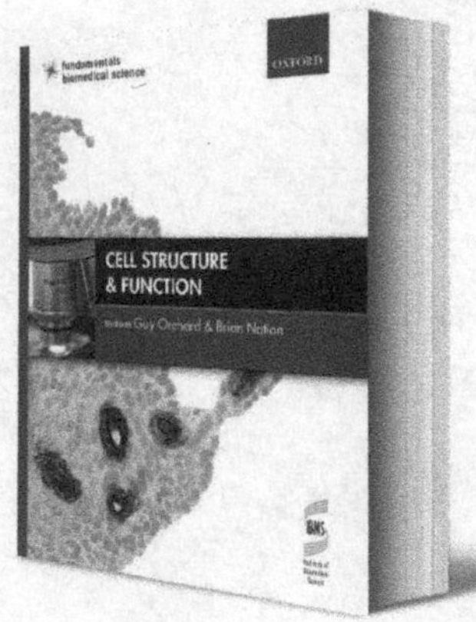
OXFORD
CELL STRUCTURE
& FUNCTION
Guy Orchard & Brian Nation

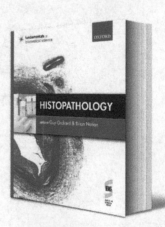
OXFORD
HISTOPATHOLOGY
Guy Orchard & Brian Nation

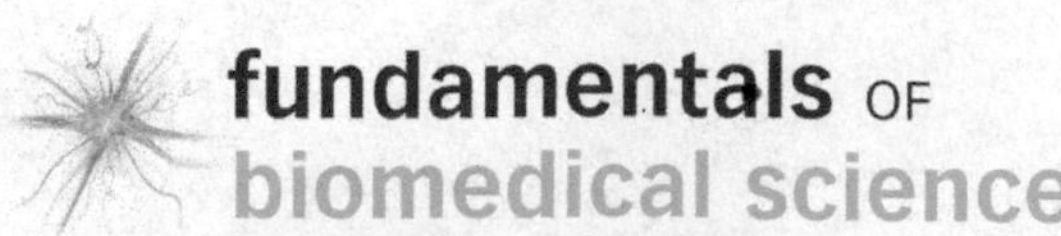
fundamentals OF
biomedical science

Fundamentals of Biomedical Science

Clinical Immunology

Second edition

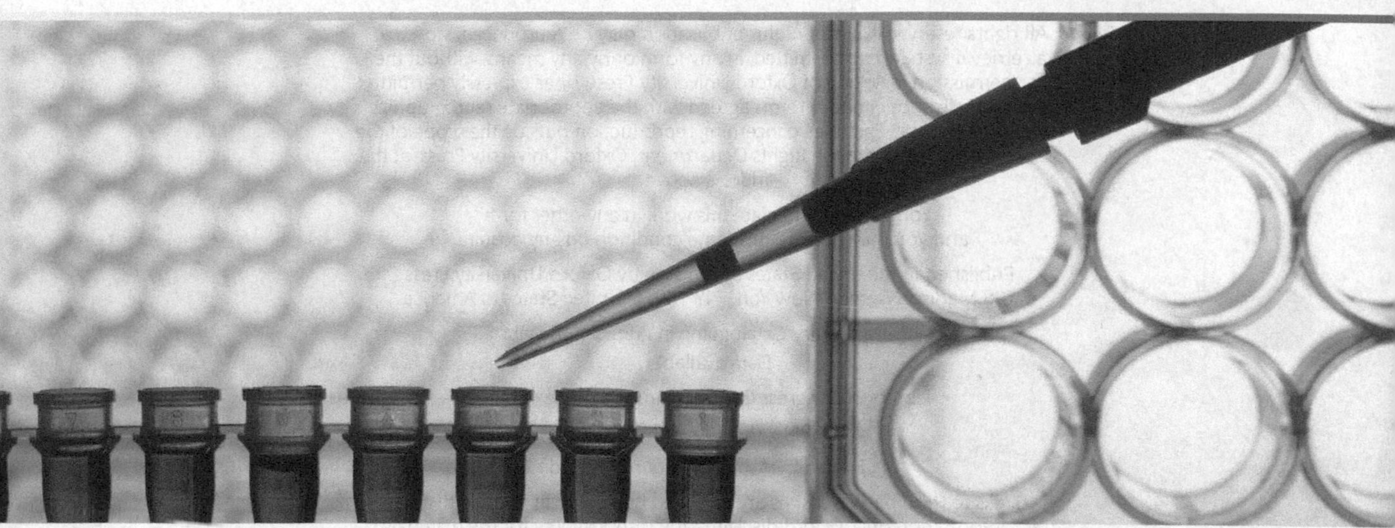

Edited by

Angela Hall
Department of Immunology, Imperial College Healthcare NHS Trusts

Chris Scott
Department of Immunology, Bart's and the London NHS Trust

Matthew Buckland
Department of Immunology, Bart's and the London NHS Trust

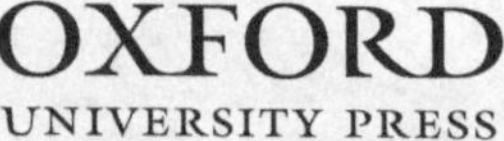

OXFORD
UNIVERSITY PRESS

Great Clarendon Street, Oxford, OX2 6DP,
United Kingdom

Oxford University Press is a department of the University of Oxford. It furthers the University's objective of excellence in research, scholarship, and education by publishing worldwide. Oxford is a registered trade mark of Oxford University Press in the UK and in certain other countries

First edition 2010

Published in the United States of America by Oxford University Press
198 Madison Avenue, New York, NY 10016, United States of America

British Library Cataloguing in Publication Data
Data available

Library of Congress Control Number: 2015948895

ISBN 978-0-19-965765-0

Printed by Ashford Colour Press Ltd.

Acknowledgement

Mr Nick Davey, Imperial College Healthcare NHS Trust, for his help in checking the HLA nomenclature.

An introduction to the Fundamentals of Biomedical Science series

Biomedical Scientists form the foundation of modern healthcare, from cancer screening to diagnosing HIV, from blood transfusion for surgery to infection control. Without Biomedical Scientists, the diagnosis of disease, the evaluation of the effectiveness of treatments, and research into the causes and cures of disease would not be possible. However, the path to becoming a Biomedical Scientist is a challenging one: trainees must not only assimilate knowledge from a range of disciplines, but must understand—and demonstrate—how to apply this knowledge in a practical, hands-on environment.

The *Fundamentals of Biomedical Science* series is written to reflect the challenges of biomedical science education and training today. It blends essential basic science with insights into laboratory practice to show you how an understanding of the biology of disease is coupled to the analytical approaches that lead to diagnosis. Produced in collaboration with the Institute of Biomedical Science, the series provides coverage of the full range of disciplines to which a Biomedical Scientist might be exposed.

Learning from the series

The *Fundamentals of Biomedical Science* series draws on a range of learning features to help readers master both biomedical science theory, and biomedical science practice.

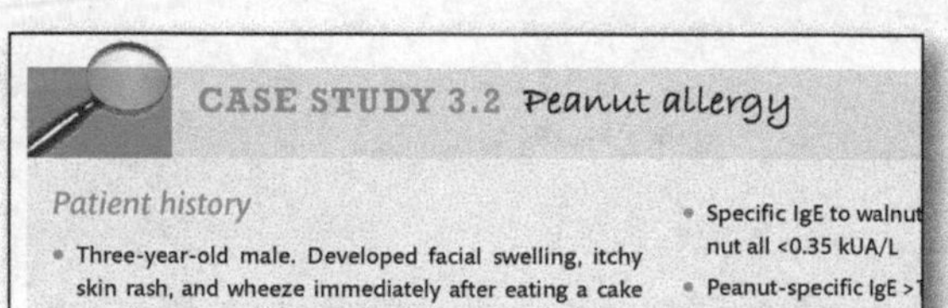

Case studies illustrate how the biomedical science theory and practice presented throughout the series relate to situations and experiences that are likely to be encountered routinely in the biomedical science laboratory.

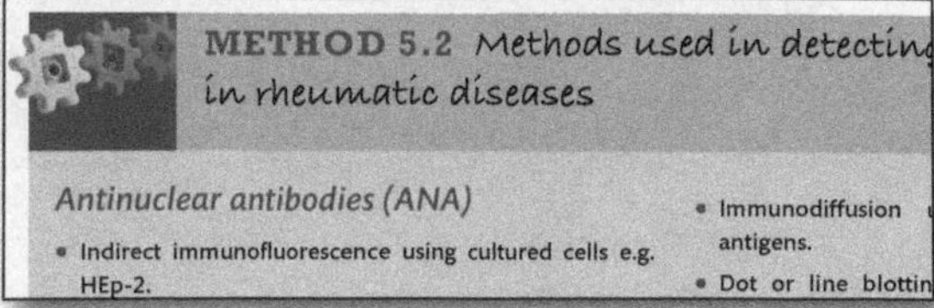

Method boxes walk through the key protocols that the reader is likely to encounter in the laboratory on a regular basis.

Clinical correlations bring relevance to the material by placing it in its clinical context.

CLINICAL CORRELATION 2.9

Are all monoclonal bands associated with myeloma?

Diseases associated with the presence of monoclonal immunoglobulin include Waldenströ macroglobulinaemia, monoclonal gammopathy of uncertain significance (MGUS), lympho chronic lymphocytic leukaemia, amyloidosis, and heavy chain disease, as well as myeloma addition benign, usually transient, monoclones may be seen in response to infection.

Key points reinforce the key concepts that the reader should master from having read the material presented, while **Summary** points act as end-of-chapter checklists for readers to verify that they have remembered correctly the principal themes and ideas presented within each chapter.

Key Point

Immunoglobulin molecules have different effector functions in different domains of the molecule.

Key terms provide on-the-page explanations of terms with which the reader may not be familiar; in addition, each title in the series features a **glossary**, in which the key terms featured in that title are collated.

However, only a minority of HCV infected patie (Ferri et al. 2002).

Cryofibrinogen

An abnormal fibrinogen that precipitates at cold temperatures and redissolves at 37 °C.

Cryofibrinogen is the result of abnormal fibrino cipitate at less than 37 °C. Ferri et al. (2002) regard ples which cause clinical symptoms indistinguisha Cryofibrinogen may also be seen in the plasma of

2.5.1 Cryoglobulin analysis

Self-check questions throughout each chapter provide the reader with a ready means of checking that they have understood the material they have just encountered; answers to self-check questions are available in the book's Online Resource Centre.

hypothyroidism (for example due to pituitary disease), and tertiary hypothyroidism (due t problem with the hypothalamus).

SELF-CHECK 7.2

Why would diseases of the pituitary or hypothalamus cause thyroid disease?

Autoimmune thyroid disease may result in an underactive thyroid (hypothyroidism) or an

Discussion questions are provided at the end of each chapter to encourage the reader to analyse and reflect on the material they have just read.

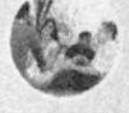

Discussion questions

9.1 Discuss the factors influencing the result of an IIF assay for anti-LKM 1 in a child.

9.2 You receive a request for 'mitochondrial antibodies please; clinically and biochemi PBC'. Your IIF result is negative for anti-mitochondrial antibody on LKS substrate. H would you proceed?

Cross references help the reader to see biomedical science as a unified discipline, making the connections between topics presented within each volume, and across all volumes in the series.

creatic islet cells, testis, oviduct, and ovary. GAD65 le for vesicular GABA production. GAD67, on the ed in the formation of cytoplasmic GABA. In the) times more abundant than GAD67 (alpha cells). s, one involved in diabetes mellitus (GAD65) and me (GAD67).

ntibodies utilizing cerebellum produces a charac- GABAergic nerve terminals of the cerebellar glo-

Cross reference

Read Chapter 7 for more information on autoimmune type 1 diabetes.

Online learning materials

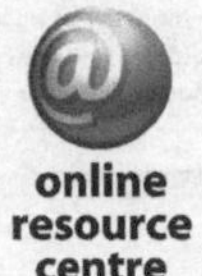

online resource centre

Each title in the *Fundamentals of Biomedical Science* series is supported by an Online Resource Centre, which features additional materials for students, trainees, and lecturers.

www.oxfordtextbooks.co.uk/orc/fbs

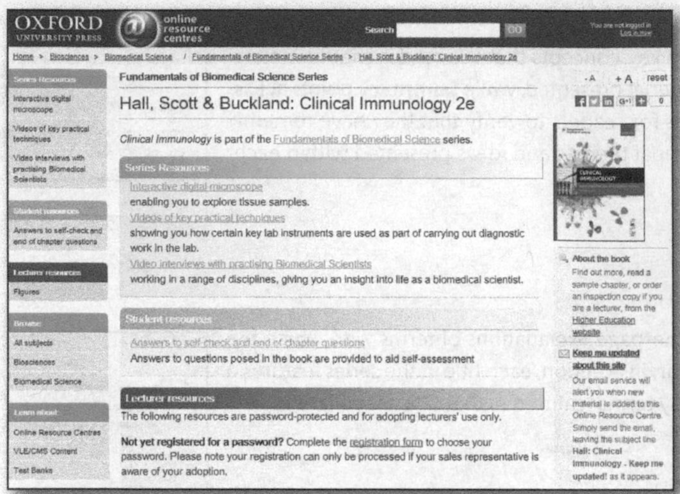

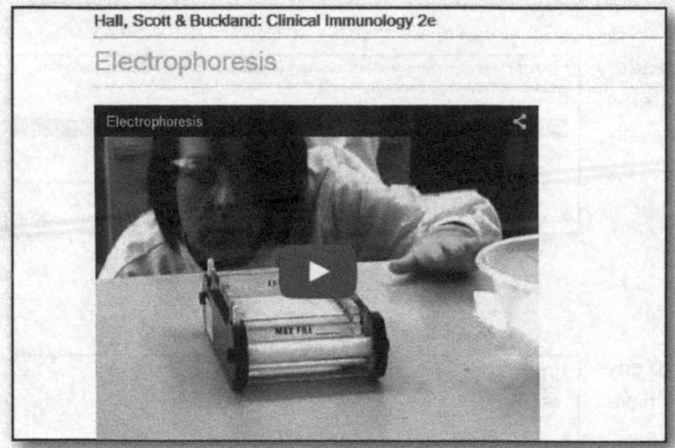

Guides to key experimental skills and methods

Video walk-throughs of key experimental skills are provided to help you master the essential skills that are the foundation of biomedical science practice.

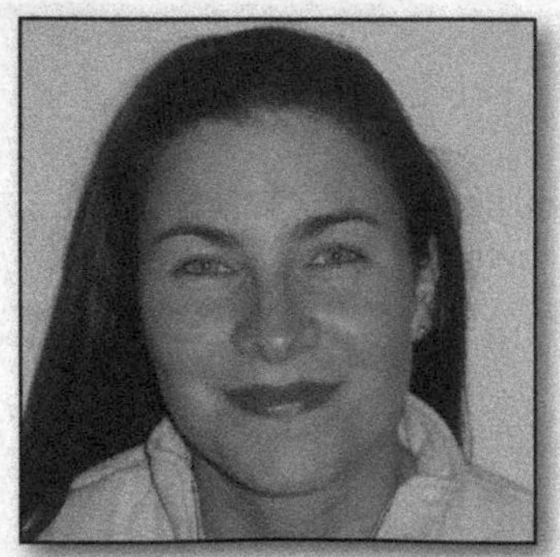

Biomedical science in practice

Interviews with practising Biomedical Scientists working in a range of disciplines give a valuable insight into the reality of work in a biomedical science laboratory.

Virtual microscope

Visit the library of microscopic images and investigate them with the powerful online micro-scope to help gain a deeper appreciation of cell and tissue morphology.

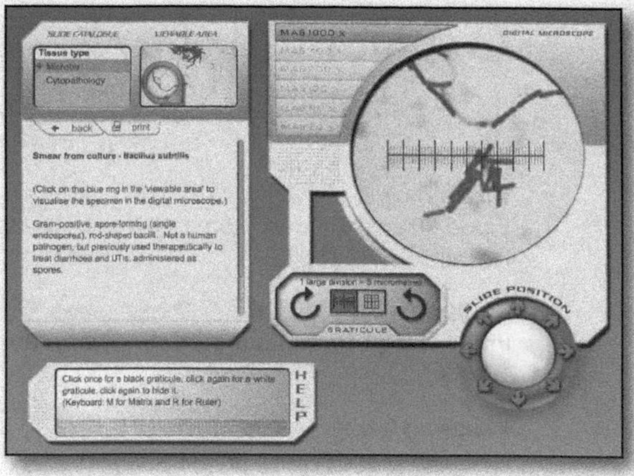

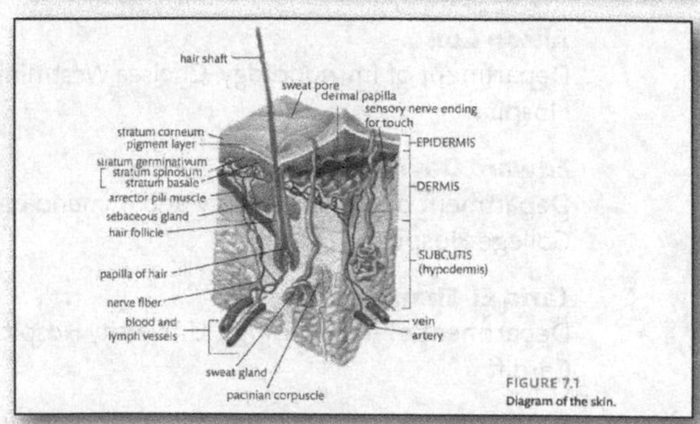

FIGURE 7.1
Diagram of the skin.

Lecturer support materials

The Online Resource Centre for each title in the series also features figures from the book in electronic format, for registered adopters to download for use in lecture presentations, and other educational resources.

To register as an adopter visit **www.oxfordtextbooks.co.uk/orc/hall2e** and follow the on screen instructions.

Any comments?

We welcome comments and feedback about any aspect of this series. Just visit **www.oxfordtextbooks.co.uk/orc/feedback** and share your views.

Contributors

Dawn Barge
Blood Sciences, Flow cytometry, Newcastle-upon-Tyne Hospitals NHS Trust

Philip Bright
Immunology and Immunogenetics, North Bristol NHS Trust

Vaughan Carter
NHS Blood and Transplant, Newcastle

Alison Cox
Department of Immunology, Chelsea Westminster Hospital

Edward Davies
Department of Clinical Allergy and Immunology, King's College Hospital

Tariq El-Shanawany
Department of Immunology, University Hospital of Wales Cardiff

Lynn Follows
Immunology Department, Sheffield Teaching Hospitals NHS Foundation Trust

Angela Hall
Department of Immunology, Imperial College Healthcare NHS Trust

Saiju Jacob
Department of Clinlcal Immunology Service, University of Birmingham

Sarah Johnston
Immunology and Immunogenetics, North Bristol NHS Trust

Stephen Jolles
Department of Immunology, University Hospital of Wales Cardiff

Abid R Karim
Department of Clinical Immunology Service, University of Birmingham

Robert J Lock
Immunology and Immunogenetics, North Bristol NHS Trust

Mo Moody
Department of Immunology, University Hospital of Wales Cardiff

B Paul Morgan
Department of Immunology, University Hospital of Wales Cardiff

Chris Scott
Department of Immunology, Bart's and the London NHS Trust

Kirsty Swallow
Immunology Department, Sheffield Teaching Hospitals NHS Foundation Trust

Phillip A Whitfield
Immunology Department, Sheffield Teaching Hospitals NHS Foundation Trust

Paul Williams
Department of Immunology, University Hospital of Wales Cardiff

David Wilson
Immunology Laboratory, Aberdeen Royal Infirmary

Online materials developed by

Sheelagh Heugh, Principal Lecturer in Biomedical Science, Faculty of Human Sciences, London Metropolitan University

Dr Ken Hudson, Lecturer in Biomedical Science, Faculty of Human Sciences, London Metropolitan University

Professor Jameel Inal, Professor of Immunology, Faculty of Human Sciences, London Metropolitan University

Contents

1

Introduction to the Clinical Immunology laboratory

Learning Objectives

After studying this chapter, you should have some understanding of:

- key aspects of immunology
- the importance of immunology in health
- the role of the Biomedical Scientist in the Clinical Immunology laboratory.

Introduction

This chapter will introduce you to Immunology and its importance in health. Immunology is one of the major Pathology disciplines. The others are Haematology, Transfusion and Transplantation science, Clinical Biochemistry, Microbiology, Histopathology, and Cytopathology. In the clinical setting, results from one discipline should be considered together with those from the other disciplines for meaningful interpretation and diagnosis. Biomedical Scientists usually specialize in one discipline but they need, at least, to have a basic understanding and to be aware of the scope of the other disciplines. This book is one in a series which aims to fulfil this need and to provide sufficient detailed information for biomedical specialists in their chosen field to be effective practitioners.

Online Resource Centre

To see video interviews with practising Biomedical Scientists, log on to www.oxfordtextbooks.co.uk/orc/fbs

In this opening chapter of this book the topics introduced are the general properties of immunology and the role of immunology as one of the biomedical sciences. It is not within the scope of this book to provide a comprehensive description of the immune system and readers are directed to more academic textbooks of Immunology for this level of detail. Instead this book provides the new Biomedical Scientist with an insight into the function of the immune system and the diagnostic techniques used to identify associated malfunctions and disorders.

By examining the key immunological principles and scientific basis of laboratory techniques, with a focus on the Biomedical Scientist's role in the diagnostic laboratory, the reader is provided with everything needed to prepare for a specialist qualification in immunology. Current tests, the rationale behind their use, the technologies employed, and the quality measures applied are illustrated by specific case studies showing how the clinician interprets the results to help the patient.

Cell-mediated immunity (cellular immunity)
Immune response mediated by cells such as T lymphocytes.

Humoral immunity
Immune response mediated by B cells and antibodies.

Innate immunity
The natural immunity that exists prior to sensitization from an antigen. It is often non-specific.

Adaptive immunity
The immunity that is acquired following sensitization with antigens.

Antibodies
Antigen-specific proteins that are produced by B lymphocytes in response to exposure to the antigen.

Antigens
Protein molecules recognized by the immune system as foreign and against which the immune system specifically reacts.

Lymphocytes
A type of white blood cell of which there are three subtypes. B cells, which give rise to humoral immunity; T cells, which give rise to cellular immunity; and natural killer cells.

Clusters of differentiation (CD)
Cell surface molecules on lymphocytes that are recognized by monoclonal antibodies to allow identification of the cell by flow cytometry.

Inflammation
A characteristic physiological response of tissues to injury. The signs of inflammation are heat, redness, swelling, and pain.

Complement
A group of blood proteins which enhance the immune response.

> **Key Point**
>
> **The result obtained from one discipline should be considered together with results from other disciplines, in order to provide meaningful interpretation and diagnosis.**

1.1 Immunology

Immunology is the branch of biomedicine concerned with the structure and function of the immune system. Immunologists study how the immune system defends the body against attack from micro-organisms and parasites, how it discriminates between self and non-self, how it deals with foreign molecules and how it recognizes and deals with neoplastic and virally transformed cells, as well as transplanted organs, cells, and proteins. They are also concerned with what happens when the immune system acts against self.

The complexity of Immunology can be quite daunting. Historically, Immunology is broken down into a description of its **cellular** and **humoral** components, then an explanation of the **innate** and the **adaptive** immune responses, before moving onto more complex subjects including immunoregulation, allergy and hypersensitivity, autoimmunity, malignancy, and immunodeficiency. This facilitates learning but the scientist must always take a more holistic approach when considering what is being done and how the results affect patients.

Immunology is a rapidly growing field with many new and exciting discoveries made each year. These enhance our understanding of health and indicate how subtle changes in the immune system have profound effects.

In the diagnostics arena immunological procedures are the basis of many haematological, microbiological, biochemical, and histopathological tests, and there is cross-over between Immunology and the other pathology disciplines. The cells, tissues, and organs of the immune system, as well as the immunologically active substances that they produce, are important to all pathologists.

The unique specificity of **antibodies** for their target **antigens** is the basis of many tests. The identification of cell surface proteins and the production of specific antibodies against them have allowed the rapid identification, investigation, and enumeration of **lymphocyte** subpopulations and the derivation of the '**clusters of differentiation**' **(CD)** classification of cells. The CD antigens are used in defining and identifying leukaemias and lymphomas. Antigen capture by antibody is fundamental to diverse techniques, including double diffusion gel-based assays, enzyme- and radio-immunoassays, nephelometry, Eli-spot assays, immunohistology, flow cytometry, and Luminex assays. Antibody/antigen technology is branching out also into other fields such as nano-engineering.

Inflammation is a key component of almost all immunological reactions. Antibody interaction with its specific antigen activates **complement**, causing increased vascular permeability and mobilization of cells, and resulting in an inflammatory infiltrate at the site of reaction. This interplay between complement, antibody, and inflammatory phagocytic cells (**macrophages**, **neutrophils**) is important for defence against infection. A deficiency in one of these components (**immunodeficiency**) predisposes the individual to repeated infections and disease.

On first exposure to an antigen, the individual becomes immunologically primed and subsequent contact with that antigen leads to secondary boosting of the immune response (**immunological memory**). This initial priming, and secondary boosting, leads to the production of antibodies and effector cells. However, in some cases, the memory reaction may be inappropriate or exaggerated causing tissue damage (**hypersensitivity**). The commonest example is **allergy**.

The immune system has evolved to recognize a diversity of foreign antigens and inevitably in doing so some lymphocytes are produced that cross-react against the body's own constituents causing **autoimmune disease**.

The **antisera** used in laboratory tests are produced by immunizing animals with the relevant, purified antigen. This results in a polyclonal antibody response from different B cell clones reacting to various determinants (**epitopes**) of the antigen. With the advent of hybridoma technology, increasingly **monoclonal antibodies** are being used. Monoclonal antibodies react with only one epitope on an antigen. They are derived from a single cell hybridized with a non-secreting myeloma cell to produce an immortalized cell line which can be cultured to produce vast quantities of monoclonal antibodies with precise reactivity. Different reporter molecules are coupled to the antibodies depending upon the assay technology to be used.

Laboratory tests differ in their sensitivity and specificity. For optimal results the cut-off points are set such that no diseased patients are test negative (false negative; **sensitivity**) and the fewest possible individuals without the disease are test positive (false positive; **specificity**). The assays described in this book are a mixture of quantitative, semi-quantitative, and qualitative. Quantitative assays usually produce precise numerical results, can be standardized against a reference preparation, and can usually be automated. Qualitative assays usually involve considerable technical expertise and interpretation can be subjective. The end-point of qualitative assays is of the positive/negative or normal/abnormal type. All Immunology laboratories strive to produce a high quality service reflected in accurate results. This is achieved through internal and external quality assurance schemes and regulation of the laboratory and personnel.

1.2 Immunology in biomedical science

Each Immunology laboratory differs in the depth and breadth of service provided according to the needs of the patients it serves and expertise of its staff. Look at Figure 1.1 to see what services can be offered by Immunology.

In the various chapters of this book you will learn more about the role of the Immunology service in diagnosis and disease management. The following chapters will describe the importance and relevance of the subject to the Immunology service.

In an era of rapidly evolving medical research and development it is hard to imagine that the original diagnostic laboratories were no more than a corner in a doctor's home, office,

Macrophages
Phagocytic cells found in the tissues that ingest, kill, and digest bacteria, foreign cells, and tissue debris. These cells also play a role in antigen presentation in the immune system.

Neutrophils
Phagocytic white blood cells that ingest and destroy bacteria as part of the innate immune response. These cells rapidly accumulate, in large numbers, at sites of infection and inflammation.

Immunodeficiency
Defects in the immune system resulting in gaps in the body's defence against pathogens.

Immunological memory
The ability of the immune system to 'recall' a previous encounter with an antigen resulting in a stronger immunological response.

Hypersensitivity
The reaction that causes reproducible signs or symptoms, following exposure to a defined stimulus, in a susceptible individual.

Allergy
A hypersensitivity reaction initiated by immunological mechanisms.

Autoimmune disease (autoimmunity)
Breakdown of tolerance, resulting in production of antibodies and/or T cells directed against own cells and tissues.

Antisera
Antibodies that are targeted against a specific antigen. Often used to identify antigens in immunological assays such as ELISA or indirect immunofluorescence (IIF).

Epitope
The region on an antigen that is recognizable by the immune system.

Monoclonal antibodies
Antibodies produced from a single clone of cells, consisting of identical molecules.

Sensitivity
The ability of an assay to correctly identify disease. The number of false negatives.

Specificity
Lack of interference from other elements other than the analyte being measured. The number of false positives.

Cross references
More precise details on the techniques used within Immunology are given in the *Biomedical Science Practice* textbook of this series.

You can look at the virtual Immunology laboratory using this link http://www.science4u.info/virtuallab/ Here you can find out what tests an Immunology laboratory can offer, hear interviews with Biomedical Scientists, and read about topics such as health and safety and training within an Immunology laboratory.

Continuing professional development (CPD)
is a process of lifelong learning, which enables you to expand and fulfil your personal and professional potential, as well as meet the present and future needs of patients and deliver health outcomes and priorities. It assures that you meet the requisite knowledge and skills levels that relate to your evolving scope of professional practice (www.IBMS.org).

Cross reference
More information on the role of Biomedical Scientists and the professional development opportunities available can be found on the website of the Institute of Biomedical Science www.IBMS.org.

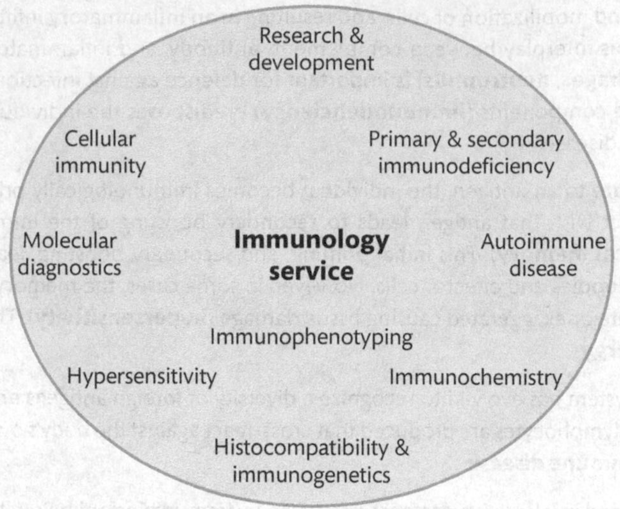

FIGURE 1.1
Breadth and scope of the immunology service.

or hospital ward with the doctor himself performing the investigations. Over 80% of medical interventions rely upon results generated in the Pathology service laboratories. The educational and regulatory requirements have grown in parallel with the development and expansion of the Pathology disciplines into independent clinical laboratory professions. Most diagnostic laboratories are found in hospitals and the majority of the professional Biomedical Scientists are employed in this setting. Those in district hospitals tend to be generalists, but in larger institutions such as the teaching hospitals, with their wider scope and increased numbers of tests, many Biomedical Scientists specialize in specific areas and departments. It is becoming common practice that Immunology laboratories will be situated within cross-disciplinary departments often linked with other pathology disciplines. This provides the opportunity for multidisciplinary trained Biomedical Scientists, who may be given the opportunity to specialize within more than one discipline.

Within the Immunology service laboratory, the specialist areas range from Immunodeficiency, Autoimmunity, Allergy and Hypersensitivity, Cellular and Humoral Immunity, Immunochemistry, Transplantation, and Malignancy. Biomedical Scientists work in all of these areas and depending upon the laboratory may be expected to rotate through the various sections. Trainee Biomedical and Clinical Scientists will have to train and work in each area to gather the knowledge, skills, and competencies to become registered professional scientists. However, training and development does not cease at registration and all scientists are required to keep up to date with advancements in their profession and to demonstrate maintenance of competencies through participation in **continuing professional development (CPD)**. Both the Institute of Biomedical Science and the Royal College of Pathologists run accredited CPD schemes. With the ability for Biomedical Scientists to become 'chartered', this provides the international recognition that Biomedical Scientists are practising science at the full professional level. Provision of accredited qualifications from the Institute of Biomedical Science gives a framework of qualifications to support advancement in career progression and demonstration of specialized, higher laboratory practice.

Biomedical and Clinical Scientists are encouraged to have a presence outside the laboratory. They should participate in **multidisciplinary team (MDT)** meetings and hospital

'**Grand Rounds**' where the results they generate are discussed with clinicians and other healthcare professionals in the context of the diagnosis and management of patients. Despite separate training pathways, there is a lot of overlap in the roles of Biomedical and Clinical Scientists especially with regard to the timely processing of samples and reporting of results. Depending upon the size and complexity of the laboratory, Biomedical Scientists predominantly take responsibility for analyses of samples and the assay platforms while the Clinical Scientists may take more responsibility for clinical liaison, validation and research and development, but at senior levels these boundaries become blurred.

Multidisciplinary team meetings (MDTs)
Whereby different groups of professionals (i.e. doctors, nurses, and scientists) meet to discuss individual patients, using the knowledge from each discipline to work towards effective diagnosis and treatments.

Grand Round
A conference in which clinicians/experts present the case studies of individual patients, or new topics in the field of medicine, and use this as an educational tool for other staff members.

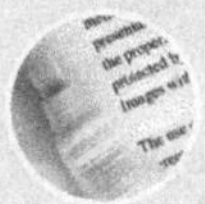

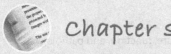

Chapter summary

- Immunology is the branch of biomedicine concerned with the structure and function of the immune system.
- Immunology is a rapidly growing field with many new and exciting discoveries made each year.
- In the diagnostics arena immunological procedures are the basis of many haematological, microbiological, biochemical, and histopathological tests, and there is a lot of cross-over between Immunology and the other pathology disciplines.
- Each Immunology laboratory differs in the depth and breadth of service provided according to the needs of the patients it serves and expertise of its staff.
- Within the Immunology service laboratory, the specialist areas range from Immunodeficiency, Autoimmunity, Allergy and Hypersensitivity, Cellular and Humoral Immunity, Immunochemistry, Transplantation, and Malignancy.

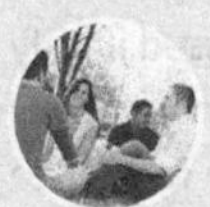

Discussion questions

1.1 What are the benefits of cross-disciplinary training?

1.2 What does the title 'chartered scientist' mean?

Answers to self-check questions are provided in the book's Online Resource Centre.

 Visit www.oxfordtextbooks.co.uk/orc/hall2e

2

Immunoglobulins

Learning Objectives

After studying this chapter you should be able to:

- outline the common features of immunoglobulin structure, function, and pathology
- describe the clinical features of monoclonal gammopathy of undetermined significance (MGUS), myeloma, cryoglobulinaemia, and multiple sclerosis (MS)
- outline the assays and techniques used to test for monoclonal gammopathy of undetermined significance (MGUS), myeloma, cryoglobulinaemia, and multiple sclerosis (MS)
- discuss the limitations of these techniques.

Introduction

This chapter describes the investigation of immunoglobulins in the clinical laboratory, both in health and in disease. In the United Kingdom, the investigations are most often performed within Clinical Chemistry or Immunology departments. Often the primary intention is to detect monoclonal gammopathies; however, there is a wealth of information to be seen using serum electrophoresis including inflammatory changes, liver disease, and renal pathology.

It is important to use both quantitative and qualitative measurement of immunoglobulins together when determining a patient's current status. A deficiency in IgA may be missed if only a qualitative screen is performed as the electrophoretic track may appear normal; conversely many low level monoclonal gammopathies will have quantitative levels within the reference range and will be overlooked if the laboratory relies solely on a quantitative screen.

This chapter describes in detail the techniques used in the clinical laboratory for the detection of immunoglobulins, their use, and their interpretation.

2.1 Immunoglobulins

Immunoglobulins are a family of proteins of the humoral immune system that bind to specific targets called antigens. They activate complement and influence effector cells such as Natural Killer (NK) cells and Mast Cells through binding to surface receptors, which activate cells or encourage phagocytosis through immune complexes. Each immunoglobulin molecule consists of two identical heavy chains designated by Greek letters γ (gamma), α (alpha), μ (mu), δ (delta), and ε (epsilon), paired with two identical light chains designated κ (kappa) and λ (lambda). The basic immunoglobulin unit consists of two heavy chains and two light chains. There are five immunoglobulin isotypes or classes named IgG, IgA, IgM, IgD, and IgE, after the corresponding heavy chain (above). The layout of two heavy chains plus two light chains structure is common to all the immunoglobulin isotypes, with differences in the number and sequence of amino acids dictating differences in size and function. IgG, IgD and IgE molecules are made up of single 4-chain units (monomers). IgA is found predominantly in a 2-unit molecule (dimer) and IgM is found as a 5-unit molecule (pentamer). In addition, IgG has four subclasses known as IgG1, IgG2, IgG3 and IgG4. IgA has two subclasses; IgA1 and IgA2.

Immunoglobulins are synthesized and secreted by plasma cells in bone marrow and lymph nodes. Plasma cells are the final stage of maturation of B lymphocytes and each plasma cell produces antibody molecules of a single isotype and antigen binding specificity (a clone). The isotype can be switched from M to G, A, or E during B cell maturation before the plasma cell stage. IgD is a cell surface molecule of unknown function and can be found in low levels in the serum.

Immunoglobulin heavy chains and light chains are produced in different regions of the endoplasmic reticulum and are assembled into a single functional molecule before secretion. However excess immunoglobulin light chains are produced, which are secreted as independent molecules. The κ free light chains circulate as monomers, whereas the λ free light chains tend to form dimers, or larger polymers. The excess light chains enter the kidneys and because of their low molecular weight they pass through the glomerulus and into the proximal tubule where they are reabsorbed and degraded into smaller peptides which are then recycled. Normally some 1–10 mg of light chains per day pass on to the distal tubule and into the urine but in **monoclonal gammopathies** the capacity of the proximal tubule can be overwhelmed and much higher levels of light chains leak into the urine.

Monoclonal gammopathy (MG)

Disease characterized by the finding of monoclonal immunoglobulin in the serum and/or urine.

The basic immunoglobulin structure consists of two heavy chains each of about 50kDa molecular weight and two light chains each of 25kDa, giving a single unit of at least 150kDa. The heavy chains have three or four constant regions or domains, depending on the isotype, and one variable domain. The constant domains are named Constant Heavy (CH) 1, 2, 3, or 4 and are so called because within them the amino acid sequence is highly conserved. They have a sub-structure of beta-pleated sheets of polypeptides cross-linked by disulphide bridges giving a barrel-like appearance. Look at Figure 2.1 to see the three CH domain model.

Cross reference

See Section 2.2 for more information on monoclonal gammopathies.

Between CH1 and CH2 is the hinge region which confers flexibility on the molecule allowing antibody binding of antigen in different planes. The hinge region varies in the number of amino acids according to the immunoglobulin isotype.

The CH1 is linked to the variable region domain VH. As the name suggests the amino acid sequence is more variable with a small hypervariable region, which is the result of shuffling of the V region genes. It is the hypervariable region which contributes to the antigen specificity of the antibody molecule.

Linked by disulphide bonds in parallel to each heavy chain (VH and CH1) is the light chain, which may be of κ or λ isotype, but never both. These are similarly divided into a constant light chain domain (CL) and one variable light chain domain (VL).

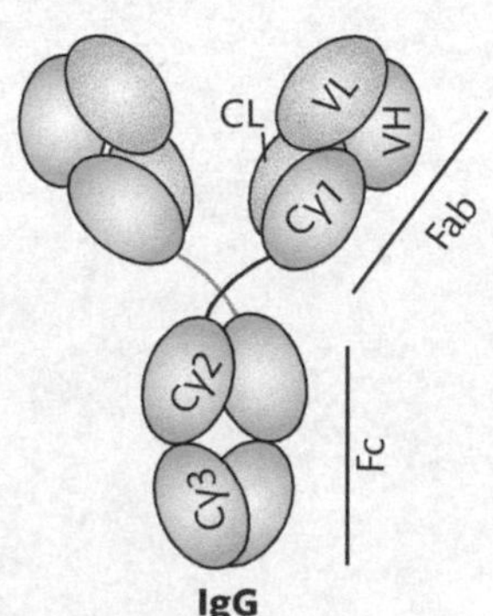

FIGURE 2.1
Structure of IgG.

Key Point

Immunoglobulin heavy and light chains are organized into barrel-like domains.

Complementarity determining region (CDR)
A short amino acid sequence found in the variable region of an immunoglobulin.

Cross reference
Look at Chapter 4 to read more about complement.

As with the heavy chain VH domain, the VL domain has hypervariable regions, differing in sequence to the VH hypervariable region. The hypervariable regions are also referred to as **complementarity determining region (CDR)** and on both heavy and light chains they are located in three zones of about five amino acids each in position 25, 50, and 75 approximately. It is the combination of the heavy and light chain CDRs which give the antibody its specificity, and since the two arms are identical the molecule has two antigen binding sites.

When an immunoglobulin binds to antigen, this causes a conformational change in the hinge region which exposes the C1q binding site in CH2 which then leads to the classical pathway activation of the complement sequence. IgA does not have this function and is unable to activate complement.

The CH3 domain acts as a ligand for IgG receptors found on cells of the immune system such as neutrophils and natural killer cells.

The structure of immunoglobulin was elucidated by using enzymes to digest and fragment the molecule. The enzyme papain digests the immunoglobulin molecule at the N terminus of the interchain disulphide bonds releasing the antigen binding arms as separate units known as Fab, or 'fragments antigen binding', and the paired CH2 and CH3 domains known as Fc, or 'fragments crystallizable'. The enzyme pepsin digests immunoglobulin molecules at the C terminus of the interchain disulphide bonds leaving both antigen binding arms linked as a single unit known as $F(ab)_2$ or 'fragment antigen binding ×2'. The remaining CH2 and CH3 domains of the immunoglobulin heavy chain are degraded to small peptides.

Key Point

Immunoglobulin molecules have different effector functions in different domains of the molecule.

2.1.1 Immunoglobulin IgG

IgG follows the three CH domain model described in Section 2.1. Physicochemically, the principal differences between the four IgG subclasses is the number of amino acids which constitute the hinge region and the interchain disulphide bonds linking the heavy chains at this point. The key properties of the four IgG subclasses are listed in Table 2.1.

IgG is an immunoglobulin which can be found in the plasma and extracellular spaces. IgG1 and IgG3 antibodies are produced as a result of exposure to T cell dependent antigens such as viral protein, whilst IgG2 antibodies are produced in response to polysaccharide antigen in adults. In children a limited IgG1 response to polysaccharide antigens is produced, as little IgG2 is produced in the first 2 years of life. Children under 2 years of age may present with pneumococcal infections and do not produce a good response to the formalin inactivated pneumococcal vaccines. The newer protein conjugated vaccines direct an IgG1 response to the peptide and are highly effective from early infancy. It is common practice to test for the presence of the IgG subclasses in patients with recurrent bacterial infection and normal total IgG, but a true deficiency of one of the IgG subclasses is rare and it is more clinically relevant to measure antibody responses to pneumococcal antigens.

IgG4 is produced in response to extracellular parasites and multiple exposures to protein antigens. This latter characteristic is exploited clinically to desensitize individuals who have an IgE-mediated hypersensitivity to insect venoms. The IgG4 anti venom can block the IgE–venom interaction.

TABLE 2.1 Features of the IgG subclasses.

	IgG1	IgG2	IgG3	IgG4
Serum concentration (adults, g/L)	3.2–10.2	1.2–6.6	0.2–1.9	0–1.3
Hinge region amino acids	16	12	62	12
Interchain bonds	2	4	11	2
Half-life (days)	21	21	7	21
Complement activation	++	+	+++	0
FcRII & III binding	++++	+	+++	+
Antigen	Peptide	Polysaccharide	Peptide	Peptide
Placental transfer	+++	+	++	+

NB: In adults, IgG3 concentrations are higher in females than in males, and IgG4 higher in males than females. Ranges from Protein Reference Unit, Sheffield.

The level of IgG in newborn infants is similar to that of adults due to the active transfer of IgG1 and IgG3 across the placenta. This maternal IgG is catabolized during the first 6 months of life and declines to about 3 g/L or lower as the infant's own synthesis of IgG commences. Adult levels of immunoglobulins (IgG) are not attained until about 15 years of age.

Cross reference

See Section 3.15 in Chapter 3 on IgG antibodies for more information on immunotherapy.

Cross reference

Refer to Section 11.3 in Chapter 11 for the clinical correlations associated with low immunoglobulins caused by the absence or loss of function of B cells.

CLINICAL CORRELATION 2.1

IgG4-related disease (G4RD)

IgG4-related disease is the name given to a fibroinflammatory condition characterized by the formation of swellings characterized by storiform fibrosis with infiltrates of lymphocytes and IgG4-positive plasma cells and often, although not always, by an increased serum IgG4 concentration. It has been linked with Type I autoimmune pancreatitis, but can affect any organ. The diagnostic criterion and more information on IgG4 disease can be found in Pieringer et al. (2014).

Laboratory IgG subclass assays have been developed to be able to measure the very low levels seen in IgG deficiency, and patients with G4RD and elevated IgG4 levels may give falsely low results in these assays due to antigen excess (see Section 2.3). Laboratories need to be aware and have verified procedures in place to detect this.

2.1.2 Immunoglobulin IgA

IgA has a CH1–3 heavy chain structure which can be seen in Figure 2.2. It represents about 15% of plasma immunoglobulin but it is the most abundant immunoglobulin in the tissues. This is because it is the principal immunoglobulin of the gastrointestinal tract, the respiratory tract, and the mucosal surfaces. Its native configuration is that of a dimer linked across CH2 and CH3 by a joining or J chain. In the mucosal compartment this complex is further enveloped by a molecule called secretory component (SC), which protects the immunoglobulin from proteolytic enzymes. IgA consists of two isotypic subclasses, IgA1 and IgA2, but they are rarely measured as distinct entities.

IgA deficiency is the commonest immunoglobulin deficiency occurring in 1:500–700 Caucasian individuals in the UK, many of whom are asymptomatic. However, some patients are prone to

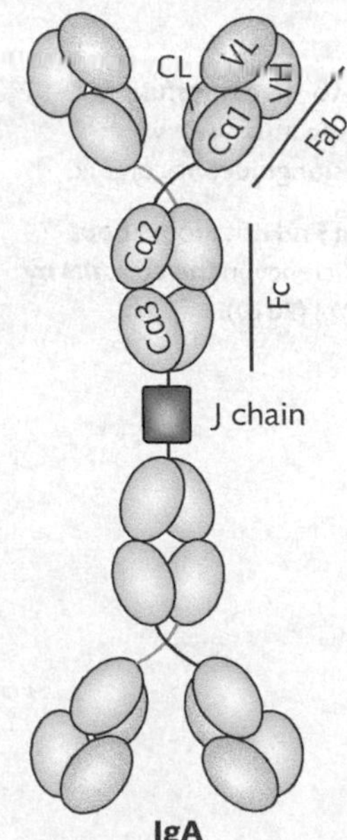

FIGURE 2.2
Structure of IgA.

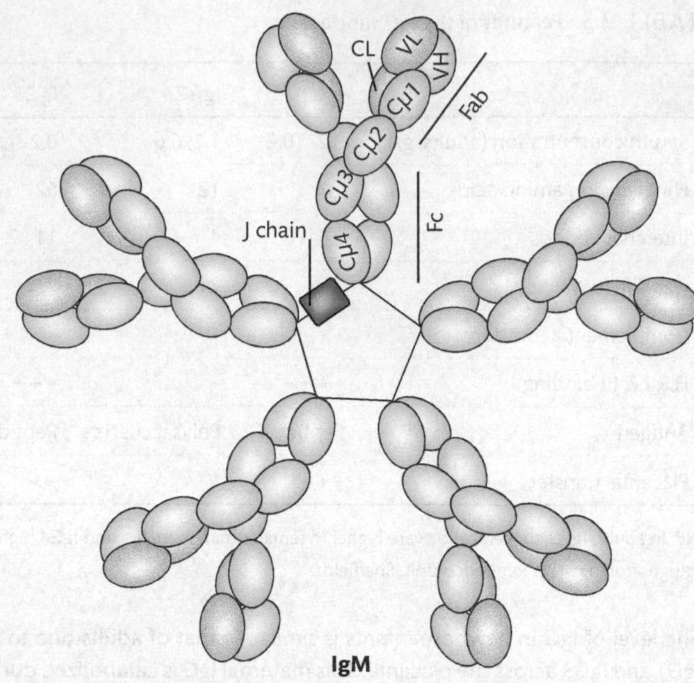

FIGURE 2.3
Structure of IgM.

chest infections and a host of associated clinical conditions including coeliac disease, autoimmune endocrinopathies, and pernicious anaemia.

Cross reference

Look at Chapter 7 to read in more detail about the organ-specific autoimmune diseases such as coeliac disease, autoimmune endocrinopathies, and pernicious anaemia.

If a patient has an IgA deficiency, the patient may go on to develop antibodies against IgA which can be IgG, IgM, or IgE class. Only a small minority of patients with IgA deficiency are at risk of developing severe allergic reactions to blood components due to the presence of donor IgA. Those at most risk have severe IgA deficiency (<0.07 g/L), often with anti-IgA antibodies in their plasma. Even then, most such patients do not react to blood transfusion. Patients with no history of severe reactions to blood transfusion should be transfused with standard blood components.

Cross references

For up-to-date transfusion policy see http://www.transfusionguidelines.org.uk.

You can find out more about IgA deficiency in the editorial by Owen Yel (2010).

2.1.3 Immunoglobulin IgM

IgM has a configuration of four CH domains, with five IgM molecules arranged together linked by a J chain, giving a molecular weight of 1×10^6 kDa, which can be seen in Figure 2.3. IgM is predominantly an intravascular immunoglobulin comprising about 10% of the plasma immunoglobulin. Upon binding to antigen, IgM readily activates the classical complement pathway and because it has up to ten binding sites it will crosslink and form large immune complexes. Isolated IgM deficiency is relatively rare indeed and is much more likely to be due to suppression by a lymphoproliferative disease or drugs than a primary immunodeficiency. When it does arise patients may paradoxically benefit from IgG replacement therapy.

2.1.4 Immunoglobulin IgE

IgE has a four CH domain structure and a molecular weight of 195kDa, shown in Figure 2.4. Its concentration is less than 1% of plasma immunoglobulin and because of this it is measured in the laboratory by different methods to the other immunoglobulins and has different reportable units. The primary function of IgE is to bind to mast cells via high affinity receptors in response to parasitic worm infestations. Upon binding with the parasite, IgE changes its conformation and triggers the mast cell to discharge its cocktail of proteolytic enzymes, histamine, and tryptase onto the parasite. IgE production is genetically determined and atopic individuals produce higher levels which correlate with an increased susceptibility to developing allergies in addition to asthma, eczema, and hay fever. Thus, mast cell bound IgE is also responsible for type 1 hypersensitivity allergic responses due to mast cell degranulation. Occasionally similar reactions can occur due to basophil degranulation because of surface bound IgE with a similar function.

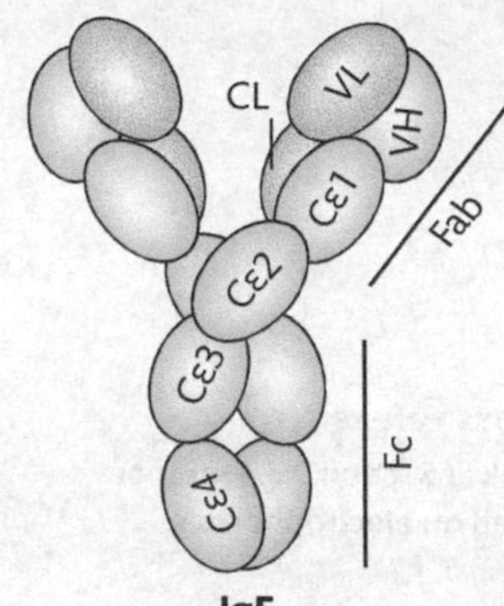

FIGURE 2.4
Structure of IgE.

CLINICAL CORRELATION 2.2

Hyper IgE syndrome

Hyper IgE (Job's) syndrome is a congenital condition characterized by very high plasma IgE often of more than 50 000 kU/L. Other immunoglobulin levels appear normal.

Patients endure frequent abscesses of the skin, respiratory tract, and ears with *S. aureus*, *C. albicans*, and *S. pneumoniae* amongst other organisms. The lymphocytes of these patients show diminished responses to mitogen and antigen stimulation. The syndrome has been linked to a defect in the *STAT3* gene on chromosome 4.

Cross reference

See Chapter 3 to read in more detail about the function of IgE and its relationship with allergy.

2.1.5 Immunoglobulin IgD

IgD is composed of three CH domains and has a molecular weight of 175kDa, shown in Figure 2.5. The majority of IgD is integral to the B cell membranes with very little detectable in plasma. Indeed a normal individual may have no detectable plasma IgD.

Many reference ranges have been reported for IgD, commonly in mg/L (Vladutiu 2000) but as there is currently no international mass standard for IgD, the results can be reported as U/ml traceable to British Research standard 67/37 with a reference range of 0–100 U/ml.

CLINICAL CORRELATION 2.3

Hyper IgD syndrome

Hyper IgD syndrome (HIDS), one of the periodic fevers, is characterized by sudden onset pyrexia of over 38.5 °C, abdominal pain, vomiting with or without diarrhoea, and skin rashes. About 80% of patients have an IgD level of greater than 100 U/ml, thus 20% of patients have IgD levels within the reference range. The underlying genetic defect is mutations of the *MVK* gene leading to mevalonate kinase deficiency (MKD).

The condition usually commences before the age of three and 60% of patients are of Dutch or French heritage.

Table 2.2 shows the immunoglobulin reference ranges for adults. It is important to note that reference ranges for immunoglobulins are age related. You should look up your local laboratory's reference ranges for children and the elderly.

TABLE 2.2 Reference ranges for immunoglobulins in adults (18–60 years).

Isotype	Adult reference range
IgG	6.0–16.0 g/L
IgA	0.8–4.0 g/L
IgM	0.5–2.0 g/L
IgD	0–100 kU/L
IgE	0–81 kU/L

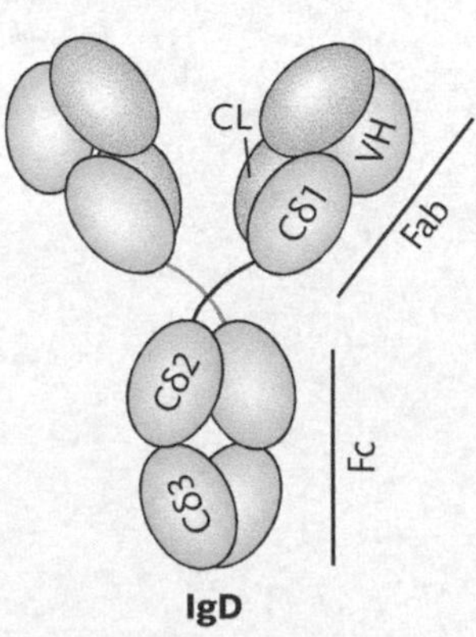

FIGURE 2.5
Structure of IgD.

2.2 The monoclonal gammopathies

Total plasma immunoglobulin is the product of millions of plasma cell clones in bone marrow and lymph nodes. Plasma cell clone reproduction is limited by homeostasis to produce the required amount of immunoglobulin for the required length of time to eliminate an infection. On occasion a plasma cell clone may undergo chromosomal translocations, escape from this control, and reproduce itself millions of times over. Not only does the cell replicate itself but it secretes its programmed immunoglobulin isotype in such large amounts that a discrete band is seen on electrophoresis. Since it is the product of a single cell clone it is referred to as a monoclonal immunoglobulin, the presence of which in a patient is described as a monoclonal gammopathy (MG).

Cross reference

Look at Section 2.3.4 for more detail on electrophoresis.

Monoclonal gammopathy can be divided into two groups. The most common presentation is as a coincidental finding during investigation of an unrelated pathology. The patient does not have symptoms attributable to the MG, the monoclonal band is less than 30 g/L, and the bone marrow has less than 10% plasma cells. This is a condition termed **monoclonal gammopathy of undetermined significance (MGUS)**. The incidence of MGUS increases with age, being 1% in the over fifties rising to 10% in the over eighties, and with a higher incidence in African-Caribbean patients. The majority of patients will die with MGUS rather than of MGUS, however 1% per year transform into the second or malignant form of MG known as **myeloma.** MGUS patients should have a sample analysed at least annually to identify and treat those who progress to myeloma.

Monoclonal gammopathy of undetermined significance (MGUS)

Monoclonal gammopathy in which the monoclonal quantification and clinical features do not meet the diagnostic criteria for any specific disease.

CLINICAL CORRELATION 2.4

What is myeloma?

Myeloma (also multiple myeloma) is a disease associated with a malignant monoclonal proliferation of bone marrow plasma cells, characterized by lytic bone lesions, plasma cell accumulation in the bone marrow, and the presence of monoclonal immunoglobulin in serum and/or urine. Clinical features include bone pain, anaemia, infections, renal failure, and possible hyperviscosity syndrome. Laboratory findings include increased serum calcium, low haemoglobin, raised mean cell volume (MCV), and increased erythrocyte sedimentation rate (ESR). 5% of myeloma patients have no identifiable serum monoclone but do have monoclonal free light chains in their urine, whilst in 1% of patients neither a serum nor a urine monoclone can be detected.

Key Point

Monoclonal gammopathy of undetermined significance (MGUS) must be monitored at least annually as 1% of patients per year evolve into myeloma.

The symptoms of myeloma are of insidious onset, and are often due to the organ system most affected by the disease. Thus the patient may present with renal failure, anaemia, severe bone pain, spontaneous fractures of long bones, or collapsed vertebrae. Bone damage is due to the breakdown of the homeostatic control of bone remodelling by osteoclasts and osteoblasts. Osteoclasts dissolve bone and in the myeloma patient their activity is upregulated in the region of the myeloma cells, as there is an imbalance in the regulatory system. Patients often present with bone pain, which may be severe. As bone is lost the patient is at risk of spontaneous fractures, particularly in long bones, ribs, or vertebrae, and this may lead to admission to

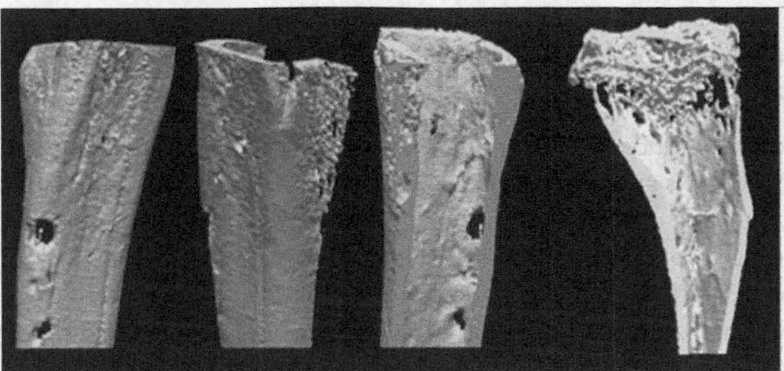
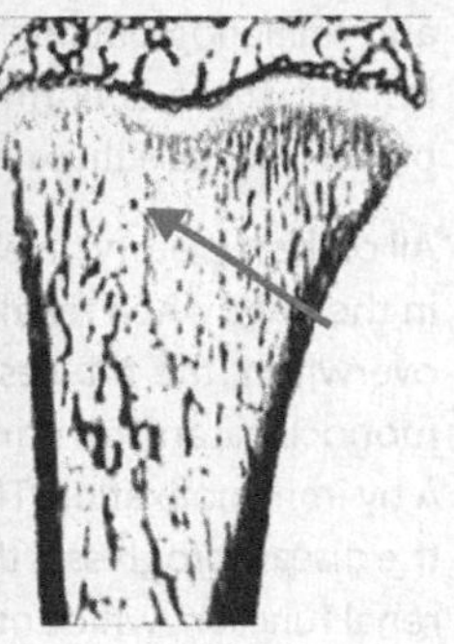

FIGURE 2.6
Osteolytic lesions in multiple myeloma.

orthopaedic wards (see Figure 2.6). Loss of bone leads to high plasma calcium levels leading to renal failure and drowsiness.

The laboratory characteristics of myeloma have common features but are not uniform in all patients and are in part dictated by the type of protein secreted by the abnormal plasma cells. Whole immunoglobulin molecule myeloma (heavy and light chain combined) is the most common with 60% of cases of IgG and over 20% of IgA isotypes. IgD myeloma represents 1% of patients and IgE myeloma is very rare. IgM myeloma is extremely rare, but has been reported (Dierlamm et al. 2002).

CLINICAL CORRELATION 2.5

Macroglobulinaemia

The condition Waldenström's macroglobulinaemia is a clonal disease of a pre-plasma cell called a lymphoplasmacytoid cell, producing monoclonal IgM. These lymphoid cells infiltrate bone marrow, suppressing normal plasma cell production, and leading to immune paresis. Patients often have high levels of monoclonal IgM leading to hyperviscosity syndrome. Type 1 cryoglobulin may be seen.

Immune paresis
Suppression of normal immunoglobulin production by a malignant bone marrow plasma cell clone.

About 10% of myelomas are of κ or λ light chain only. Large quantities of monoclonal light chain may be produced but when renal function is good much of this is rapidly cleared in the urine, and it may not readily give rise to a visible band on serum electrophoresis (SEP), or there may be a small band with the same mobility as one of the beta or alpha bands. Upon finding a monoclonal light chain the laboratory must exclude the possible presence of IgD and IgE heavy chains by immunofixation. Light chain myelomas very often have immune paresis.

Cross reference
You can read more about cryoglobulins in Section 2.5.

Cross reference
See Section 2.3 for more information on how immunoglobulins are quantified and to find out more about serum electrophoresis.

CLINICAL CORRELATION 2.6

What is immune paresis?

Immune paresis is the suppression of normal immunoglobulin production by the malignant cell clone. Low immunoglobulin results may be the only sign of the presence of a small serum free light chain or an IgD monoclone. This is why it is important to perform immunofixation on samples from adults with low immunoglobulin results even if no abnormal electrophoretic band can be seen.

Cross reference
Look at Section 2.3.7 for more information on immunofixation.

Less than 1% of myelomas apparently do not secrete a monoclonal immunoglobulin. On bone marrow examination there are large numbers of plasma cells (greater than 10% of nucleated bone marrow cells), which by staining with either fluorescein or enzyme conjugated anti-immunoglobulins demonstrate their cytoplasm is packed with one immunoglobulin isotype. These abnormal plasma cells lack the mechanism to secrete their immunoglobulin product and are thus named non-secretory myelomas.

All of the secretory myelomas produce excess free light chains, much of which is rapidly cleared in the urine when renal function is good. Free light chains may be produced in quantities that overwhelm the tubules and appear in urine as overflow **proteinuria**. These light chains are monoclonal and on urine electrophoresis (UEP) form discrete bands which can be typed as κ or λ by immunofixation. The monoclonal light chains are referred to as **Bence Jones proteins**. As the disease progresses the renal tubules suffer increasing damage and loss leading to worsening renal function, which may be the presenting clinical feature.

Proteinuria

The presence of protein in the urine. Proteins filtered through the kidney glomeruli should be actively reabsorbed in the tubules and so proteinuria should normally be absent or minimal.

Bence Jones proteins

Monoclonal light chains found in the urine of patients with renal failure; named after the English physician Henry Bence Jones (1813-1873), who described some of their physicochemical properties in 1847.

Examples of IgG, IgA, and IgM heavy chain only monoclones have been described, but these are rare. The monoclone often appears on serum electrophoresis as a smear of protein immunostaining for the heavy chain in question.

The UK Nordic myeloma forum guidelines suggest IgG and IgA isotype monoclones are over 30 g/L, however IgD myeloma monoclones are usually of less than 10 g/L. The concentration of the monoclonal immunoglobulin is a reflection of the size of the abnormal plasma cell clone, and it is used as the principal monitor of the success or failure of treatment, which makes it the archetypal tumour marker. Myelomas usually, but not always, have immune paresis which may lead to repeated infections requiring antibiotic support.

Quantification of patients' monoclonal immunoglobulins is most accurately by densitometry or capillary zone electrophoresis (CZE), as described in Sections 2.3.6 and 2.3.9. Immunochemical methods, described in Section 2.3, use polyclonal antisera calibrated against polyclonal standards. Monoclonal immunoglobulins often lack some of the epitopes present on normal immunoglobulin and therefore bind differently to the polyclonal anti-immunoglobulin antisera, giving results which are not accurate.

Cross reference

You can read the guidelines for MGUS in Bird et al. (2014).

CLINICAL CORRELATION 2.7

What is a monoclonal immunoglobulin?

Immunoglobulins are produced by B lymphocytes (plasma cells), with each B lymphocyte producing a specific immunoglobulin. Proliferation of a single (mono) B lymphocyte will produce a 'clone' of those lymphocytes and an associated increase in the serum level of the associated immunoglobulin. All those immunoglobulin molecules will have identical amino acid sequences and identical electrophoretic mobility and so will form a band on an electrophoresis pattern. All the molecules in a monoclonal immunoglobulin (MIg, M-protein, paraprotein) will have identical heavy and light chains (see Section 2.1 for immunoglobulin structure). Immunofixation identifies the heavy and light chain components of the sample and so can determine whether an electrophoretic band is monoclonal or not.

Biclonal is the term used for two monoclones present in the same serum.

Paraprotein

An abnormal (usually monoclonal) protein seen in a monoclonal gammopathy such as MGUS or myeloma.

2.3 Quantification of immunoglobulins

2.3.1 Measurement of serum immunoglobulins

In serum, IgG, IgA, and IgM are amenable to measurement by simple antibody:antigen (Ab:Ag) immune complex formation assays such as nephelometry and turbidimetry. Due to the low levels in serum, IgD is usually measured by radial immunodiffusion or ELISA. IgE is usually assayed by labelled immunoassays such as ELISA or chemiluminescence. Radial immunodiffusion methods are available for IgG, IgA, and IgM but are rarely used in UK laboratories. The most important requirements for either methodology are to maintain **antibody excess** in the reaction mixture and to be aware of when **antigen excess** may occur and how to deal with it. The assays must, therefore, be validated by the manufacturer to use the optimum amount of antibody, dilution of sample, and volume of sample.

Antibody excess
The state in an antibody/antigen mixture where the concentration of antibody exceeds that of antigen.

Antigen excess
The state in an antibody/antigen mixture where the concentration of antigen exceeds that of antibody.

In antibody excess the fixed amount of antibody binds antigen, and because of the two binding sites per molecule and the polyclonal nature of antibody, it cross-links to other antigen molecules forming a three-dimensional lattice immune complex in the diluent buffer. In increasing antigen concentration more of the antibody is consumed in the immune complex. At the equivalence point the amounts of antibody and antigen are equal, the immune complex lattice formation is maximal, and the immune complex forms and redissolves at an equal rate. The addition of more antigen creates an antigen excess condition where the antibody's binding sites become occupied by single antigens and cannot cross-link. Thus the lattice structure begins to break apart and redissolve. With increasing antigen excess the lattice will redissolve completely. The states of antibody and antigen excess were defined by Heidelberger and Kendall in the 1930s and are described by the bell curve named after them. This is shown in Figure 2.7. It is the amount of immune complex lattice formation that the optical systems in nephelometry and turbidimetry measure, and if the lattice is reduced by antigen excess then a false low result will be produced.

There are various strategies to minimize the interference from antigen excess. All analysers dilute the sample prior to the assay, and will redilute samples giving a signal higher than the highest calibrator value. Nephelometers are more sophisticated than turbidimetric systems and they may produce calibration curves with a very broad dynamic range that extends well into the predicted antigen excess zone. A pre-reaction analysis may also be used wherein a small amount of the sample is mixed with the standard volume of antibody and the reaction is monitored for a few seconds. If lattice formation proceeds rapidly this may be due to very high antigen concentration and the assay is stopped and processed at a higher dilution of the sample.

Key Point

You must understand the principle of antigen excess and how the individual analysers deal with this in the routine laboratory setting.

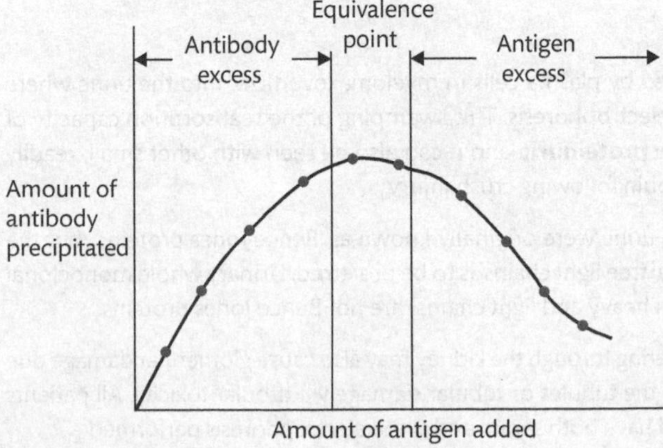

FIGURE 2.7
The Heidelberger–Kendall curve.

Nephelometry is the measurement of light scattered by particles, and has been adapted as immunonephelometry to measure light scattered by immune complexes formed in a small optical cuvette. When the wavelength of the incident light is smaller than the immune complex then forward angle light scatter predominates. This is known as Mie scattering and it maximizes the amount of light scattered to the optical detector, which is located at an angle from the light path. Increasing scattered light is directly proportional to the antigen concentration.

In turbidimetry, the optical system measures the light transmitted as apparent absorbance, or optical density. The amount of light passed through the reaction mixture is inversely proportional to the antigen concentration.

For optimal performance, both immunonephelometry and immunoturbidimetry include polyethylene glycol (PEG) in the reaction mixture. This high molecular weight polymer is highly hygroscopic and is thought to remove water molecules from around the antibody and antigen, bringing the two closer together and allowing the formation of measurable immune complexes in a few minutes.

All assay systems for immunoglobulin rely on the use of international reference material to standardize instrument calibration. For IgG, IgA, and IgM this is known as ERM-DA470K/IFCC and all assays used in clinical laboratories must state that the calibration standard in use is derived from this. There is no agreed international standard for IgG subclasses and IgD but British Research standard 67/37 is widely adopted.

Key Point

Use of calibration material traceable to the International Reference Protocol (IRP) ERM-DA470K/IFCC helps to standardize results between laboratories.

Laboratories must not rely on immunoglobulin quantification to detect the presence of monoclonal bands on the assumption that all significant monoclones will give results higher than the normal range or exhibit immune paresis. There are many examples of clinically significant monoclones, particularly light chain and IgD isotypes, and most MGUS cases, where the total immunoglobulin assay results are well within the normal range. Only by combining immunoglobulin quantification with serum electrophoresis and immunofixation can the presence of a monoclone be ruled out.

2.3.2 Urine electrophoresis and Bence Jones proteins

Excess free light chains produced by plasma cells in myeloma 'overflow' into the urine where they can be detected by urine electrophoresis. This swamping of the reabsorption capacity of renal tubules is called **overflow proteinuria** and it can also be seen with other small, readily filtered proteins such as myoglobin following crush injury.

Overflow proteinuria

Proteinuria caused by glomerular filtration of levels of protein which exceed the reabsorption capacity of the renal tubules.

Monoclonal free light chains in urine were originally known as 'Bence Jones proteins', but the more specific name 'monoclonal free light chains' is to be preferred. Urinary whole monoclonal immunoglobulins (i.e. with both heavy and light chains) are not Bence Jones proteins.

Monoclonal free light chains filtering through the kidney may also cause glomerular damage due to deposition of the proteins in the tubules or tubular damage via tubular toxicity. All patients with suspected myeloma should have both serum and urine electrophoresis performed.

Urine monoclonal free light chains are not necessarily indicative of myeloma or malignant disease (Beetham 1979), but where laboratory data is indicative, new serum or urine free light chain monoclones should be telephoned urgently to the requesting source.

2.3.3 Measurement of free light chains

In recent years, assays for the measurement of serum κ and λ free light chains (SFLC) have become available, and are usually reported together with a serum free light chain (κ:λ) ratio. These assays have been developed for nephelometric and turbidimetric systems. Both assays use antibodies to antigenic determinants on light chains which are normally hidden by the partner heavy chain. This allows measurement of the concentration of free light chains in monoclonal gammopathies and it is a particularly suitable assay for diseases which express free light chains only, i.e. light chain myelomas and amyloidosis. The assays also detect free light chain in many samples from patients classified as non-secretory myeloma thus potentially giving the clinicians a diagnostic and monitoring marker for some examples of this disease. Measurement of free light chains also provides a useful marker for the risk of progression to myeloma by MGUS patients. If the MGUS patient has an abnormal κ:λ free light chain ratio then they are at least 2.6 times more likely to develop myeloma than if the ratio is normal.

SFLC assays require care and experience in use and interpretation. Results are expressed in mg/L and patients with light chain myeloma are sometimes measured with apparently 60 000 mg/L, i.e. 60 g/L, when the electrophoresis strip clearly shows a monoclonal band by densitometry of perhaps 3–4 g/L. The assays are acknowledged to be non-linear and susceptible to antigen excess, due to the limited number of antigenic epitopes on an abnormal monoclonal light chain. Analytical protocols are provided with the commercial kits for the instruments for which the assay is configured in an effort to address these issues. However the controls provided in the kits have target levels of less than 100 mg/L, which is well below the levels seen in myeloma patients. When using these assays, laboratories should consider producing their own high level controls from pooled patient material.

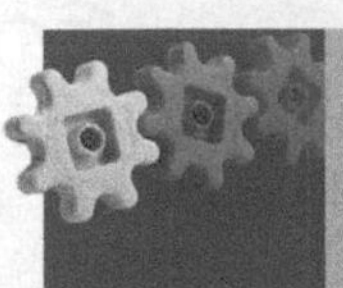

METHOD 2.1 *Quality control procedures for measuring serum immunoglobulins*

Laboratories must establish an internal quality control (IQC) procedure using samples of known concentration and the standard deviation about that target concentration. Using the statistical models and rules developed by James Westgard (Westgard and Groth 1979) the laboratory can apply rules for multiple levels of immunoglobulin concentration and reject runs which exceed these limits. Internal control runs must be performed and recorded before and after each batch of patient samples. Look at Figure 2.8 which shows an example of a Levy-Jennings chart.

External quality assessment (EQA) is achieved by the laboratory assaying samples sent from a central body and reporting the results as if they were patient material. In the UK the National External Quality Assessment Scheme (UK NEQAS) for specific proteins provides this service, dispatching three samples per month to participating laboratories. UK NEQAS provides a report on the participant's performance of the assay compared to other laboratories, performance trends, and differences between assay providers.

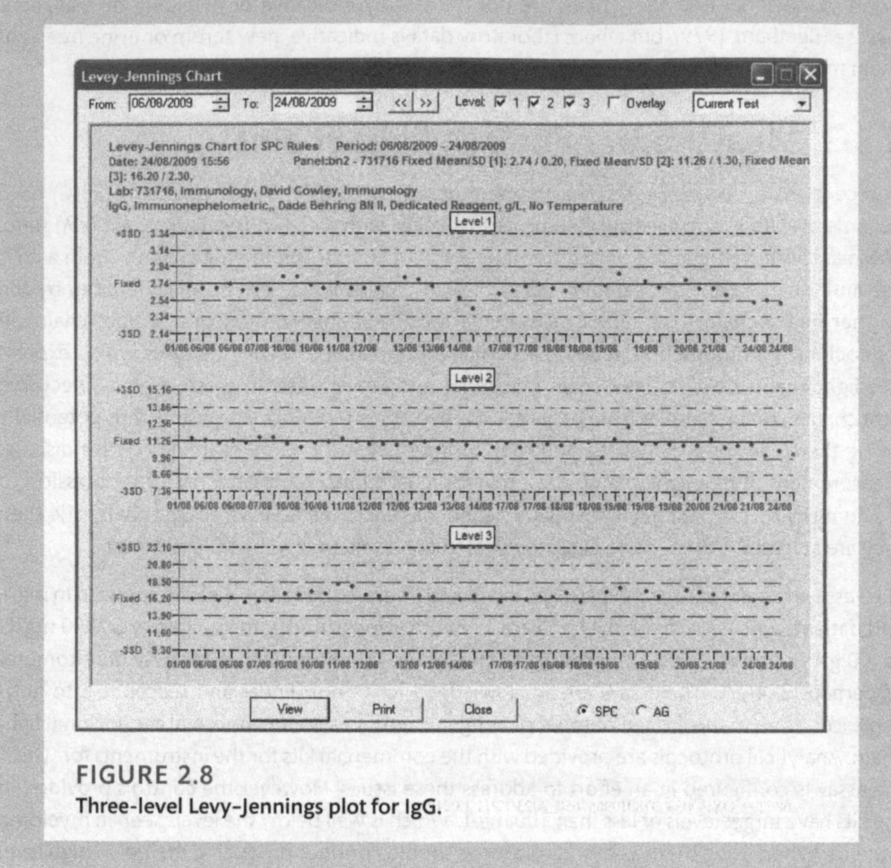

FIGURE 2.8
Three-level Levy-Jennings plot for IgG.

2.3.4 Electrophoresis

Together with serum immunoglobulin measurement, serum and urine electrophoresis form the primary screen for monoclonal gammopathy. Monoclonal immunoglobulin usually produces an abnormal banding pattern on electrophoresis.

Electrophoresis is a technique which uses an electric field to separate molecules according to their electric charge. Most hospital laboratories use automated or semi-automated electrophoresis systems which make analysis faster and simpler. The semi-automated systems use gel electrophoresis techniques, whilst the fully automated systems are usually capillary zone electrophoresis (CZE). Semi-automated techniques require significant manual input, so it is important to understand how the method works and how to get the best results from it, whereas CZE is more 'press-and-go'. However, both technologies require an understanding of the same two concepts: the isoelectric point and how it relates to the behaviour of proteins in solution, and electroendosmotic flow.

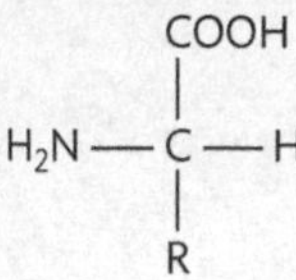

FIGURE 2.9
General structure of an amino acid.

The isoelectric point (pI)

Amino acids are the building blocks of protein and have a general structure as shown in Figure 2.9. When amino acids are placed in solution they form ionic species. Whether an amino acid becomes positively or negatively charged depends upon the nature of the amino acid R group, and the pH of the solution.

When a whole protein is placed in solution, its net charge is the sum of the charges on its component amino acids. The isoelectric point (pI) is the pH at which the protein net charge is zero. The pI for any given protein is constant and specific for that protein.

When the solution is acidic relative to the pI the protein will gain protons from the solution and, if an electric field is applied, the protein will migrate towards the cathode. When the solution is basic relative to the pI the protein will donate protons to the solution and will migrate towards the anode.

Most gel systems use an alkaline buffer. At these pH levels all serum proteins have a net negative charge and should move towards the anode.

Electroendosmotic flow

Electroendosmosis (sometimes called electro-osmosis or endosmosis) is an effect caused by the use of an immobile support medium which has a negative charge relative to that of a mobile solution. When an electric field is applied to the system the relatively positive ions in the solution begin to flow towards the cathode. The flow strength increases as the charge difference between the two phases (mobile and immobile) increases, and also as the voltage increases.

Cross reference

For a more complete explanation of electrophorectic techniques, see Keren (2003).

2.3.5 Gel protein electrophoresis

Method

Online Resource Centre

To see an online video demonstrating agarose gel electrophoresis, log on to www.oxfordtextbooks.co.uk/orc/fbs

Separation occurs within a gel (usually agarose on a plastic support) which is loaded with buffer pH 8.6.

Sample is applied between the anodal and cathodal ends of the gel. The amount of protein applied to the gel is determined by the concentration of protein in the sample and length of time the sample is allowed to diffuse into the gel.

As the electrophoresis buffer is alkaline relative to the pI of the serum proteins, the proteins become negatively charged. When an electric field is applied the proteins begin to move towards the anode. This may be at different velocities depending on the net negative charge of the protein.

However, the agarose gel is negatively charged relative to the buffer, and this sets up an electroendosmotic flow of positive buffer ions towards the cathode. For protein molecules with low net negative charge their pull towards the anode is weaker than the pull of the electroendosmotic flow and, like poor swimmers in a strong current, they are carried towards the cathode.

After electrophoresis the gel is dried and stained with a protein selective stain.

By using a protein selective stain the molecules of interest, i.e. immunoglobulins, can be visualized without excessive interference from other serum components, such as hormones, metabolites, and ions.

A 'normal' serum **protein electrophoresis** pattern shows six major fractions. There are five bands–Albumin, alpha-1, alpha-2, beta-1, and beta-2–and a non-banded gamma region. These are shown in Figures 2.10a and 2.10b. Table 2.3 lists some of the proteins that are found in each of the major fractions.

A 'normal' urine protein electrophoresis pattern shows only an albumin band, which can be seen in Figure 2.11.

Protein electrophoresis

The separation of the protein molecules within a solution (usually serum, urine, or CSF) as a result of their differing motilities within an electric field.

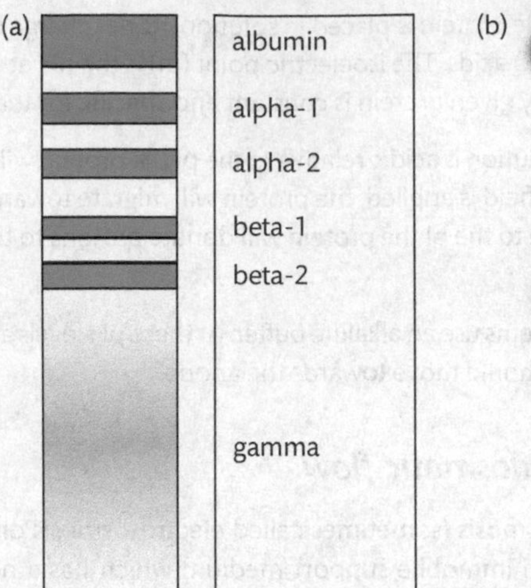

FIGURE 2.10
(a) Diagrammatical representation of serum protein separation in gel electrophoresis; (b) normal serum protein electrophoresis.

TABLE 2.3 Proteins found in the regions of protein electrophoresis.

Region	Major proteins present
Albumin	Albumin
α_1	α_1-Antitrypsin, $\alpha_1$acid glycoprotein
α_2	α_2-Macroglobulin,$_1$haptoglobin
β_1	Transferrin
β_2	C3
γ,	Immunoglobulins (γ-globulins)

FIGURE 2.11
Normal urine protein electrophoresis.

SELF-CHECK 2.1

Why it is important to use a protein selective stain in electrophoresis?

Technical points to note

The gel

- Gels packaged in excess buffer require 'blotting' before use—excess surface buffer can interfere with sample application.
- To prevent distortion of migration, gels need to be uniform. Care should be taken when handling gels and, ideally, gels with obvious defects should not be used.
- Voltage application generates heat. This heat needs to be removed, and one way of achieving this is a Peltier plate—an electrical device which can provide or remove heat. If the system uses a Peltier plate it is important that the gel has a uniform contact with the plate so that optimal heat transfer can occur.

Sample preparation

- Serum should be used in preference to plasma, as plasma contains fibrinogen. Haemolysed and lipaemic samples should be also be avoided. Early morning urine is preferred as it has a higher protein concentration.
- Urine electrophoresis methods need to be able to detect protein fractions down to approximately 10 mg/L. If this cannot be achieved using neat urine, then urine samples should be concentrated before application using an ultrafiltration membrane with a cut-off of <10 kDa, to ensure no free light chains are lost. Sample is loaded onto the membrane and water is either absorbed through the membrane by absorbent pads, or liquid may be pulled through the membrane by centrifugation. Concentration should occur until albumin is visible.
- CZE has few advantages to offer over other systems for urine electrophoresis; however, if CZE is used urine requires concentration and desalting. Desalting improves electrophoretic resolution and is achieved by dialysis.

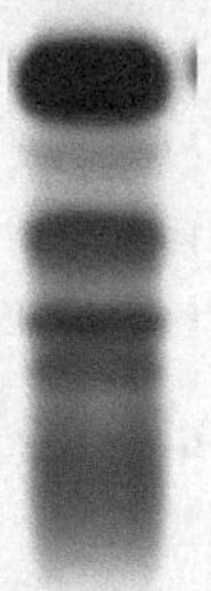

FIGURE 2.12
An example of sample 'overloading' on gel electrophoresis.

Sample application

- Sample is applied to the gel surface via an 'application device' which allows consistent application of a number of samples simultaneously. It is important that sample is not overloaded onto the gel, the result of which can be seen in Figure 2.12.
- Conversely, crystals in urine can impede the flow of sample onto the gel and result in under-application, as can cryoglobulin in serum samples.

Staining

- The first step is to fix the proteins within the gel using an acidic solution. Some systems have separate fix and stain solutions, others have a combined fix/stain. If the acid fixative is reused then its pH will increase over time due to contamination with alkaline gel buffer. To maintain good staining it is important to replace the fix solution at the recommended intervals.
- Amido black and acid violet are the most frequently used stains. Amido black is usually used for serum protein electrophoresis staining, whilst the more sensitive acid violet stain is used for urine protein electrophoresis and for immunofixation. An ideal stain binds linearly to protein, meaning that the amount of protein present is directly related to the stain intensity. This allows the quantification of bands within the gel by **densitometry**.
- Following staining the gel is 'destained' a number of times to remove background staining, thus enhancing the contrast between the stained proteins and clear gel.

Densitometry
The quantitative measurement of optical density.

Reading protein electrophoresis gels

A textbook can only give an introduction to reading gels. The only way to learn to read gels is by reading them routinely in a clinical laboratory.

- Before starting to read, prepare your environment:
    - sit in an area with good lighting and (ideally) no distractions
    - find a piece of clean white paper to place behind the gel—this will help show up changes in stain density (some people prefer yellow for reading urine gels).
- Check that any internal quality control samples on the gel have run correctly.

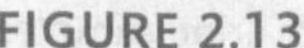

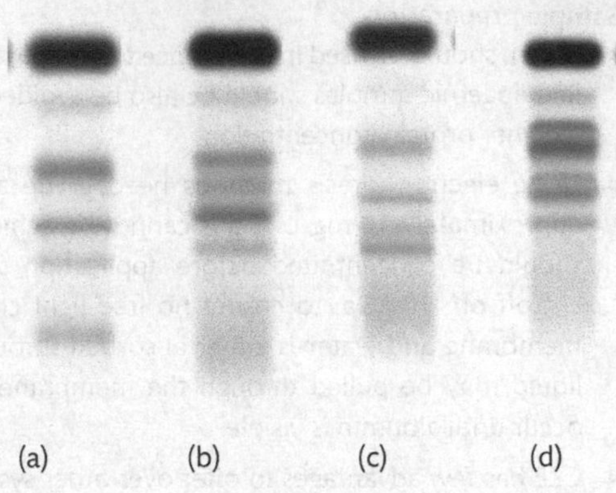

FIGURE 2.13

(a) A strip from a sample containing a monoclonal immunoglobulin; (b) a sample with haemolysis; (c) a sample with fibrinogen; (d) a sample with lipaemia. These show patterns which can be mistaken for a monoclone.

Serum

- Depending which system is being used, there may be five or six regions. (In higher resolution systems the β region can be split.) Note whether there are five (six) regions.
- Note whether the staining in each region is lower than normal, normal, or greater than normal. (**Note:** this may not be as easy as it sounds since stain intensity can vary significantly between gels. The usual method is to assess the average intensity for that region over the whole gel and use this as 'normal' for that gel.)
- Note whether there are any extra bands present and where they are in relation to the named regions.

Figure 2.13 shows a strip from a sample containing a monoclonal immunoglobulin and samples with haemolysis, fibrinogen, and lipaemia. These show patterns which can be mistaken for a monoclone.

Table 2.4 details some of the major electrophoresis patterns seen in the laboratory setting.

Using these observations, together with the knowledge of how protein levels alter in disease and information from other blood tests, a final decision can be reached about whether further investigation for monoclonal gammopathy is required. A sample showing an unexplained banding pattern together with immune paresis or with raised IgA or IgM levels should be sent for **immunofixation.**

Immunofixation

Process in which a specific antibody is used to 'fix' antigens within a gel after electrophoresis by means of the formation of antibody-antigen complexes. After removing unfixed molecules by washing and then staining the fixed complexes, the presence or absence of specific molecules in the original sample can be demonstrated.

Key Point

Raised immunoglobulins are seen in many different diseases, for example raised IgA in heavy drinkers with renal dysfunction, or raised IgM in primary biliary cirrhosis (PBC). Depending on the clinical reasoning for performing electrophoresis, immunofixation may not be performed.

Cross reference

You can read more about IgM in PBC in Chapter 9.

Urine

- Note whether there is an albumin band present.
- Note whether there are any other bands present.

TABLE 2.4 **Proteins found in the regions of protein electrophoresis.**

A. Single region with altered staining intensity	
Absent α_1 band	Associated with α_1-antitrypsin deficiency, or with an α_1-antitrypsin variant with altered electrophoretic mobility.
Absent β_2 band	Usually seen in aged samples. C3 is converted to C3c, which runs in the β_1 region.
Reduced γ region	May be associated with reduced immunoglobulins, but may be normal (e.g. in young children). **Need to measure immunoglobulins to assess properly**.
Increased γ region	May be associated with increased polyclonal immunoglobulins (e.g. in infection or chronic disease) but may be artefact due to overstaining. **Need to measure immunoglobulins to assess properly**.
β-γ bridging	Increased staining under the β_2 band is known as β-γ bridging. Seen in liver disease and associated with raised polyclonal IgA and (sometimes) IgM. **Need to measure immunoglobulins to assess properly**.
B. Altered intensity in several bands	
Acute phase response	Decreased albumin, increased α_1(↑ α_1-antitrypsin), increased α_2(↑ α_2-macroglobulin and haptoglobin), normal/decreased β_1 (↓ transferrin), normal/increased β_2(↑ C3), normal/increased γ.
Chronic inflammatory pattern	As acute phase response but with additional increased γ region.
Cirrhotic pattern	Albumin, α_1, α_2, β_1, and β_2 bands all decreased due to reduced protein production by the liver with an increased γ region.
Nephrotic pattern	All regions are reduced due to protein loss through the kidney, particularly albumin and the γ regions. The α_2 band is normal or increased as α_2-macroglobulin is too large to be lost in this way. A reduction may be seen in the β band as transferrin is lost, but C3 may be raised.
C. Extra bands present[a]	
Bisalbuminaemia	Bisalbuminaemia is an inherited abnormality of albumin in which both normal albumin and an albumin variant are produced. The variant has a different electrophoretic mobility, but may migrate either above or below the normal band. Bisalbuminaemia has no clinical significance.
Fibrinogen	If plasma is tested rather than serum, an extra band due to fibrinogen (the protein from which the fibrin clot is formed when blood coagulates) is seen below the β_2 band. A fibrinogen band may obscure a monoclone in this region.
Haemoglobin-haptoglobin	Free haemoglobin in blood is scavenged by haptoglobin. The haemoglobin–haptoglobin complex has an electrophoretic mobility different from that of free haptoglobin and this shows as an extra band in the region between the α_2 and β_1 bands. It is most commonly seen in haemolysed samples.
Lipoprotein	All samples contain lipoproteins, but they are not usually detectable on gel electrophoresis. In patients with raised lipoprotein levels extra bands with a distinctive shape may be seen in the α and β regions.
Monoclonal immunoglobulin	Bands due to monoclonal immunoglobulins can migrate between the α_2 band and the end of the γ region. Their intensity can vary significantly, and small monoclones can easily 'hide' under the normal bands. It is recommended to measure IgG, IgA, and IgM on samples for serum electrophoresis, as abnormal immunoglobulin levels with a normal electrophoresis pattern may suggest a concealed monoclonal band.

[a] Extra bands are not necessarily abnormal, but they need to be investigated and accounted for.

The staining patterns seen on urine electrophoresis are much more variable than those seen on serum and any sample showing either no albumin bands or bands in addition to albumin should be investigated further by immunofixation (see Section 2.3.7).

2.3.6 Capillary zone electrophoresis

Method

Separation occurs in a liquid buffer (pH~10—the exact pH depends upon the analyser used) flowing through a fused silica capillary tube. A set volume of sample is then aspirated and introduced into the anodal end of the capillary.

The buffer is alkaline relative to the pI of serum proteins, so the proteins donate protons to the buffer and become negatively charged. When an electric field is applied the proteins remain at the anode. However, the interior of the capillary has a strong negative charge relative to the buffer, and the application of a high voltage creates a strong electroendosmotic flow of buffer ions to the cathode. The pull of this flow is much stronger than the attraction to the anode and so the proteins begin to move cathodally. Proteins with the lowest net negative charge at pH 10 have the weakest attraction to the anode. They travel rapidly in the electroendosmotic flow and reach the cathode first. Proteins with the highest net negative charge at pH 10 have the strongest attraction to the anode. This retards their movement and they reach the cathode later as shown in Figure 2.14.

An ultraviolet detector at the cathodal end of the capillary detects the proteins as they pass by using peptide bond UV absorbance at 214nm. From this, a plot of absorption versus time—an electropherogram—can be constructed. A 'normal' serum protein electropherogram shows the same six major fractions as gel electrophoresis: five bands—albumin, alpha-1, alpha-2, beta-1, and beta-2—and a non-banded gamma region. Look at Figure 2.15a, whilst urine shows only a trace of albumin, shown in Figure 2.15b.

Technical points to note

Buffer

- Different buffers are used for different applications. Ensure you are using the correct buffer and that the system has been primed before use.

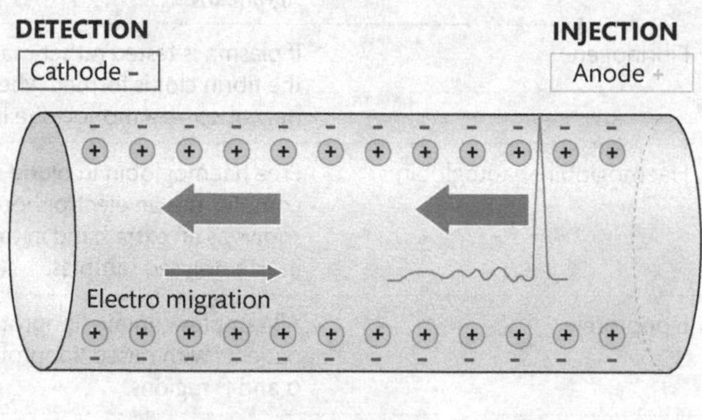

FIGURE 2.14
Protein migration towards the cathode.

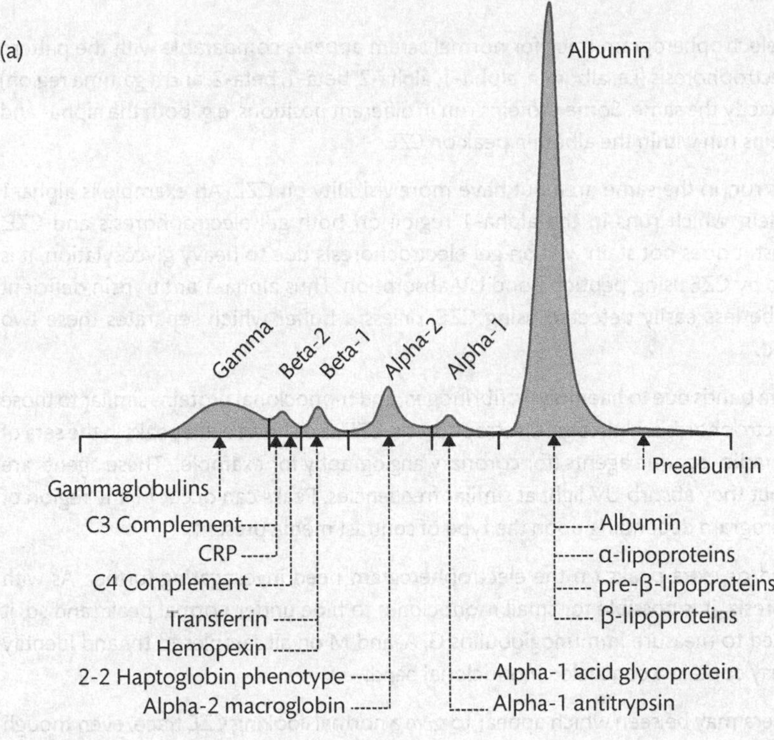

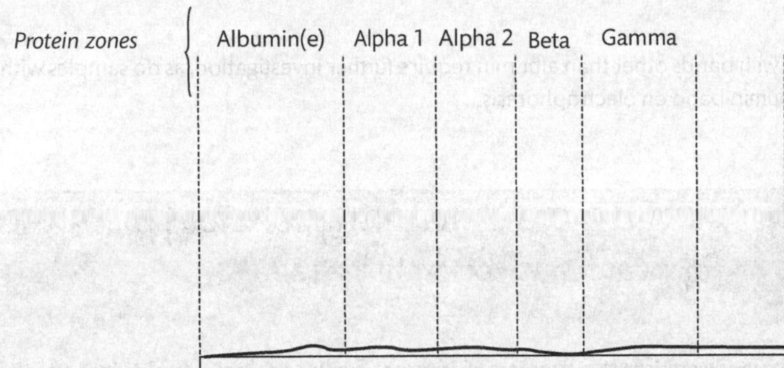

FIGURE 2.15
(a) Normal serum protein electropherogram; (b) normal urine electropherogram.

Sample application and separation

- Urine samples may need special preparation—e.g. desalting—before testing.
- Unlike gel electrophoresis, where each sample has its own individual section of gel, the capillaries in CZE analysers are washed and then prepared for the next sample. It is important to follow cleaning and maintenance protocols to ensure that the capillaries remain clean and give good performance.

Reading protein electropherograms

As with reading protein electrophoresis gels, the only way to become proficient at reading electropherograms is through practice.

Serum

Although the electropherogram trace for normal serum appears comparable with the pattern seen on gel electrophoresis (i.e. albumin, alpha-1, alpha-2, beta-1, beta-2, and a gamma region) they are not exactly the same. Some proteins run in different positions, e.g. both the alpha- and beta-lipoproteins run within the albumin peak on CZE.

Some proteins run in the same area but have more visibility on CZE. An example is alpha-1 acid glycoprotein which runs in the alpha-1 region on both gel electrophoresis and CZE. However, whilst it does not stain well on gel electrophoresis due to heavy glycosylation, it is easily detected by CZE using peptide bond UV absorption. Thus alpha-1 antitrypsin deficient samples may be less easily detected using CZE, unless a buffer which separates these two proteins is used.

CZE shows extra bands due to haemolysis, fibrinogen, and monoclonal proteins similar to those seen on gel electrophoresis. Unlike gel electrophoresis, CZE also shows extra peaks in the sera of patients given radio-opaque agents (for coronary angiography for example). These agents are not proteins, but they absorb UV light at similar frequencies. Peaks can occur in any region of the electropherogram depending upon the type of contrast media present.

All unusual and/or extra peaks on the electropherogram need investigating further. As with gel electrophoresis, it is possible for small monoclones to hide under normal peaks and so, it is recommended to measure immunoglobulins G, A, and M on all samples to try and identify those which may contain a concealed monoclonal band.

Occasionally, sera may be seen which appear to give a normal-looking CZE trace, even though immunofixation then shows there to be a significant monoclone present. These can often be identified by abnormalities in immunoglobulin quantitation.

Urine

All samples with bands other than albumin require further investigation, as do samples without a visible albumin band on electrophoresis.

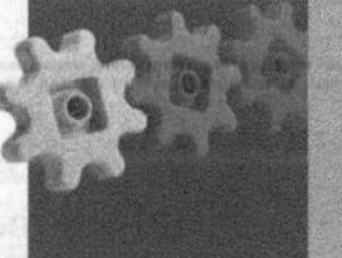

METHOD 2.2 Quality control procedures for protein electrophoresis

Electrophoresis requires the running of internal quality control samples just as other laboratory tests do. It is recommended to run a known paraprotein of known concentration in parallel.

UK NEQAS for Immunology runs a scheme for monoclonal protein identification which includes serum and urine protein electrophoresis and also serum and urine monoclone identification and quantification.

SELF-CHECK 2.2

What sample (or samples) would you run as internal quality controls for serum and urine electrophoresis, and why?

2.3.7 Immunofixation

The primary purpose of immunofixation ('fixing') is to identify the presence and determine the isotype (the heavy and light chains present) of a monoclonal immunoglobulin in a sample. The technique uses gel electrophoresis followed by reaction with antisera against heavy and light chains. However, it can also be used to determine the presence/absence of any protein for which a specific antiserum is available. Immunofixation is the only way of determining the presence of a small monoclone under a normal electrophoretic band.

Not all samples showing abnormalities require immunofixation. For example, samples from patients with a known, obvious monoclonal band do not need fixing every time a serum is received in the laboratory unless there is a significant change, such as another band appearing. Similarly, a haemolysis pattern obtained from a haemolysed sample does not need investigation unless other pathology test results suggest that there may also be a monoclone present.

CLINICAL CORRELATION 2.8

Why is it important to type the monoclone?

- **Certain diseases are associated with certain monoclone types for example, IgM monoclones are associated with Waldenström's macroglobulinaemia.**
- **Certain monoclone types, such as an IgD monoclone, are associated with a poorer prognosis.**
- **The presence of co-migrating monoclones with different isotypes can be identified by immunofixation.**
- **There are different clinical correlations with free κ and free λ light chains. Free λ light chains are associated with AL amyloidosis. Free κ light chains are associated with light chain deposition disease. Prognosis of these two diseases are different, therefore it is important to know the type of free light chain.**

Method

Immunofixation has four stages:

1. **Electrophoresis:** each sample is run in a number of identical lanes (usually six).
2. **Antisera application:** a general protein fixative (usually acid) is applied to lane 1 to give a reference track and then specific antisera are applied to the other protein lanes. If a corresponding antigen is present in the sample, immune complexes form between it and the antiserum. These complexes lodge ('fix') within the gel matrix. The usual protocol for initial immunofixation is fixative, anti-G, -A, and -M heavy chains, anti-κ and anti-λ light chains.
3. **Wash:** all unfixed proteins are washed from the gel.
4. **Stain:** all the fixed proteins are stained with a sensitive stain, such as acid violet.

By comparing the proteins fixed in each lane, the constituents of an electrophoretic band can be identified and its mono- or polyclonality determined. Undefined bands may be seen in the γ region associated with chronic inflammatory states such as infection or autoimmune disease. See Figure 2.16 for examples of immunofixation.

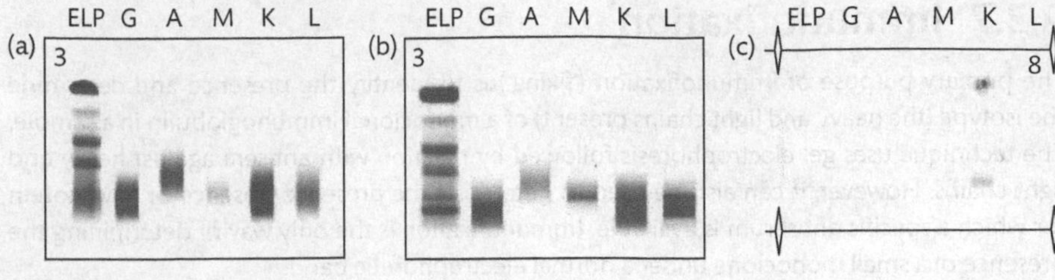

FIGURE 2.16
(a) Normal serum immunofixation; (b) serum bi-clone IgGλ and IgMλ; (c) urine κ free light chain.

Technical points to note

Electrophoresis

- Immunofixation is more sensitive than electrophoresis alone and so serum samples are usually diluted before application. Immunofixation is subject to antibody/antigen excess effects so the dilution factors need to be chosen carefully. Urine samples can be applied neat or concentrated. The concentration factor usually depends upon the urine total protein level.

Antisera application

- Ensure any devices for applying antisera are clean and dry so that there is no carryover between tracks.
- Immunofixation is capable of giving false negative results due to antibody or antigen excess. In these situations only small immune complexes are formed. These cannot fix within the gel and are washed out with the other non-fixed proteins. Antigen excess shows as a 'cut-out' hole in the middle of the band. This is shown in Figure 2.17. To confirm this, the serum can be diluted and retested. However, if you have to dilute the sample, either to reduce the likelihood of antigen excess occurring (e.g. if a large monoclone is present or because the immunoglobulin level is raised overall) then there is a possibility of 'diluting out' any small monoclones which might also be present. Complete investigation may sometimes require testing at a number of different sample dilutions.
- Immunofixation can also appear to give false positive results if the antisera reacts with other serum components in addition to its main target—for example an anti-λ antisera which also reacts with fibrinogen. Laboratories need to be aware of these—check the package insert—and confirm band identity with a second antiserum if necessary.
- Occasionally, there is some difficulty in detecting IgA λ paraproteins, as the λ light chains do not stain. Sometimes changing the anti-λ source to another commercial company resolves this.

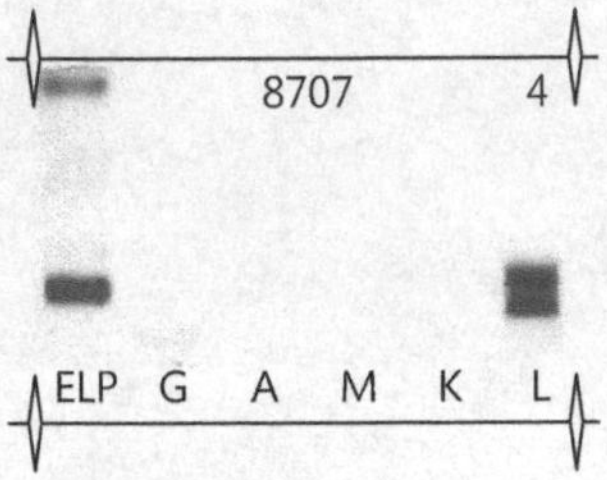

8707 4

ELP G A M K L

FIGURE 2.17
Antigen excess on immunofixation. See how the band in the λ lane has its centre 'cut out'.

Immunofixation interpretation

Serum

- Bands in the individual antisera lanes must line up with those in the reference lane and must match the pattern seen on electrophoresis. Whole monoclones are most common, free light chain monoclones are not uncommon, and heavy chain only monoclones are rare but possible.
- IgA paraproteins tend to have a tight band; IgA heavy chain monoclones can appear like a smear due to the fragmented heavy chain.
- Immunofixes showing a possible free light chain monoclone must have IgD and IgE monoclones excluded (usually by further immunofixation with IgD and IgE antisera).
- Where raised polyclonal immunoglobulin is present it may not be possible to identify small monoclones against the deeply stained background, commonly seen in viral infections. Repeat at a higher dilution if necessary.

- Some IgM monoclones may precipitate at the application point and not separate electrophoretically. Pre-treatment with 1M dithiothreitol (DTT) reduces polymerization by interrupting disulphide linkages between the molecules and can resolve the problem in most cases. DTT is less toxic than 2-mercaptoethanol which was traditionally used for this purpose.

Urine

Bands in the individual antisera lanes must line up with those in the reference lane and must match the pattern seen on electrophoresis.

2.3.8 Immunotyping by CZE

Immunotyping by CZE is the equivalent of immunofixation, but is currently limited to detection of IgG, IgA, IgM, and free light chain monoclones.

Method

Incubating the serum with specific antiserum (anti-IgG, anti-IgA, anti-IgM, anti-κ light chain, or anti-λ light chain), either attached to a bead or in fluid phase, will remove or alter the mobility of the corresponding peak.

The electropherogram obtained for each supernatant is compared with that for non-treated serum. If a monoclone is present, a peak will be seen on the untreated electropherogram. If the monoclone is caused by one of the five isotypes tested, the supernatant from that well will show an electropherogram with the peak missing. The isotype of this well can then be assigned to the monoclone. Monoclonal peaks will show subtraction of the peak in electropherograms corresponding to a single heavy and a single light chain antiserum, whilst polyclonal peaks will have partial subtractions with both light chain antisera and potentially more than one heavy chain antiserum. This is shown in Figure 2.18.

Technical points to note

- If the monoclonal fraction does not totally disappear on the antisera patterns then a higher serum dilution may be required.
- Some small clones (<5 grams) are not easily detectable by CZE immunotyping—especially if there is a polyclonal background. In these cases it may be better to use gel-based methods instead.

Interpretation

- The detected monoclonal peak must be located at the same migration distance as the suspected monoclonal fraction seen in the reference lane.
- Samples which appear to have more than one monoclonal component should be pretreated with a depolymerizing agent and retested to exclude polymerization. This tends to be an issue in hyperviscosity syndrome associated with IgA and IgG3 myelomas.
- Traces showing a possible free light chain monoclone should have IgD and IgE monoclones excluded. This will usually require immunofixation with IgD and IgE antisera as immunosubtraction for IgD/IgE is not yet commercially available.

2.3.9 Densitometry

When a monoclonal immunoglobulin is present it requires quantification. Initial quantification can give information about prognosis in some diseases and serial measurements can be used to assess disease progression and therapy effectiveness. Densitometry is used because

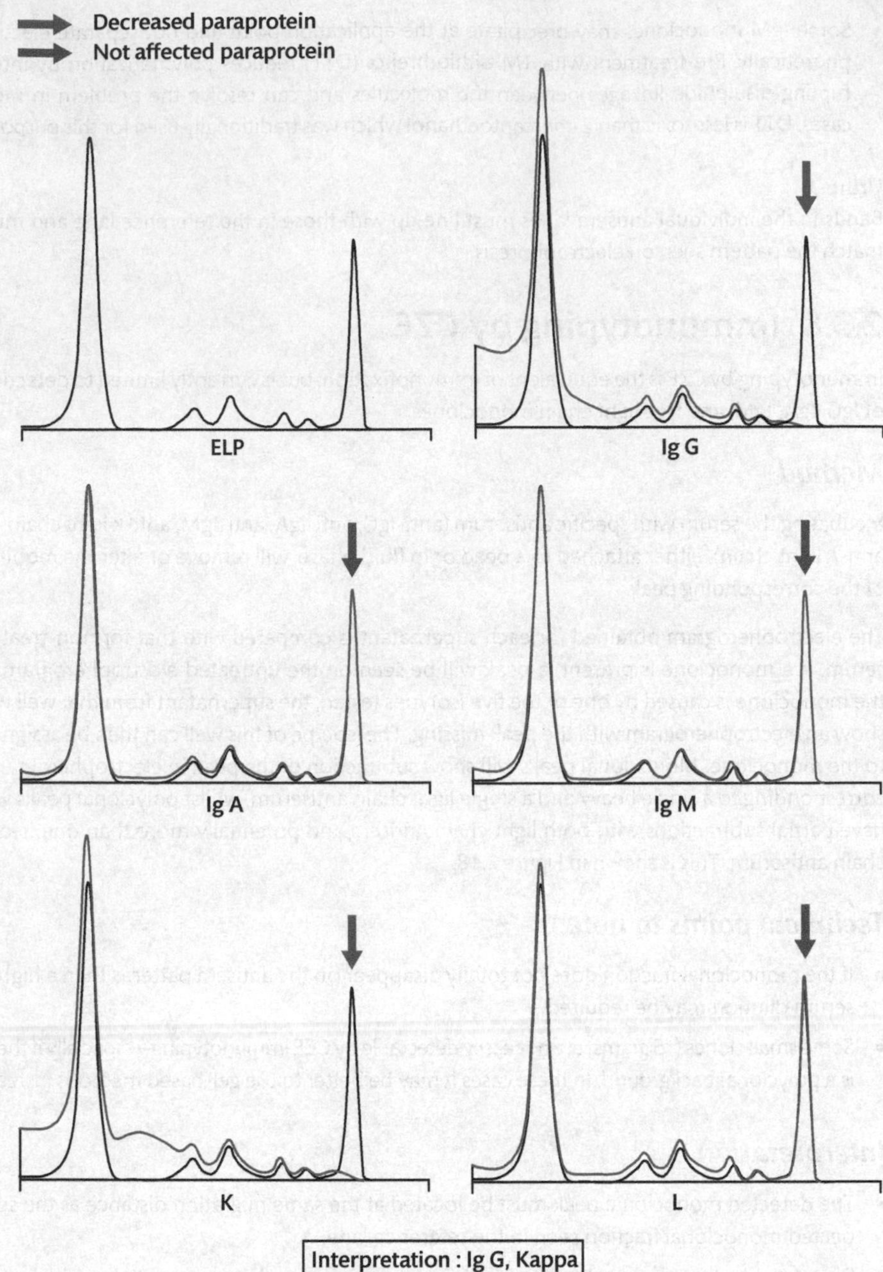

FIGURE 2.18
An example of subtraction showing an IgG κ monoclone.

it allows monoclones to be quantified individually and specifically. This is not the case with immunoglobulin measurements where monoclonal and polyclonal immunoglobulin cannot be separated and multiple monoclones cannot be quantified separately.

Method

When light is passed through an electrophoresis strip, the amount of light absorbed by the gel at any point is related to the intensity of the stain (the wavelength chosen depends upon the stain used). A plot of absorbance over the length of the electrophoresis strip gives the densitometric scan for that sample. Originally this required a densitometer with different light filters for different stains, but it is more usual now to use simple flat-bed scanners with software conversion of the signal into that expected from a densitometer.

If a linear stain has been used then the stain intensity is directly related to the amount of protein in the strip and the area under the scan is equal to the sample total protein. By dividing the scan using 'gates', the percentage of the total protein in an area can be calculated. If the serum total protein is measured the monoclone percentage protein can be converted into a monoclone quantification. The plot of UV absorbance against time in the CZE electropherogram is directly comparable with the densitometric plot of light absorbance against gel length and is used to quantify monoclonal peaks in the same way. Look at Figure 2.19 to see a densitometric scan.

Technical points to note

- Flat-bed scanners pick up artefacts. Ensure the back of the gel and the scanner plate are free of stain deposits, dust, hairs, etc. before scanning. When analysing the scans, be aware of bands on the scan which are not on the gel. Such artefactual bands are common with urine scans but can also occur with serum.
- There is a non-linear relationship between dye-binding and protein concentration at high monoclone concentrations.
- Despite the ability of densitometry to gate monoclonal bands individually, the quantification may still not be totally specific for the monoclone. Where a relatively small monoclone overlays a polyclonal background a significant proportion of the monoclonal quantification will be polyclonal in origin.

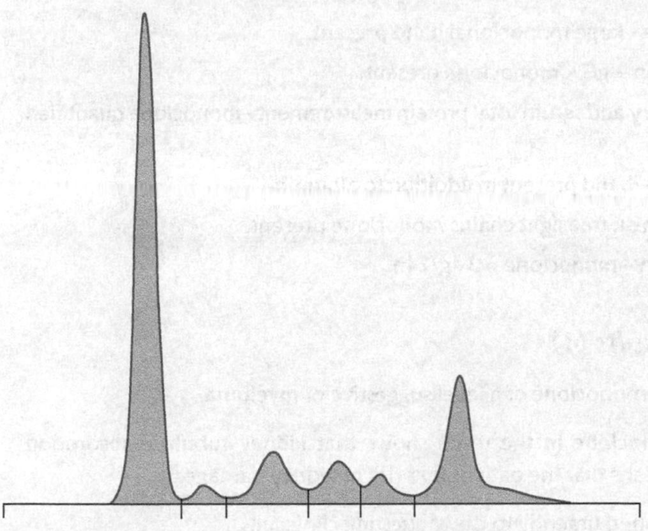

Serum protein electrophoresis

Fractions	%	Ref. %	Conc.	Ref. Conc.
pre-albumin	56.7		21.66	39.00–46.00
alpha-1	2.3		0.88	0.90–1.70
alpha-2	9.7		3.71	5.00–7.00
beta-1	6.5		2.48	4.00–6.00
beta-2	4.3		1.64	1.00–3.00
gamma	20.5		7.83	5.00–11.00

FIGURE 2.19 **An example of a densitometric scan.**

- Where a monoclone underlies a normal band (e.g., beta-2) it is not possible to quantify the monoclone specifically. Quantification involving subtraction of a nominal value for a normal background band and reporting of the 'corrected' value, or only reporting the area of the peak above the normal band, introduces errors. In this case the whole beta-2 band should be quantified and then a comment added to the results to say that the quantification includes the normal proteins of the beta-2 region.
- Total protein is commonly measured by standard biuret method, but different total protein methods can give different results and this can have an effect on monoclone quantification.
- Gating strategies differ between laboratories. It is important that all staff in a given laboratory use the same gating strategy so that results between sequential patient samples are consistent and comparable.

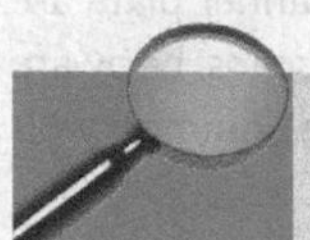

CASE STUDY 2.1 Myeloma

Patient history

A 77-year-old male presenting to GP with back pain and anaemia.

Serum and 24-hr urine samples sent for electrophoresis–?myeloma.

Results (1)

- **Serum electrophoresis–large monoclonal band present.**
- **Serum immunofixation–IgG κ monoclone present.**
- **Scanning densitometry and serum total protein measurement–monoclone quantified at 30g/L.**
- **Urine electrophoresis–band present in addition to albumin.**
- **Urine immunoflxation–κ free light chains monoclone present.**
- **Scanning densitometry–monoclone = 0.4g/24h.**

Scanning densitometry (densitometry)
The determination of the density of stain along a protein electrophoresis strip by means of light absorption. If the stain density is linear in relation to the amount of protein present, the densitometric scan can be used to determine the amount of protein in a given area, e.g. within a monoclonal band.

Significance of results (1)

The patient has a serum monoclone of a level suggestive of myeloma.

The presence of a monoclone in the urine shows that kidney tubule reabsorption is overwhelmed, and means that the patient is at risk of kidney damage.

The results were telephoned urgently to the requesting clinician.

Results (2)

- **Bone marrow trephine and aspirate showed BM plasma cells >20%.**
- **Skeletal survey showed no lytic bone lesions.**

Significance of results (2)

The patient has two out of the three diagnostic features of multiple myeloma.

2.3.10 Monoclone reporting

Having identified and quantified the monoclone a report can be issued to the requesting clinician. All new serum monoclones should have a comment added to the report to suggest that urine electrophoresis be performed if a urine sample has not already been sent. Some results may require clinical staff input or telephoning to the requesting source for urgent attention. This should be protocol driven within the laboratory but may include results for new large monoclones, new light chain monoclones, and >50% increases in monoclone quantification.

CLINICAL CORRELATION 2.9

Are all monoclonal bands associated with myeloma?

Diseases associated with the presence of monoclonal immunoglobulin include Waldenström's macroglobulinaemia, monoclonal gammopathy of uncertain significance (MGUS), lymphoma, chronic lymphocytic leukaemia, amyloidosis, and heavy chain disease, as well as myeloma. In addition benign, usually transient, monoclones may be seen in response to infection.

2.4 Cerebrospinal fluid and isoelectric focusing

2.4.1 Cerebrospinal fluid (CSF)

CSF is the fluid that surrounds the brain and spinal cord and protects them from impact. It also bathes the brain in electrolytes and proteins, although its protein content is low (0.15–0.5g/L) compared with that of plasma. Normally 80% of CSF protein is derived from plasma via ultrafiltration across the blood–CSF barrier, 18% is synthesized within the CSF area, and 2% is released due to cell breakdown. Filtration of protein from the plasma to the CSF is selective, with low molecular weight proteins passing through more readily than those with higher molecular weight. The amount of any individual protein filtered into the CSF is therefore dependent on its molecular mass and relative serum concentration. Thus the concentration of albumin in the CSF is approximately 225 times less than that in plasma (200 mg/L v. 45 000 mg/L) whilst that of immunoglobulin IgG is 500 times less (20 mg/L v. 10 000mg/L) due to its higher molecular weight. In healthy individuals all the immunoglobulin IgG within the CSF will be plasma-derived. In certain diseases however cells migrate across the blood–brain barrier, and where those cells are lymphocytes the CSF may include locally produced (intrathecal) IgG. By comparing the IgG composition of paired serum and CSF, this intrathecal synthesis can be detected by the presence of banding patterns (oligoclonal bands) in the CSF which are not present in serum. Normal electrophoresis is not sufficiently sensitive for this, but a variant of electrophoresis called isoelectric focusing is.

CLINICAL CORRELATION 2.10

Diseases associated with intrathecal IgG synthesis and oligoclonal banding

- **Multiple sclerosis (MS).**
- **Viral infections such as meningitis, encephalitis, and subacute sclerosing panencephalitis (SSPE).**
- **Neurosyphilis.**

- **Bacterial meningitis.**
- **Systemic lupus erythematosus (SLE).**
- **Sarcoidosis.**

Diffusion ratio

When no intrathecal synthesis is present the ratio of serum and CSF albumin and IgG should be approximately constant. A diffusion ratio between the proteins can be calculated:

$$\frac{\text{Serum Alb}\ [\text{g/L}]}{\text{Serum IgG}\ [\text{g/L}]} \times \frac{\text{CSF IgG}\ [\text{mg/L}]}{\text{CSF Alb}\ [\text{mg/L}]} = \text{Diffusion Ratio}$$

Where intrathecal synthesis is present, the CSF IgG level will be higher than expected from the serum concentration, and the diffusion ratio will increase. A value of >0.7 indicates possible intrathecal synthesis.

However, the diffusion ratio can be insensitive and may give a value ≤0.7 even when isoelectric focusing shows patterns indicating intrathecal synthesis. That is why IgG oligoclonal band detection by isoelectric focusing is the reference method for MS diagnosis.

2.4.2 Isoelectric focusing (IEF)

IEF is an electrophoretic technique in which the gel is permeated with chemicals (called ampholines) which migrate to set up a pH gradient through the gel when the electric field is applied. The molecules in the sample move through the gel according to their electric charge as before, but that charge alters as the molecules pass through the pH gradient. When the molecules reach their individual isoelectric point (pI)—the pH at which the net molecular charge is zero—they stop migrating. This increases the resolution which can be achieved and means that molecules with similar pI values (which would run together on normal electrophoresis) can be separated.

Technical points to note

- Paired serum and CSF samples should be run side by side. Interpretation is not possible without a concurrent serum sample. If a serum is not taken at the same time as the CSF then a sample taken within 7 days is acceptable.
- For comparability, serum and CSF samples need similar IgG levels. To achieve this serum samples should be diluted before application.
- CSF should usually be applied neat, but samples with a raised CSF IgG level may be difficult to interpret. Dilution to ~50mg/L (with similar for the serum sample) can help.
- IgG in CSF can be unstable and banding patterns can deteriorate over time. Small samples are more prone to this deterioration. Multiple freeze-thawing should be avoided.
- IEF electrophoresis is a high-voltage technique. A large amount of heat is produced during the process and this heat must be removed effectively for good resolution to be achieved.

After IEF, a staining technique is required which is both sensitive and specific for IgG. One option is immunoblotting: blotting the proteins from the gel onto a nitrocellulose membrane and then using a two-stage immunoenzyme technique for visualization. Another is immunofixation with IgG followed by immunoenzyme staining.

Interpretation

There are five recognized 'patterns' which are shown in Figures 2.20 and 2.21.

- Pattern 1 shows normal diffuse polyclonal IgG in both CSF and serum.
- Pattern 2 shows oligoclonal banding in the CSF but polyclonal IgG in the serum, indicating intrathecal IgG synthesis. This pattern is seen in MS.
- Pattern 3 shows oligoclonal banding in both CSF and serum, but with extra bands in the CSF which are not seen in the serum. This indicates the presence of systemic inflammation, but with additional intrathecal synthesis. This pattern is seen in MS, SLE, sarcoidosis, and central nervous system (CNS) infection.
- Pattern 4 shows identical oligoclonal banding in the CSF and serum, indicating systemic disease such as Guillain–Barré syndrome, HIV infection, or another chronic inflammatory state.
- Pattern 5 also shows identical banding in CSF and serum and is associated with the presence of a serum IgG monoclone. The multiple bands are due to isomers of the monoclone which have small charge differences, as glycosylation alters the charge and molecular weight, and therefore move differently. These isomers are resolved by IEF but show as a monoclone on normal electrophoresis.
- **Note**: it is impossible to distinguish patterns 2, 3, and 4 without a concurrent serum sample.

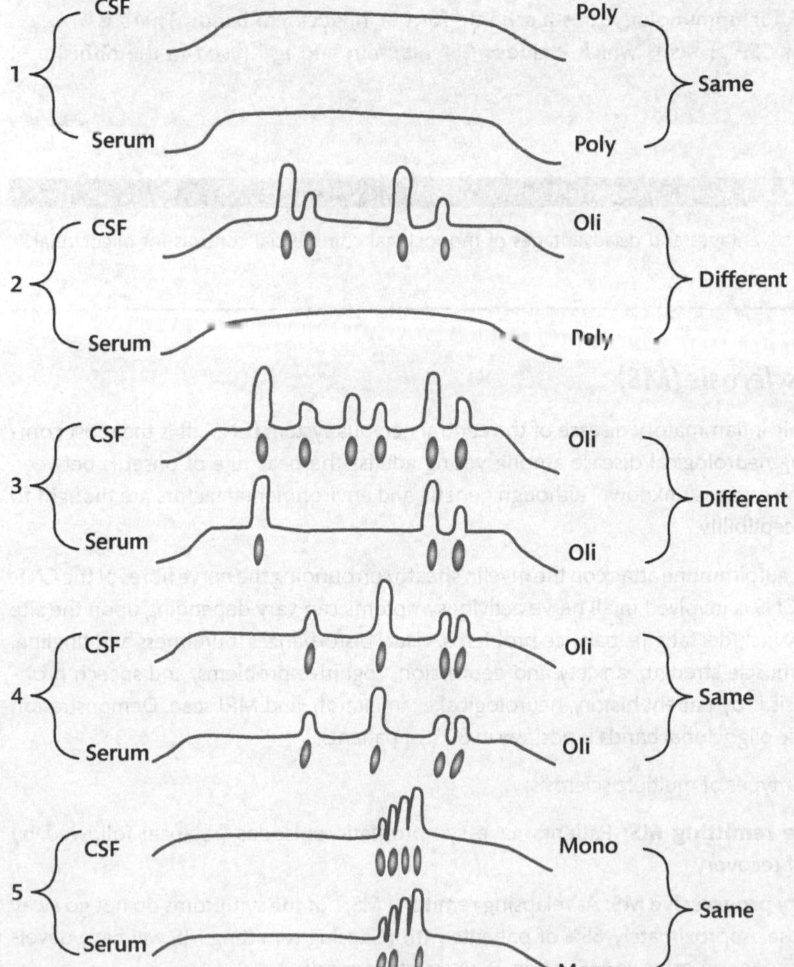

FIGURE 2.20
The five recognized patterns of isoelectric focusing shown diagrammatically.

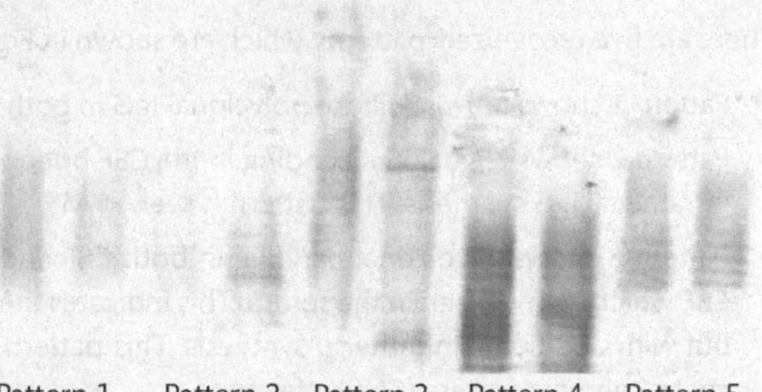

FIGURE 2.21
The five recognized patterns of IEF on a completed nitrocellulose membrane.

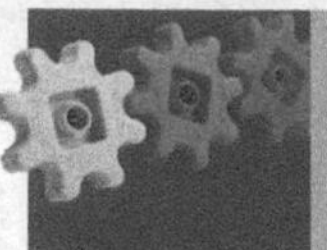

METHOD 2.3 Quality control procedures for oligoclonal bands

Because oligoclonal banding patterns 2, 3, and 4 may be unstable, commercial controls are usually monoclonal.

UK NEQAS for Immunology runs a scheme for CSF oligoclonal bands. There is also a scheme for CSF proteins which includes CSF albumin and IgG (used in the diffusion ratio).

SELF-CHECK 2.3

What are the advantages and disadvantages of monoclonal commercial controls for oligoclonal banding?

Multiple sclerosis (MS)

MS is a chronic inflammatory disease of the central nervous system (CNS). It is the most common disabling neurological disease among young adults—the peak age of onset is between 20 and 40. The cause is unknown, although genetic and environmental factors are thought to influence susceptibility.

In MS there is autoimmune attack on the myelin sheath surrounding the nerve fibres of the CNS. Because the CNS is involved in all nerve activity symptoms can vary depending upon the site affected. They include: fatigue, balance problems, visual disturbances, numbness and tingling, pain, loss of muscle strength, anxiety and depression, cognitive problems, and speech problems. Diagnosis is by patient history, neurological examination, and MRI scan. Demonstration of CSF-specific oligoclonal bands is positive in 80% of patients.

There are four types of multiple sclerosis:

- **Relapsing remitting MS:** Patients have symptomatic episodes (relapse) followed by periods of recovery.
- **Secondary progressive MS:** As relapsing remitting MS, but the symptoms do not go away after relapse. Approximately 65% of patients with relapsing remitting MS will have developed secondary progressive MS within 15 years of diagnosis.

- **Benign MS:** As relapsing remitting MS but patients have very few relapses, complete or near complete recovery after relapse, and minimal disability.
- **Primary progressive MS:** Patients show worsening symptoms and increasing disability from the outset.

2.5 Cryoglobulins

Cryoglobulins are immunoglobulins which precipitate at less than 37 °C and then redissolve completely at 37 °C. The propensity to precipitate can occur at any point below 37 °C and varies markedly between individuals. The clinical consequences can also be apparent at any point below 37 °C.

Cryoglobulin
Abnormal immunoglobulins (IgG or IgM) that precipitate when serum is cooled.

Raynaud's phenomenon
Spasm of the tiny artery vessels supplying the blood to the extremities during periods of low ambient temperature.

The clinical presentation of cryoglobulin includes purpura, weakness, and arthralgia in over 80% of patients. More than 30% have **Raynaud's phenomenon**, wherein the capillaries of the body's extremities become occluded as the ambient temperature falls, leading to tissue ischaemia and the possible loss of fingers and toes. Renal disease in the form of mesangio-capillary glomerulonephritis is also seen in some 30% of cases of cryoglobulin. Cryoglobulin may be the cause of false results in full blood counts. Haematology analysers often count cryoglobulin complexes as leukocytes or platelets giving abnormally high results.

Wintrobe and Buell first reported cryoglobulin in 1933. The classification discussed here is that of Brouet et al. (1974) which divides cryoglobulins into three types:

- **Type 1 cryoglobulins:** Type1 cryoglobulins are comprised solely of monoclonal immunoglobulin and are invariably associated with a monoclonal gammopathy such as myeloma or Waldenström's macroglobulinaemia. Most are IgM, some IgG, and rarely IgA. The cryoprecipitation occurs within a few hours of storing the patient plasma at 4 °C and is due to the abnormal structure of the pathological monoclone, which cannot maintain the colloid state in the cold. They account for some 10% of cryoglobulins.
- **Type 2 cryoglobulins:** Type 2 cryoglobulins consist of a mixture of immunoglobulins of different isotypes. There is usually one monoclonal immunoglobulin directed against the Fc portion of IgG, usually IgM κ. They are seen in hepatitis C virus (HCV) infections and Sjögren's syndrome, and account for approximately 60% of cryoglobulins.
- **Type 3 cryoglobulins:** Type 3 cryoglobulins are a mixture of polyclonal immunoglobulins, usually polyclonal or oligoclonal IgM and IgG. The IgM acts as a rheumatoid factor (RF) and binds to the Fc portion of IgG. They are seen in viral and bacterial infections and some autoimmune disorders. They account for approximately 30% of cryoglobulins.

Types 2 and 3 cryoglobulins can take up to a week to fully form when a plasma sample is stored at 4 °C, but the clinical significance of a cryoglobulin that takes up to a week to form at 4 °C is debatable.

Using the most sensitive serological assays as many as 80% of mixed cryoglobulins are positive for antibody to HCV although this varies with the population under study and the methods employed. Furthermore polymerase chain reaction (PCR) studies reveal HCV RNA in the purified cryoprecipitate. Hepatitis C infection has been associated with autoimmune disease such as autoimmune hepatitis (AIH). Anti-immunoglobulin RF is produced as part of the antiviral immune response to enhance the clearance of virus:antivirus complexes, thus explaining the coexistence of HCV in the immunoglobulin precipitate and RF. HCV infects lymphocytes and has been associated with non-Hodgkin's lymphoma, a B cell dyscrasia. Lymphoma may develop in the mixed cryoglobulinaemia patients who are followed up long term and it is possible that the monoclonal IgM type 2 variant is a precursor of lymphoma. When viewed from the perspective of HCV infection, depending on the population in question, as many as half of the HCV patients have detectable cryoglobulin without the associated clinical symptoms. However, only a minority of HCV infected patients will develop clinical cryoglobulinaemia (Ferri et al. 2002).

Cryofibrinogen
An abnormal fibrinogen that precipitates at cold temperatures and redissolves at 37 °C.

Cryofibrinogen is the result of abnormal fibrinogen molecules native to plasma, which precipitate at less than 37 °C. Ferri et al. (2002) regard these as false positive, but there are examples which cause clinical symptoms indistinguishable from cryo-precipitable imunoglobulins. Cryofibrinogen may also be seen in the plasma of normal individuals.

2.5.1 Cryoglobulin analysis

Sample collection for cryoglobulin analysis, referred to as the pre-analytical phase, is of crucial importance to obtain a valid result. The precipitation occurs at less than 37 °C and at ambient temperature in a non-anticoagulated sample tube some of the cryoglobulin will be bound up in the fibrin clot and lost to analysis. Lack of control of the temperature in the pre-analytical phase is the most important factor in failing to detect a cryoglobulin. The following protocol for the collection of cryoglobulin samples is recommended.

Sample collection

The venepuncture is performed in a warm room. Place about 250 ml of water at 37 °C into a vacuum flask or a Dewar flask. A sample without anticoagulant and an EDTA blood tube are labelled with the patient's details using a ballpoint pen and these are then pre-warmed by placing them in a plastic bag in the 37 °C flask. Similarly the syringe or vacuum phlebotomy system must be pre-warmed, again by placing them in a plastic bag in the 37 °C flask. Alternatively the clinic could have a stock of tubes and blood drawing equipment in a 37 °C incubator ready for use.

Once the blood is obtained it must be placed in the 37 °C flask at once and forwarded to the laboratory without delay. On receipt the laboratory must check the temperature of the water, which must be not less than 37 °C and not more than 40 °C. If these limits are exceeded the samples must be rejected.

The laboratory must then transfer the samples to a 37 °C waterbath/incubator and left to clot for minimum one hour. Centrifuge the samples at 37 °C to separate the serum and EDTA plasma. Very few laboratories have a centrifuge with a verified 37 °C option, thus the samples should be transferred to a 37 °C incubator or water bath and allow the red cells to sediment by gravity over several hours. Samples received in the afternoon of the working day can be safely left overnight at 37 °C, but it should be acknowledged that they will not be suitable for certain tests which may be requested subsequently. Two labelled secondary tubes for each of the serum and plasma samples are prepared, one set of which is transferred to a refrigerator at 4–6 °C and the other pair are kept at 37 °C. These are then left for not less than 3 days and up to 7 days.

Sample analysis

The analytical phase of cryoglobulin analysis begins with the visual examination of the samples. The samples incubated at 37 °C should be reviewed first in order to establish the background turbidity, if any. The samples at 4 °C are then examined. If there is no precipitate or turbidity then the test is negative and no further action is required. If precipitate or turbidity is seen or suspected then further analysis is required.

Type 1 monoclonal immunoglobulin cryoglobulins can precipitate within a few hours. As well as precipitating they may occasionally form a solid gel with little or no free fluid. These may completely liquefy when put back in an incubator at 37 °C for a few minutes. Because of the gel formation further analysis is difficult, as it is not possible to wash the cryoglobulin and remove uninvolved protein. Since these are due to pathological monoclones they can be investigated by the usual serum electrophoresis and immunofixation procedures maintained at 37 °C.

Cryoprecipitate can appear as flocculates or a fine precipitate covering the bottom of the EDTA plasma sample only.

Any type of cryoglobulin seen requires further investigation. A refrigerated centrifuge must be pre-chilled to 4 °C. Centrifuge the samples to form a pellet and mark the tube to indicate the fluid level. Transfer the supernatant fluid to a labelled clean tube for possible use later. The cryoglobulin pellet is resuspended in 0.15M saline solution pre-chilled to 4 °C and centrifuged again. The saline supernatant is discarded and the wash cycle repeated at least three times. Maintaining the cryoprotein at 4 °C throughout this phase of the analysis is essential. This includes taking care not to handle the bottom of the tube containing the cryoprecipitate with one's fingers as heat can be transferred. The recommended number of washes varies in laboratories but it should be pointed out that each wash cycle will lose a little of the cryoprotein.

The hallmark of cryoglobulin is to precipitate at less than 37 °C and redissolve at 37 °C. At the end of the wash cycle the cryoglobulin is resuspended in 0.15M saline to its original volume and placed overnight at 37 °C. Precipitate which has not redissolved is not cryoglobulin but is likely to be lipid or fibrin in nature and therefore the test for cryoglobulin is negative. If incubation at 37 °C has dissolved the cryoglobulin then it must be characterized further by immunofixation. The total protein content of the dissolved cryoglobulin is typically small, e.g. <1 g/L, thus it is advisable to use the same highly sensitive immunofixation protocol as used for urine Bence Jones protein analysis. Type 2 cryoglobulin presents most frequently as an IgM κ monoclone with polyclonal IgG κ and IgG λ staining. Type 3 cryoglobulin on immunofixation typically reveals polyclonal IgM and IgG staining. Cryofibrinogen can be detected with anti-fibrinogen on immunofixation.

Quantification of cryoglobulin can be attempted but there is no standardization. The total protein content of the washed cryoglobulin can be determined by using the same assay as that for urine total protein. Alternatively the IgG, IgA, and IgM content of the washed cryoglobulin can be determined, although the variables in the washing process and the lack of references ranges make this difficult to interpret.

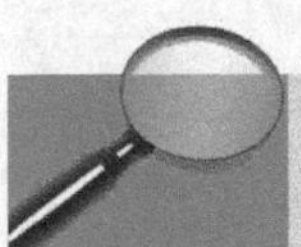

CASE STUDY 2.2 Cryoglobulin

Patient history

A 32-year-old male presented with vasculitis, purpura of the lower limbs, and arthralgia.

The clinical history revealed a 7-year past of intravenous drug abuse.

Routine bloods taken for urea and electrolytes (U&E), liver function test (LFT), and full blood count (FBC).

Results (1)

LFT

- **Serum total protein 66 g/L (NR 63–79 g/L).**

- Serum albumin 28 g/L (NR 35–48 g/L).
- Globulin 38 g/L (NR 18–36 g/L).

FBC

The haematology analyser revealed abnormally high figures for the red and white cell counts. On examination of the blood film the cell counts were estimated to be low.

Significance of results (1)

The presence of cryoglobulin was postulated to be the cause of the high analyser cell counts as cryoprecipitates are known to pass through the cell count apertures and trigger a signal to the analyser.

Samples were then sent for the investigation of cryoglobulin and, in view of the history of drug abuse; the patient was tested for antibodies to hepatitis B (HBV), hepatitis C (HCV), and human immunodeficiency virus (HIV).

Results (2)

Cryoglobulin analysis demonstrated a large cryoglobulin which typed as an IgM κ monoclone with polyclonal IgG. This complex had a total protein content of 15 g/L.

- Rheumatoid factor 1200 IU/mL (NR 0–15 IU/ml).
- HCV Ab—present.
- HCV RNA—detectable.

Significance of results (2)

The results are consistent with a type 2 cryoglobulinaemia.

The HCV infection was treated with pegylated interferon alpha over 6 months. During this time the FBC, U&E, and LFT were analysed at monthly intervals. The FBC was tested following warming of the sample to 37 °C on all occasions. The clinical chemistry results were always reported from samples at ambient temperature and the results were consistently similar to the original sample. The presence of the large monoclonal IgM suggests that the serum total protein and globulin levels were grossly underestimated due to the cryoprecipitation at ambient temperature which was removed by centrifugation in the clot. Unfortunately this was not pointed out to the clinicians or the clinical chemistry laboratory.

After 6 months treatment the patients' symptoms had significantly resolved. The HCV RNA was no longer detectable and the cryoglobulin analysis showed a markedly reduced IgM κ monoclone in a background of polyclonal IgG.

In summary cryoglobulins may be classified as one of three types, the first and least common of which is solely monoclonal Immunoglobulin associated with a B cell dyscrasia. The mixed cryoglobulins, types 2 and 3, can be distinguished on immunofixation by the presence or absence of monoclonal IgM with polyclonal immunoglobulin. Type 2 and 3 are associated with hepatitis C infection; around half of patients will have a cryoglobulin but only a minority will have symptoms associated with cryoglobulinaemia.

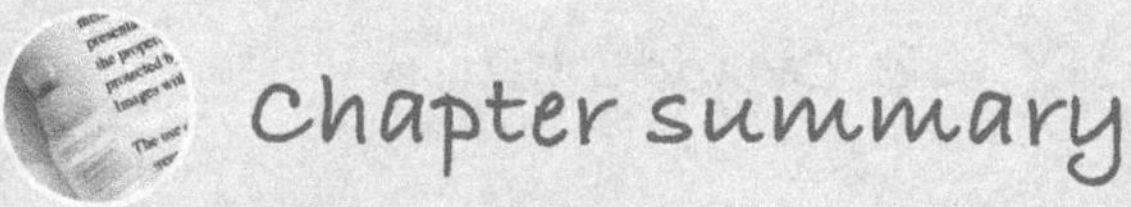

Chapter summary

- Immunoglobulins are key effector molecules in adaptive immunity with a two identical heavy chain and two identical light chain template structure.
- Clonal expansion of plasma cells produces monoclonal gammopathies which may be benign or malignant.
- Monoclonal gammopathies present a measureable band on electrophoresis which can be used to monitor the size and progress of the tumour.

- Monoclonal free light chains can overflow into the urine where they are known as Bence Jones proteins.
- Recently assays have been developed to measure monoclonal free light chains directly in serum.
- Immunoglobulins, and fibrinogen, may spontaneously precipitate at temperatures below 37 °C leading to the formation of cryoprecipitates.
- Although standardization of the assay is poor they have been classified into four subtypes: cryoglobulin types 1, 2, or 3 and cryofibrinogen.
- Intrathecal synthesis of IgG is an important diagnostic feature of multiple sclerosis.
- Due to the low level of protein in cerebrospinal fluid the analysis requires the use of isoelectric focusing enhanced by immunoblotting or immunofixation.

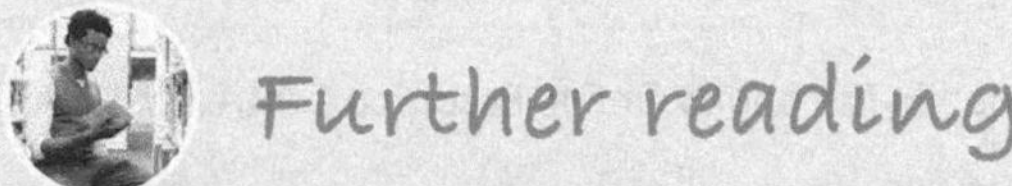

Further reading

- Andersson M *et al.* (1994) *Cerebrospinal fluid in the diagnosis of multiple sclerosis: a consensus report*. *J Neurol Neurosurg Psychiatry*, **57**, 897–902.
- Bird JM *et al.* (2014) *Guidelines for the diagnosis and management of Multiple Myeloma on behalf of the BCSH & UK Myeloma Forum*. www.bcshguidelines.com.
- Dispenzieri A *et al.* (2009) *International Myeloma Working Group guidelines for serum-free light chain analysis in multiple myeloma and related disorders*. *Leukaemia*, **23**, 215–24.
- Johnson S *et al.* (2006) *Guidelines on the management of Waldenström's macroglobulinaemia*. *Br J Haematol*, **132**, 683–97.
- Keren D (2003) *Protein Electrophoresis in Clinical Diagnosis*. Arnold, London.
- Lilic D, Sewell WAC (2001) *IgA deficiency: what we should—or should not—be doing*. *J Clin Pathol*, **54**, 337–38.
- Milford Ward A Sheldon J Rowbottom A Wild GD Milford Ward A, Sheldon J, Rowbottom A, Wild GD (2007) *Protein Reference Unit Handbook of Clinical Immunochemistry*. 9th Edition, PR Publications, Sheffield.
- Miller D *et al.* (2008) *Differential diagnosis of suspected multiple sclerosis: a consensus approach*. *Mult Scler*, **14**, 1157–74.
- Smith A, Wisloff F, Samson D (2005) *Guidelines on the diagnosis and management of multiple myeloma*. *Br J Haematol*, **132**, 410–51.
- UK Myeloma Forum (2004) *Guidelines on the diagnosis and management of AL amyloidosis*. *Br J Haematol*, **125**, 681–700.
- UK Myeloma Forum and Nordic Myeloma Study Group (2009). *Guidelines for the investigation of newly detected M-proteins and the management of monoclonal gammopathy of undetermined significance (MGUS)*. *Br J Haematol*, **147**, 22–42.
- Yel L (2010) *Selective IgA deficiency*. *J Clin Immunol*. **30** (1), 10–6.

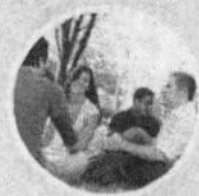

Discussion questions

2.1 Immunoglobulin molecules are composed of highly conserved subunits. Name the subunits and describe their structure.

2.2 Which of the heavy chain domains is concerned with:

a) complement activation

b) opsonization

c) antigen binding?

2.3 What are the effector roles of each of the IgG subclasses?

2.4 How does antigen excess lead to falsely low results in nephelometry and turbidimetry?

Answers to self-check questions are provided in the book's Online Resource Centre.

Visit www.oxfordtextbooks.co.uk/orc/hall2e

3

Allergy

Learning Objectives

After studying the chapter you should be able to:

- outline the immunological basis of allergy
- describe the major clinical features of allergic disease
- describe the clinical and laboratory techniques used to diagnose allergy
- discuss the advantages and limitations of these techniques
- outline the role of flow cytometry in determining basophil activation
- explain how mediators released during an allergic reaction can be used when investigating allergy
- discuss the use of allergen-specific IgG tests in hypersensitivity reactions.

Introduction

The incidence of allergy in developed countries is increasing. In the United Kingdom the incidence of common allergic diseases has trebled in the last 20 years to become one of the highest in the world. It is estimated that approximately one third of the population has an allergy. This, along with diagnostic and therapeutic developments, is impacting significantly on clinical and laboratory practice. This chapter provides an overview of how clinical and laboratory investigations come together to provide accurate diagnoses leading to effective management and enhanced quality of life.

3.1 Allergy terminology

Allergy is an exaggerated response to substances common in the environment that are usually harmless. The European Academy of Allergy and Clinical Immunology (EAACI) and the World Allergy Organization (WAO) have defined allergy as a hypersensitivity reaction initiated by immunological mechanisms. However, the term is more frequently restricted to the description of Type I (IgE-mediated) immediate hypersensitivity reactions.

TABLE 3.1 Gell and Coombs (1963) classification of hypersensitivity.

Type	Antigen	Mechanism
I Immediate hypersensitivity	Soluble antigen	IgE-mediated mast cell and basophil degranulation leading to release of vasoactive mediators
II Cytotoxic antibody	Cell or matrix associated antigen or cell-surface receptors	IgG- and IgM-mediated cell destruction by antibody-dependent cell-mediated cytotoxicity or by complement
III Immune complex	Soluble antigen	Antibody–antigen complex deposition leading to complement activation and inflammation
IV Delayed-type hypersensitivity	Soluble antigen or cell-associated antigen	T_H1-mediated cytokine release leading to macrophage recruitment and activation

Hypersensitivity describes the reaction that causes reproducible signs or symptoms, following exposure to a defined stimulus, in a susceptible individual. A hypersensitivity reaction can be mediated by various immune cells or antibodies. In type I hypersensitivity the antibody responsible for the reaction belongs to the Immunoglobulin E (IgE) isotype class and is driven by T_H2 cells. All other hypersensitivity reactions, mediated by antibodies of other immunoglobulin classes or various cells, are known as non-IgE-mediated hypersensitivity. There are four types of hypersensitivity as defined by Gell and Coombs (1963); these are briefly listed in Table 3.1.

Cross reference

You can get more information about how allergic responses are generated in Section 3.3.

Some individuals have a genetic tendency to develop allergic diseases such as asthma, hay fever, or eczema. These individuals with **atopy** usually have exaggerated IgE antibody responses to commonly occurring allergens. It may be an individual or familial tendency and usually develops in childhood or adolescence. Non-atopic individuals who have similar exposure to allergens do not produce a prolonged IgE antibody response. Atopic individuals usually present with eczema and/or asthma as well as allergy. Some individuals will only produce IgE in the target organ (e.g. respiratory tract) and local allergic rhinitis (LAR) without systemic atopy is also known as **entopy**.

Atopy

A genetic predisposition to produce prolonged IgE antibody responses to commonly occurring allergens.

Entopy

Localized mucosal allergic disease in the absence of circulating allergen-specific IgE.

Atopy causes raised total IgE levels and positive skin prick tests and specific IgE (sIgE) tests to common environmental allergens. Entopy is associated with positive allergen provocation tests, but negative skin prick or IgE tests.

Cross reference

You can read more about skin prick tests, specific IgE tests and total IgE in Sections 3.5.2, 3.6, and 3.11.

3.2 Allergens

The antigens that induce immune responses which cause allergy are termed **allergens**. Most allergens are of biological origin, for example, pollens, animal hair and dander, mites, moulds, or plant and animal derived foods. Allergens are predominantly proteins and display considerable heterogeneity in molecular size, composition (glycosylation), and conformational structure. Low molecular weight chemicals can act as **haptens** (a complex of a small molecule with a carrier, usually protein) which can behave as allergens and bind to IgE antibodies, for example, the β-lactam ring of penicillin binds to albumin in the body to provoke an allergic response in some individuals.

Allergens

The antigens that induce immune responses which cause allergy.

3.3 Allergy mechanisms

An allergic response can be broadly divided into two phases that can be seen in Figure 3.1.

a) An induction phase in which the immune system forms IgE antibodies in response to initial exposure to the allergen. The induction phase can also be referred to as the early phase response.

b) A reactive phase in which an allergen binds to IgE molecules present on Fc receptors on mast cells (in tissues) and basophils (in the blood), causing the cells to release pre-formed or rapidly synthesized mediators. The reactive phase can also be referred to as the late phase response.

3.3.1 Induction phase: sensitization

When an allergen comes in contact with the immune system for the first time it is captured and processed by antigen presenting cells (APC). Presentation of the allergenic epitope, in association with MHC class II and co-stimulatory molecules, to T cells then occurs. Depending upon the nature of the APC, characteristics of the allergen, levels of allergen exposure, activation of toll-like receptors, and cytokine microenvironment, T cells can differentiate into distinctive sub-populations. These sub-populations are distinguished on the basis of their predominant cytokine profile. In allergy, T_H2 lymphocytes (IL-4; IL-5; IL-13 producers) are pivotal in signalling B lymphocytes to produce IgE antibodies. These allergen-specific IgE antibodies are

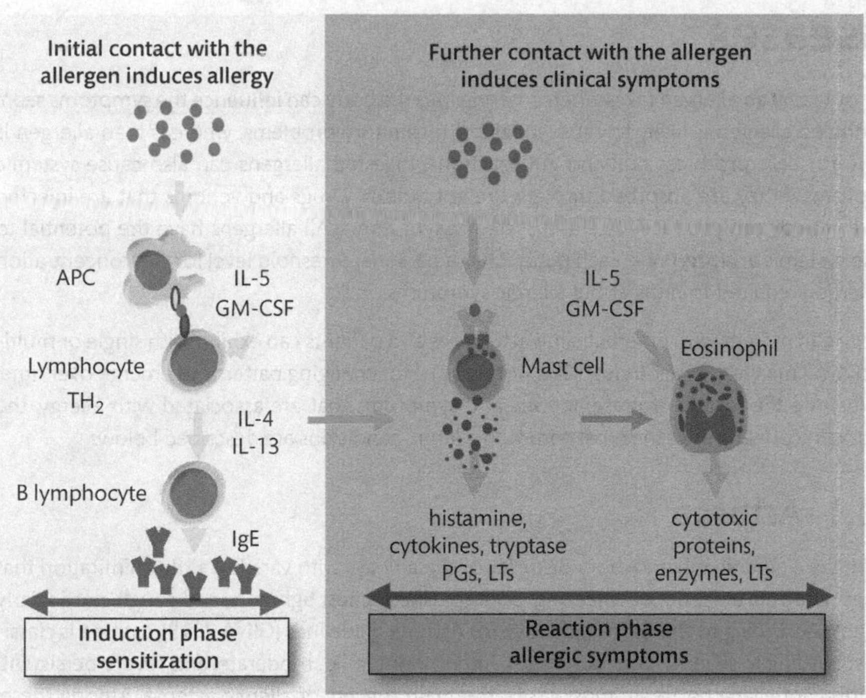

FIGURE 3.1

Diagrammatic representation of the induction and reactive phases of an allergic reaction showing the interaction between cellular and soluble components. APC: antigen presenting cell; IL: interleukin; GM-CSF: granulocyte macrophage stimulating factor; PAF: platelet activating factor; PGs: prostaglandins; LTs: leukotrienes.

released into the circulation and bind to high affinity IgE Fc receptors (FcεRI) on the surface membranes of basophils and mast cells. The binding and concentration of specific IgE antibodies on the surface membranes 'sensitizes' the cells and allows faster responses to the allergen in the reactive phase.

3.3.2 Reactive phase: allergic response

The reactive phase occurs upon subsequent exposure to allergen. It begins with allergen cross-linking specific IgE molecules on the surface of the sensitized mast cells and basophils. This results in release of potent pre-formed mediators (histamine; heparin; proteases) from the cells. In addition, synthesis of a second set of chemical mediators (leukotrienes; prostaglandins; thromboxanes; chemotactic factors) occurs. These mediators are released into the tissues several hours after the reaction. The actions of both sets of mediators result in the characteristic features of allergic reactions: vasodilation, increased mucus production, swelling, and itch. How these features present in different forms of allergic disease is described in Section 3.4.

SELF-CHECK 3.1

Can you describe the immunological mechanisms which give rise to allergic symptoms?

3.4 Clinical features of allergic diseases

The route that an allergen takes when entering into the body can influence the symptoms seen. An inhaled allergen is likely to cause localized respiratory problems, whereas if an allergen is eaten it usually produces oral and gut reactions. Ingested allergens can also cause systemic symptoms if they are absorbed through the gut quickly. Drugs and venoms that are injected into the body can produce local and systemic symptoms. All allergens have the potential to cause systemic **anaphylaxis**. Each patient has a personal threshold level for the concentration of allergen required to bring about allergic symptoms.

Anaphylaxis
occurs when there is widespread mast cell activation causing a potentially fatal reaction

Allergy can present with different clinical features and patients can exhibit with single or multiple clinical manifestations. Indeed, it is not unusual for changing patterns to emerge over time. To illustrate the variety of presentations and symptoms that are associated with allergy, the major clinical features of the most common allergic conditions are described below.

3.4.1 Asthma

Asthma is a chronic inflammatory disorder of the airways with variable airflow limitation that causes recurrent episodes of wheezing, breathlessness, chest tightness, and cough, particularly at night. According to the Global Initiative for Asthma guidelines (GINA 2015), asthma is classified according to severity into four stages: intermittent, mild, moderate, and severe persistent. The inhalant allergens are, in most cases, the main triggers of allergic asthma. Among these, house dust mites, storage mites, grass pollen, and pet dander are the most frequent, either alone or in combination. Occasionally, foods, drugs, hymenoptera venoms, and chemical allergens can cause allergic asthma. Interestingly, the major allergen of house dust mites is the faeces and most people with suspected bird allergy turn out to be allergic to house dust mites that thrive in the cages.

CLINICAL CORRELATION 3.1

Asthma guidelines

Further information about the diagnosis and management of asthma can be found in National Institute of Health and Care Excellence (NICE) quality standard 25 (QS25) and The British Guideline on the Management of Asthma by The British Thoracic Society and Scottish Intercollegiate Guidelines Network (www.sign.ac.uk)

3.4.2 Rhinitis

Rhinitis is the most prevalent respiratory disease affecting more than 15% of the UK population. Most cases are IgE-mediated. Nasal itching, blockage, watery rhinorrea, loss of sense of smell, and frequent sneezing are the major symptoms of rhinitis. Allergic rhinitis induced by pollen during the spring and summer seasons is known as hay fever. The major allergens in rhinitis are the same as mentioned previously for asthma. Any patient affected by allergic rhinitis should be studied for asthma and vice versa.

3.4.3 Rhinoconjunctivitis

Allergic rhinitis accompanied by watery and itchy eyes is referred to as allergic rhinoconjunctivitis. In most cases, treatment of the nasal symptoms also improves the allergic conjunctivitis.

3.4.4 Urticaria

In urticaria the hypersensitivity reaction that occurs in the skin is characterized by a raised itchy rash. It is often referred to as nettle rash or hives. Urticaria, which has an allergic basis, is usually triggered by food and drug allergens.

3.4.5 Angioedema

Angioedema is frequently associated with urticaria. Whilst urticaria affects the epidermis producing a superficial erythema, angioedema impacts the deeper dermal level, inducing skin swelling. Drugs, foods, and insect stings are the most common allergens inducing angioedema. Non steroidal anti-inflammatory drugs (NSAIDs) and angiotensin-converting enzyme (ACE) inhibitors are groups of drugs that may induce episodes of urticaria/angioedema. ACE inhibitors induce non-allergic bradykinin dependent angioedema and many other drugs such as NSAIDS cause angioedema via IgE independent degranulation of mast cells also called **anaphylactoid** reactions.

Anaphylactoid
Immediate systemic reactions, with the same clinical features as anaphylaxis, but not mediated by allergen-specific IgE.

3.4.6 Eczema

Eczema describes a local erythematous inflammation of the skin. When related to other allergic clinical manifestations it is known as atopic eczema. Special attention should be paid to atopic eczema that appears in early childhood and is induced by foods such as cow's milk and eggs. This is because most of the affected children will develop respiratory allergy in later years. Close contact with various metals and chemicals may result in a delayed local eczema that appears after 48–72 hours of the contact. This is known as contact dermatitis and is a type IV hypersensitivity response.

Cross reference

There are different causes of angioedema. Another common type seen in the Clinical Immunology laboratory is hereditary angioedema (HAE) caused by a problem with the complement cascade. You can read in more detail about this in Chapter 4.

3.4.7 Anaphylaxis

Anaphylaxis is the most severe allergic reaction and involves more than one bodily system: skin, respiratory system, blood, cardiovascular system, or gastrointestinal tract. It can be life-threatening and fatalities occur if adrenaline is not promptly administered. Almost

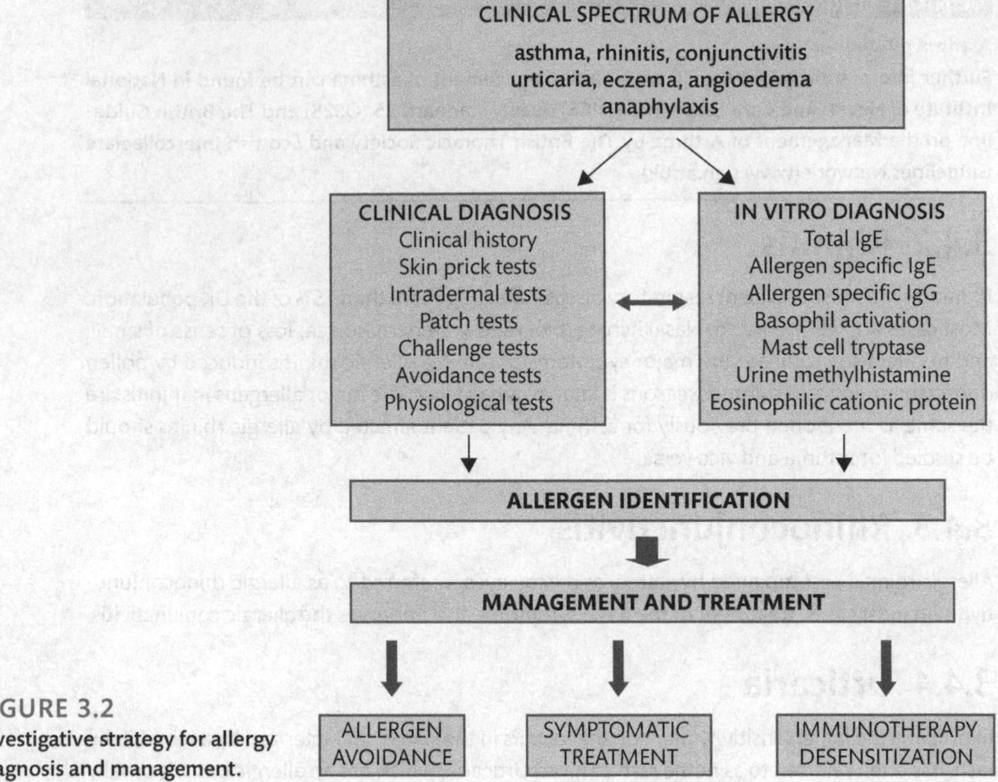

FIGURE 3.2
Investigative strategy for allergy diagnosis and management.

universally, patients experiencing an anaphylactic attack report a 'feeling of impending doom'. Many allergens can induce anaphylaxis but the most frequent are:

- foods: peanuts, tree nuts, and shellfish
- drugs: antibiotics, muscle relaxants, and pain killers
- venoms: Hymenoptera (bees and wasps)
- latex.

Establishing an accurate diagnosis is crucial for patient management and treatment. This is achieved through both clinical and laboratory investigations. The various elements of the investigative strategy are shown in Figure 3.2 and described in detail in Sections 3.5 and 3.6.

Key Points

- **Allergy is a systemic disease.**
- **Allergy patients can present with single or multiple manifestations.**
- **Clinical symptoms can change over time.**

3.5 Clinical diagnosis

3.5.1 Clinical history

Taking an accurate clinical history is the most important tool for diagnosis of allergic diseases. This includes collecting information about the type of symptoms, time of onset of reaction, frequency and duration, day–night variation, shape, size, and distribution of any skin lesions, occurrence in relation to different triggers and conditions, exercise, food and drug intake, personal and familial history, type of work and hobbies, relationship to the menstrual cycle, quality of life, and concurrent therapy.

Depending on the type of allergy under investigation a number of specific points should be queried.

- For respiratory allergy, it is important to know whether symptoms are seasonal or perennial and if the patient identifies any triggers (animals, dust, or work place).
- In food allergy, it should be established whether the reaction is different depending if the food is raw or cooked. It may be useful for the patient to keep a food diary if the causative allergen is not immediately apparent, as some foods contain 'hidden allergens' or it could be due to cross contamination by other foods.
- In suspected drug allergy, the lapsed time between drug intake and the onset of symptoms should be noted and whether the patient has taken the same drug before and after the allergic episode.

A number of *in vivo* tests can also be used to aid diagnosis and these are described below.

3.5.2 Skin prick test

Skin prick testing is the 'gold standard' diagnostic method in the allergy clinic. It is useful for the diagnosis of most IgE-mediated allergies. The test takes advantage of the presence of mast cells in the skin. If the patient has specific IgE present on the mast cell surface it will cause degranulation and local tissue swelling when the causative allergen is present. The selection of allergens to test is determined according to the clinical history. Most allergens can be obtained from commercial sources. Sometimes the suspected allergen is not available and testing is performed directly using the suspected product which is applied to the skin, removed, and the skin pricked with a lancet. It is important to check that the patient is not taking antihistamines as this will diminish the sensitivity of the test and may give false negative results.

BOX 3.1 Hidden allergens

Hidden allergens are common in foods and medications. They are ingredients that may be used in small quantities and can be easily overlooked when investigating allergy. Common hidden allergens include: polyethylene glycol (PEG), soya, milk, nuts, wheat, and eggs. The term can also be used to describe substances used during food or drink production, such as sulphites. Case Study 3.1 will show you how we can investigate for allergy to hidden allergens.

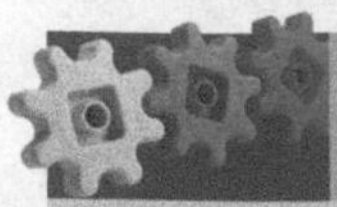

METHOD 3.1 Skin prick testing

- Liquid allergen drops are placed on the volar aspect of the forearm and pricked with a 1mm lancet.
- Histamine is used as a positive control and saline as a negative control.
- The position of each allergen used is recorded so that results can be correctly identified.
- A positive reaction is identified by a wheal (red, raised lump) and flare (red, inflamed area) around the site of the skin prick (Figure 3.3a).
- Wheal size is measured after 15 minutes. A reaction is considered positive when the wheal is at least 3mm in diameter and equal to or greater than the wheal formed by the positive control.

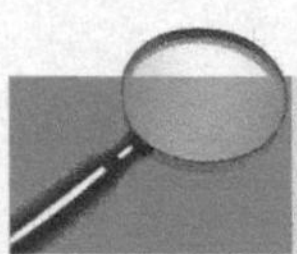

CASE STUDY 3.1 Hidden allergen

Patient history

- 40-year-old male. Suffered tongue swelling, urticarial rash, and brief loss of consciousness following a steroid injection for a heel complaint.
- Patient was transferred to Emergency department where he received adrenaline to relieve the symptoms. Later referred to an allergy clinic for further investigations.
- Known to be allergic to penicillin but this was not used. No history of other allergic reactions.
- Skin prick tests to a selection of different steroids were performed, including the drug used: depo-medrone (active steroid ingredient is methylprednisolone).
- Specific IgE tests to steroids are not available, therefore unable to use this method of investigation.

Results (1)

- Skin prick tests to hydrocortisone, prednisolone, and methylprednisolone were all negative.
- Skin prick test to depo-medrone positive.

Significance of results (1)

- Patient did not react to the steroid ingredient of the injection as the methylprednisolone skin test was negative.
- The ingredient list of depo-medrone was checked to determine what other substances it contained.
- Other ingredients included polyethylene glycol (PEG), sodium chloride, and myristyl-gamma-picolinium chloride. The results of the initial skin tests prompted the allergy clinic to carry out skin tests to these substances.

Results (2)

- Skin test to PEG positive. Negative results to the other ingredients.

Significance of results (2)

- It is highly likely that the patient is allergic to PEG.

PEG is a hidden allergen that is present in a large number of substances including medications, cosmetics, and food. No previous reactions reported, therefore it was decided that an oral challenge test to PEG would be performed to determine if the patient could tolerate ingested PEG. During the challenge the patient developed facial swelling, itch, and urticarial rash. He was immediately treated with adrenaline and the challenge test deemed positive. He was advised to avoid all forms of PEG and prescribed an adrenaline auto-injector to carry at all times for emergency use. Care must be taken to check the ingredients of items such as foods and medication prior to using them and he should inform people of his allergy if he has any further medical procedures.

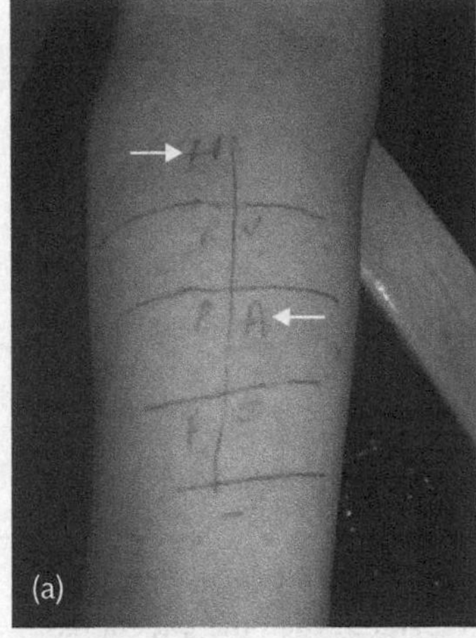

Histamine	
Rocuronium	Vecuronium
Propofol	Atracurium
Fentanyl	Saline

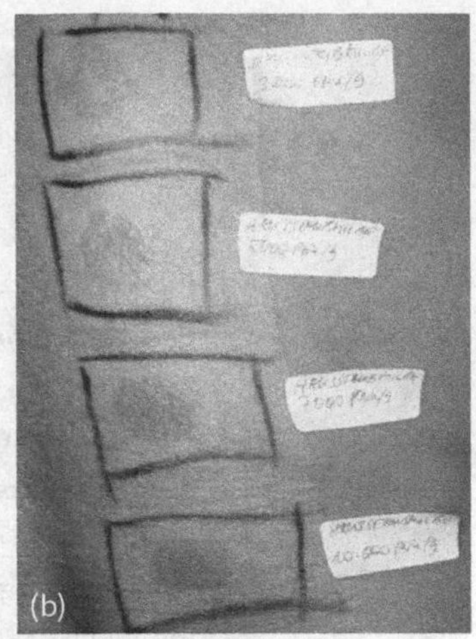

FIGURE 3.3

(a) Skin prick testing in a patient who experienced a peri-operative anaphylactic reaction. Wheal and flare reactions (arrowed) were observed for histamine (positive control) and atracurium (a muscle relaxant drug). Negative reactions were observed for saline (negative control) and other anaesthetic drugs. (b) Demarcated areas of eczematous rash following patch testing.

Figure 3.3a courtesy of Dr M. Shields.

3.5.3 Patch test

Patch tests are used for the diagnosis of contact dermatitis (Type IV hypersensitivity). The test is performed on the patient's back by applying adhesive patches containing the different suspected chemicals. After 48 hours the patch is removed and the eczematous reactions are identified. This can be seen in Figure 3.3b. Patch tests are useful in diagnosing delayed type hypersensitivity.

3.5.4 Intradermal test

Intradermal tests are usually performed when a skin prick test is negative but one of the allergens tested is still suspected to be the causative substance. A small amount of the allergen is injected under the skin. The injection site is checked after 15 minutes for signs of a reaction (swelling and redness). They are more sensitive than skin prick tests, however they can give false positive results. This test is usually carried out to a single specific allergen, rather than a range of allergens as you would do for skin prick testing. These tests are most commonly used when investigating drug or venom allergy. There is a greater risk of anaphylaxis than with skin prick testing.

3.5.5 Challenge test

Challenge or provocation tests can take a number of forms: oral, inhaled, injected, or direct contact, and the form chosen depends on the nature of the allergy. The procedure exposes the patient to progressively increasing concentrations of the allergen to a point where a normal level of exposure is reached. This is compared with the reaction observed with placebo.

Double-blind placebo controlled challenge (DBPCC) is the preferred method for both diagnostic purposes and scientific studies. However, the process is time consuming and requires specialist expertise. Consequently, open challenge (investigator and patient aware of the test substances) is more commonly undertaken. For practical reasons open tests are the first approach, particularly when the probability of a positive outcome is estimated to be low.

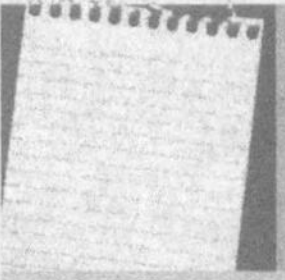

BOX 3.2 Quality control of skin tests and intradermal tests

- Clinical staff carrying out these tests should have had the appropriate training.
- Care should be taken to ensure that the skin is punctured to allow the allergen to enter the skin. Failure to puncture the skin can be a cause of false negative results.
- The positive and negative controls should always be checked.
- Atopic patients may give a positive response to the negative control showing that any positive results seen are invalid.
- Patients taking antihistamines at the time of the test may have a negative result to the positive control. In this case the tests should be repeated when the patient has stopped taking the medication.
- The wheal and flare measurements should be recorded in the patient notes for future reference.

Confirmation of occupational allergy or when the agent is known to have a modest false positive rate on non-invasive testing are indications for provocation testing.

HEALTH & SAFETY 3.1

Precautions to take during challenge tests

Careful monitoring of signs and symptoms should be made throughout the challenge testing procedure. There is a risk that the patient may have a reaction ranging from mild symptoms to full anaphylaxis. Monitoring should be carried out by trained healthcare personnel and as the procedure carries some risk, emergency treatment should be available.

Key Points

- Taking an accurate clinical history is the most important tool in allergy diagnosis.
- Skin prick tests, intradermal tests, and challenge tests can be performed in the clinic to aid in the diagnosis of allergy.

CLINICAL CORRELATION 3.2

Considerations when diagnosing allergy

- Guidelines for allergy investigations are available from a number of sources including NICE, EAACI, and the British Society for Allergy and Clinical Immunology.
- Patients often present with complicated or unclear clinical histories, therefore the approach taken when deciding which investigations to carry out may be different from patient to patient.
- Other medical conditions may restrict the tests that can be performed, for example patients that are pregnant or have poorly controlled asthma may not be offered a challenge test.

3.6 Allergen-specific IgE tests

3.6.1 History of specific IgE tests

Allergen-specific IgE antibody (sIgE) testing is the most common laboratory procedure employed in the diagnosis of allergic disease. The assays have developed significantly in the last 40 years and continue to evolve in the areas of allergen characterization, antibody detection, and instrumentation.

Originally described in the late 1960s, the radioallergosorbent test (RAST) was the first routine technique used for determining sIgE in serum. This *first generation* assay employed cyanogen bromide activated paper discs as the solid phase (allergosorbent) and used a birch pollen specific IgE calibration curve from which the levels of sIgE could be interpolated. Results were semi-quantitative and organized into classes of reactivity related to skin prick test positivity. These are described in Table 3.2.

Second generation methods, introduced in the early 1990s, offered marked improvements in assay convenience and performance. These included:

- Developments in solid phase allergosorbent materials or use of a liquid-allergen matrix resulting in enhanced antigen–antibody kinetics and assay sensitivity.
- The use of non-isotopic detection methods (spectrophotometry; fluorimetry; and enzyme-enhanced chemiluminescence).
- Reporting of quantitative sIgE results (kUA/L) standardized to a WHO International Reference preparation for total IgE.

In addition, systems became semi-automated resulting in faster turnaround times for results.

Further refinements have been introduced with *third generation* assays, most notably in the extension of the lower limit of detection, and in the availability of random access automated analytical platforms.

TABLE 3.2 Classification of allergen-specific IgE reactivities.

Class	kUA/L	Interpretation
0	<0.35	Negative
1	0.35–0.7	Weak Positive
2	0.7–3.5	Positive
3	3.5–17.5	Positive
4	17.5–52.5	Strong Positive
5	52.5–100	Strong Positive
6	>100	Strong Positive

Adapted from Milford Ward et al. (eds), *PRU Handbook of Clinical Immunochemistry*, 9th edition, 2007; reproduced with permission.

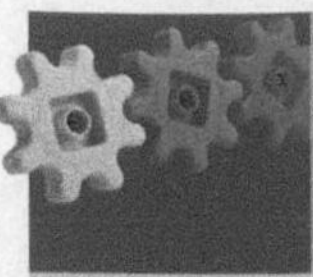

METHOD 3.2 Detection of allergen-specific IgE (sIgE)

- Patient serum is added to a solid phase allergosorbent material which contains an extract of the allergen of interest.
- If sIgE to that allergen is present in the patient sample, it will bind to the allergen.
- Unbound patient sample is washed off. Bound sIgE will remain in the solid phase material with the allergen.
- An enzyme conjugated anti-human antibody is added and binds to any sIgE present. Excess conjugate is removed by a wash step.
- The substrate to the enzyme conjugate is added.
- Colour change, or fluorescence, is measured at the detector. The amount of signal seen at the detector is directly proportional to the amount of sIgE present.
- The concentration of sIgE can be determined using a calibration curve constructed using a number of samples with known concentrations of allergen.

Online Resource Centre

To see a video demonstrating the ImmunoCAP test, log on to www.oxfordtextbooks.co.uk/orc/fbs

3.6.2 Test performance characteristics

The performance characteristics (diagnostic sensitivity/specificity; positive and negative predictive values) for sIgE tests have been widely studied. For most common food and inhalant allergens correlation of sIgE positivity with clinical features and/or skin testing reactivity is generally good.

Specific IgE antibody levels measured with different commercial assays cannot be considered as equivalent. This is largely due to variability in the composition and immunogenicity of the allergen preparations used in the assays. Therefore, when considering performance characteristics of respective assays the analytical platform on which results are obtained should be borne in mind as the results obtained from different systems may not be interchangeable This caveat also applies in the general sense that complete concordance between *in vitro* sIgE testing and skin testing cannot be expected. The former measures circulating IgE antibodies, the latter cutaneous mast cell reactivity. See Section 3.12 for information about how sIgE tests are quality controlled.

Cross references

Examples of the variation that can be seen between different assay platforms are shown in Section 3.12.2.

You can read more about allergen standardization in Section 3.7.

SELF-CHECK 3.2

Can you describe the investigative strategies used in allergy diagnosis?

3.7 Allergen standardization

Identification of specific IgE reactivity, leading to an accurate diagnosis, is dependent on the quality of the allergen extract employed. Most allergen extracts used in commercial assays are prepared by chemical extraction from raw material. The final extract contains many different substances that make up the whole allergen. Ensuring standardization of allergen preparations poses significant challenges for manufacturers because of:

- the heterogeneous mixture of allergenic and non-allergenic components in the biological material;
- the requirement to be able to extract all relevant allergens at biologically (and diagnostically) appropriate concentrations;
- variability in source material, for example, climate/pollution affecting the nature of pollens, species variability in food allergens, or contamination of source material by moulds or insect proteins.

In addition, many biological sources contain allergens with strong potential for cross-reactivity. The use of heterogeneous extracts containing cross-reactive structures may result in multiple positive and potentially clinically erroneous results in some patients.

Whilst significant progress has been made towards standardizing allergen preparations, the potential for variability remains. As a means of addressing some of these issues, purified (native) components or recombinant protein allergens are being produced and introduced into diagnostic practice.

Cross references

You can read in more detail about cross-reactivity in Section 3.8 and quality assurance in Section 3.11.

You can read more about purified and recombinant allergens in Section 3.9.

3.8 Cross-reactivity

Cross-reactivity occurs when sIgE antibodies bind to structurally similar epitopes from different species. It is a phenomenon that always needs to be considered in allergy testing. The main explanations for cross-reactivity are:

- Biochemical similarity between antigenic determinants.
- Cross-reactive carbohydrate determinants (CCD).

3.8.1 Biochemical similarity

This form of cross-reactivity occurs because sIgE antibody recognizes the same or similar antigenic determinants from a variety of allergen sources. Generally, cross-reactivity can occur when a sequence homology of >70% is present between the respective antigenic determinants. It is usually associated with allergens that are common to organisms across various taxonomic groups, for example: Family 10 of the pathogenesis related proteins (PR-10); tropomyosin; profilin; and lipid transfer proteins (LTP). Look at Table 3.3 to see a brief overview of the most common cross-reactive components.

Allergens such as birch tree pollen and fruits may be distantly related but contain components that are structurally similar, e.g. PR-10, as well as components that are specific to each (see Figure 3.4). When a patient has sIgE to a cross-reactive component it can lead to positive skin prick test and laboratory test results for all allergens containing these components. It is important to note that cross-reactive components from different sources are given different names, for example the birch tree pollen PR-10 is called Bet v 1, whereas the apple PR-10 is Mal d 1. You can read more about how allergen components are given names in Section 3.9.1.

Cross reference

Several databases are available which can be used to determine or predict allergen cross-reactivity, e.g. http://www.allergome.com/ and http://www.allergen.org/

Clinically, **oral allergy syndrome (OAS)** is a common feature of cross-reactivity between allergens found in pollen with fruit and vegetables. Similarly, multiple allergies to fish and shellfish can occur. Cross-reactivity can also occur when allergens may not appear to be of the same species, such as latex with kiwi fruit and banana and the cross-reactivity between house dust mite and shrimp. However, conserved proteins have now been identified and appropriate component allergen tests may be undertaken to resolve these clinically.

Oral allergy syndrome (OAS)

Mild oral symptoms, usually mouth tingling or itching. Patients usually have hay fever and the reaction is caused by cross-reactive PR-10 components in pollen and plant derived foods.

TABLE 3.3 Common cross-reactive allergen groups.

Allergen group	Properties	Present in	Clinical impact
PR-10 protein	Bet v 1 (Birch pollen) homologue. Degraded by heat and proteases.	Pollens and food from plant origin (e.g. fruit, nuts, and vegetables).	Highly cross-reactive. Oral allergy syndrome (OAS).
Lipid transfer protein (LTP)	Role in plant defence. Heat and protease stable.	Pollens and food from plant origin.	Can be cross-reactive (OAS) or cause specific sensitization (systemic reactions).
Profilin	Small proteins found in the cytoplasm of cells. Degraded by heat and proteases.	Pollens and food from plant origin.	Minor allergen. Can cause cross-reactivity between distantly related species. May cause OAS.
Tropomyosin	Actin-binding protein.	Mites and shellfish.	Potential cause of house dust mite–shrimp or shellfish cross-reactivity.
Cross-reactive carbohydrate determinants (CCDs)	Glycoproteins containing complex carbohydrate structures. Heat stable.	Many allergens including: plants, venoms, latex, and nuts.	Highly cross-reactive. Possible cause of false positive sIgE results. Little or no clinical significance.

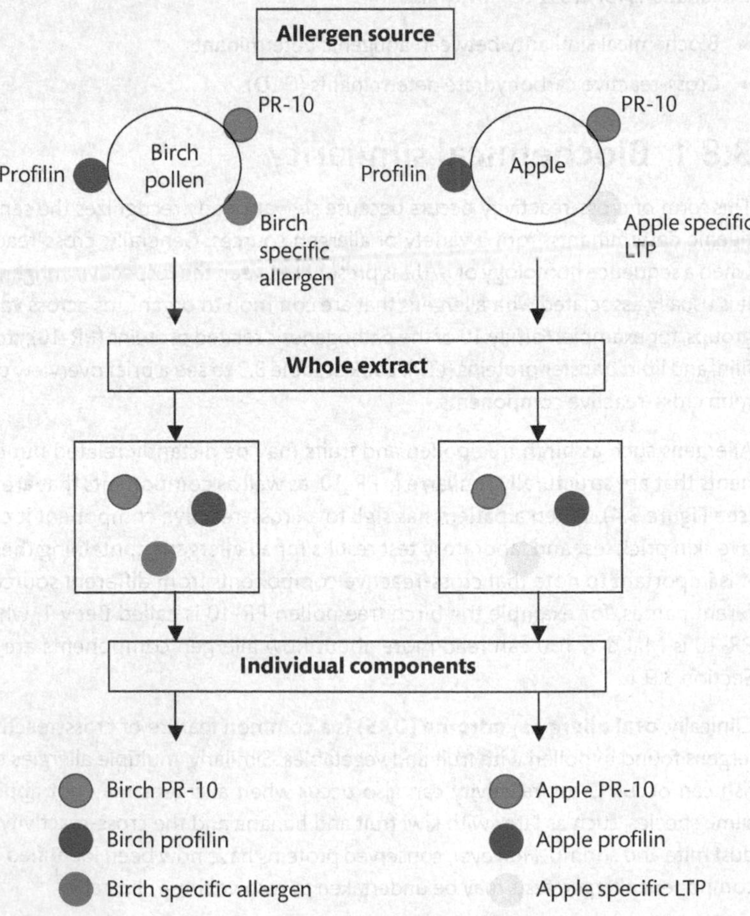

FIGURE 3.4
Components present in birch tree and apple pollen. Whole extracts contain all the components that are present. Cross-reactive components, such as PR-10 proteins and profilin, are common causes of multiple positive specific IgE results if patients are sensitized to those components. Specific allergens are also present. Testing for individual components can help to identify the agent causing sensitization.

3.8.2 Cross-reactive carbohydrate determinants

Many plant glycoproteins are composed of complex carbohydrate structures covalently bound to proteins. These carbohydrate entities share significant similarities in structure and this can result in non-specific binding to CCDs. This phenomenon can result in false positive results in sIgE assays. Suspicion of a false positive result may arise when discrepant results are obtained from sIgE assays and skin testing and/or sIgE results are not consistent with the clinical history.

As a means of establishing the likelihood of CCD false positivity, patient sera can be tested with sIgE reagents to a glycoprotein, for example bromelain (AnA C 1) or horse radish peroxidase—these are CCDs but rarely cause allergy. If these tests are positive it would suggest that CCD is responsible for other false positive results.

SELF-CHECK 3.3

How might the presence of cross-reactive allergens affect the way you interpret specific IgE results?

3.9 Component resolved diagnostics

Allergy diagnosis and treatment has further been improved by the commercial availability of purified components and recombinant protein allergens. An individual allergen component is used as the extract for the sIgE test, therefore it is known that a positive result shows that the patient has sIgE directed towards that component. The use of individual components is called component resolved diagnostics (CRD).

These individual allergens can provide valuable information about patterns of cross-reactivity in patients. They can also show if a patient is sensitized to components, which can indicate that they are more likely to suffer from severe reactions when exposed to that allergen. See Figure 3.4.

3.9.1 Nomenclature of allergen components

Many allergen components have been described and an internationally agreed form of nomenclature has been developed as a means of standardization and classification. The nomenclature system, established by the International Union of Immunological Societies (IUIS) Allergen Nomenclature Sub-committee, assigns allergens according to the following scheme.

> **Cross reference**
> Comprehensive lists of recognized allergens can be found at http://www.allergome.com and http://allergen.org/Allergen.aspx

The first 3 letters are from the plant's genus, followed by the first letter of the specific name and the number indicating the order of discovery of the allergen. An example is the major pollen allergen of the birch tree (Bet*ula* v*errucosa*) which is named *Bet v 1*.

3.9.2 Use of allergen components for clinical decisions

Table 3.4 shows allergen components of peanut that can be tested as a screening panel. The panel comprises peanut-specific allergens that are linked with severe reactions and cross-reactive components. Testing for these allergens can help make decisions about how to treat the patient. For example if they were positive for Ara h 2 (linked to severe reactions) they might be told to avoid all nuts and given injectable adrenaline for emergency use. However if they were positive to Ara h 8 (a PR-10) you may want to question them further about OAS symptoms

TABLE 3.4 Peanut allergen components.

Protein	Common name	Biological function
Ara h 1	Storage protein (7S vicilin)	7S vicilin-like globulins. Peanut specific.
Ara h 2	Storage protein (2S albumin, conglutin)	Trypsin inhibitor (inhibits trypsin which is used in digestion). Peanut specific.
Ara h 3	Storage protein (11S globulin, glycinin)	11S globulins, trypsin inhibitor. Peanut specific.
Ara h 5	Profilin	Actin-binding protein
Ara h 8	PR-10	Ribonucleases (degradation of RNA).
Ara h 9	LTP	Lipid transfer proteins (movement of fatty acids and phospholipids between cell membranes).

and carry out further testing to check if this positive result was due to cross-reactivity. Similar component panels can be used to check for allergens other than those found in peanuts, including other nuts, and PR-10 proteins to check for OAS and latex components.

Cross reference

Look at Case Study 3.3 for an example of how oral allergy syndrome can be investigated.

New components are continually being identified and added to the number of tests available in the clinical diagnostic laboratory.

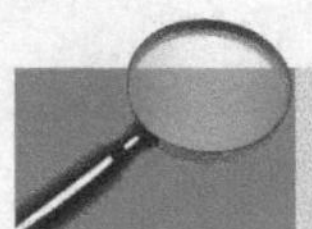

CASE STUDY 3.2 Peanut allergy

Patient history

- 3-year-old male. Developed facial swelling, itchy skin rash, and wheeze immediately after eating a cake containing nuts whilst at a birthday party.
- Treated with adrenaline and antihistamines in Emergency department.
- He has eaten nuts previously without any symptoms and is not on any medication.

Results

- Skin testing to a panel of nut allergens gave the following results:
- Negative to walnut, hazel nut, cashew nut, and brazil nut
- Positive to peanut (6×6mm wheal and 10×10mm flare)
- Negative control gave no wheal and flare, positive control gave a 4×4 wheal and 6×6 flare
- Specific IgE to walnut, hazel nut, cashew nut, and brazil nut all <0.35 kUA/L
- Peanut-specific IgE >100 kUA/L

Significance of results

- The clinical presentation, skin test results, and specific IgE results led to a diagnosis of peanut allergy.
- Advice was given to avoid all nuts and foods containing nuts. Although the patient only tested positive to peanut, contamination of other nuts and nut products with peanut is common. Therefore the general advice given is to avoid all nuts.
- An adrenaline auto-injector was prescribed and the parents were trained how to use this correctly. It was suggested that the child should wear medic alert jewellery.

Key Points

- **Allergen proteins are heterogeneous in size, degree of glycosylation, and conformation.**
- **Cross-reactivity between different allergens is common, and caused by biochemical similarity or sharing of cross-reactive carbohydrate determinants.**
- **Component resolved diagnostics can be used to determine the disease eliciting components of a given allergen.**

SELF-CHECK 3.4

What do you understand by the term component resolved diagnostics?

3.10 Microarray-based allergy testing

Based on the development of DNA microarray technology in the 1990s, the application of protein microarrays in allergy testing is now emerging. This advancement has coincided with the use of component resolved diagnostics. Microarrays allow for multiple component allergen tests to be carried out at the same time.

The assays are based on immobilization of allergen proteins (purified or recombinant) on to glass slides or silicon chips. The surfaces of these supports are treated to ensure stability and appropriate orientation of the proteins. The allergens are 'spotted' robotically in a distinctive pattern or array. When serum is applied to the slide/chip, each micron-sized spot becomes a reaction site for an antigen–antibody reaction. Bound IgE is then detected by a fluorescently labelled anti-human IgE antibody and fluorescence measured using a microarray scanner. Fluorescence images are analysed by customized software which relates fluorescence intensity of the respective spots to values derived from a calibrator serum which is incorporated in the assay. Results are reported semi-quantitatively: kUA/L or in classes.

See Figure 3.5 for an example of how a microchip may appear. Testing each allergen multiple times on the chip acts as a form of quality control as it checks for consistency in fluorescence between each spot. Some microchips also have in-built quality control spots which emit a known amount of fluorescence when a sample comes into contact with them. If the control spots fail to meet the set criteria, the software will reject that particular microarray and the test will have to be repeated.

Using allergen microarrays, sIgE reactivities to a large number of allergens, using very small volumes (microlitre amounts) of serum is feasible. Currently available microarrays have a standard panel of components including PR-10s, LTPs, profilins, and species-specific components, all from a large number of different sources. In future it may be possible to custom make microarrays to target different groups of patients, for example, those that present with possible oral allergy syndrome.

Work is required to establish the diagnostic characteristics of these assays in relation to third generation immunoassays and to demonstrate economic benefits. Specialist skills are also required to interpret the results with respect to the clinical history. A pitfall of using microarrays is that, as a range of allergens are tested, there may be unexpected positive results to allergens

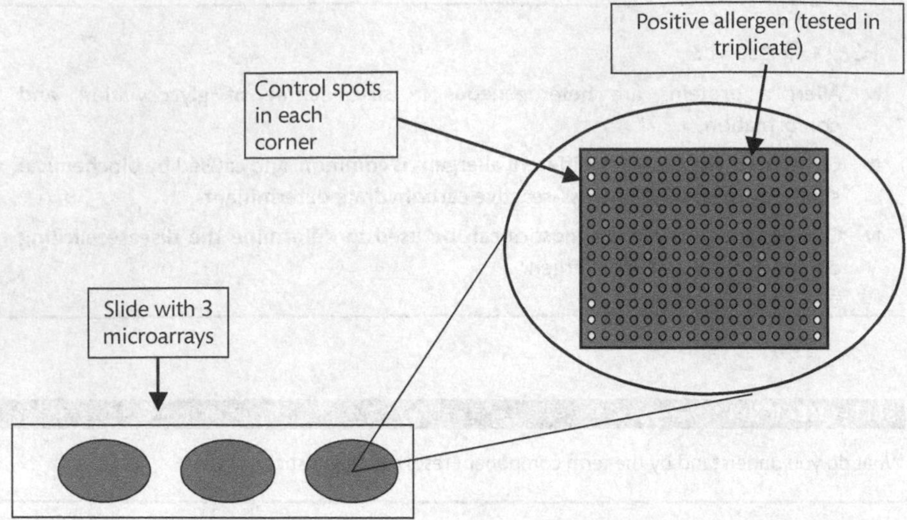

FIGURE 3.5
A slide with three microarrays. On each of these microarrays there are 49 allergens all tested in triplicate. Control spots (yellow) are present in each corner to ensure that sample has been placed across the whole test area. Positive results lead to fluorescence (shown in green) of the spots. A more intense fluorescent signal indicates a higher level of specific IgE antibodies to that allergen.

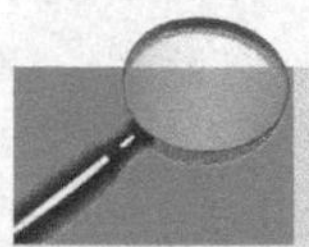

CASE STUDY 3.3 Oral allergy syndrome (OAS)

Patient history

- 66-year-old female. Referred to allergy clinic by GP after having complained of lip and throat itching and mild lip swelling after eating apples.
- The patient is able to eat cooked apple pies without symptoms.
- Previously had lip tingling after eating pears and peaches.
- Hay fever in early spring.

Results (1)

- Skin prick tests to tree pollen, apple, peach, and pear were all positive. Negative to grass pollen.
- Specific IgE results:
- Tree pollen 4.5 kUA/L
- Apple 14.2 kUA/L
- Peach 0.72 kUA/L
- Pear 0.8 kUA/L
- Grass pollen <0.35 kUA/L.

Significance of results (1)

- Positive skin tests and specific IgEs to tree pollen and a range of different fruits.
- Patient has relatively mild symptoms that are limited to the mouth. She is also able to eat cooked apples without any reaction. These features suggest possible oral allergy syndrome.
- Individual components of tree pollen and fruits were tested as part of a component resolved diagnosis screening panel for oral allergy syndrome.

Results (2)

- Bet v 1 (Birch tree pollen PR-10) 10.2 kUA/L
- Pru p 3 (Peach LTP) <0.35 kUA/L
- Bet v 2 (Birch tree pollen profilin) <0.35 kUA/L
- Pru p 1 (Peach PR-10) 6.9 kUA/L
- Pru p 4 (Peach profilin) <0.35 kUA/L.

Significance of results (2)

- Positive results to the cross-reactive PR-10 proteins.
- Based on the clinical history and test results the patient was diagnosed with oral allergy syndrome.

The lady was told that she could continue to eat fruits that she had no symptoms or minimal symptoms with. Fruits that she has more severe symptoms with, such as apples, should be avoided in the raw form. She was advised to take antihistamines to minimize hay fever symptoms and also to take them when she has symptoms with fruits, if required.

that had not been considered in the clinical history. A clinical decision has to be made in these cases about whether the test result should be pursued.

3.11 Total IgE measurements

Whilst detection of allergen-specific IgE antibodies has an important role in allergy diagnosis, measurement of total serum IgE is of very limited value. Total IgE levels are age dependent and, as with all normal ranges, the levels may differ between different populations. Total IgE ranges used in the UK are shown in Table 3.5. They can vary widely in allergic and non-allergic individuals. There is no clear cut-off level to indicate allergic disease. High levels of sIgE may occur when the total IgE concentration is within the normal range. Alternatively, high levels of total IgE (>1000 kU/L) may give rise to false positive sIgE results, so measuring total IgE may be helpful if non-specific positivity is suspected.

CLINICAL CORRELATION 3.3

Total IgE

Total IgE measurements can be useful in a number of non-allergic conditions such as:

- **parasitic infections**
- **immunodeficiency (e.g., hyper IgE syndrome, Wiskott-Aldrich syndrome, or Omenn's syndrome)**
- **vasculitis (Churg-Strauss syndrome)**
- **IgE myeloma.**

SELF-CHECK 3.5

In what circumstances are total IgE measurements useful?

TABLE 3.5 Age-related serum total IgE levels (kU/L).

Age	Median	95th centile
Newborn	0.5	5
3 months	3	11
1 year	8	29
5 years	15	52
10 years	18	63
15 years	22	75
Adult	26	81

Adapted from Milford Ward et al. (eds), *PRU Handbook of Clinical Immunochemistry*, 9th edition, 2007; reproduced with permission.

3.12 Quality assurance of laboratory allergy tests

Good laboratory practice will incorporate the use of both internal quality control (IQC) and external quality assurance (EQA) schemes.

3.12.1 Internal quality control (IQC)

Internal quality control for sIgE assays relies on the inclusion of sera and/or commercial preparations of known sIgE concentrations in the assay. IQC should be tested daily, prior to reporting patient results. They should be at levels covering the entire calibration curve; however, it is important that one of the internal controls should be at a concentration close to the assay clinical decision point of 0.35 kUA/L. Assay verification is undertaken by monitoring results on Levy–Jennings plots and by applying Westgard rules.

The extensive range of allergens for which tests are available presents a particular difficulty for quality control of the sIgE assays. There is a limited repertoire of standardized sIgE commercial preparations and laboratories have difficulty in obtaining sufficient quantities of patient sera covering a complete range of specificities. Thus, it is common practice for laboratories to incorporate a limited number of sera with sIgE positivity to the most clinically appropriate allergens. Inconsistency in allergen extract preparations may result in batch-to-batch variability and so results for IQC should be monitored carefully.

3.12.2 External quality assessment (EQA)

External quality assessment (EQA) refers to a programme of inter-laboratory proficiency testing. Such programmes are available from commercial companies or independent providers. Proficiency testing provides a benchmark of accuracy of results reported by clinical laboratories. The schemes also enable laboratories to assess their performance with other laboratories using similar or different analytical systems.

In the United Kingdom the principal scheme is organized by the United Kingdom National External Quality Assessment Service (UK NEQAS). For allergy, two programmes are offered:

1. UK NEQAS for Total IgE.
2. UK NEQAS for allergen-specific IgE. Distributions are made up from a panel of sera containing 15 common or clinically relevant sIgE allergens.

Cross reference

UK NEQAS offer a web-based educational tool (www.immqas.co.uk). In the allergy section, you can select your level of expertise and then navigate through a series of allergy results, interpret them, and complete case reports. Completed assessments are compared with peer group responses and can be logged on a personal achievement folder.

Figure 3.6 shows an example of EQA cumulative results from approximately 250 laboratories (reporting 10 different methods) for specific IgE reactivity to four allergens in a single serum sample. All columns indicate the distribution of values for all methods; coloured columns represent the cumulative results reported by approximately 50 laboratories using the same assay platform. You can see from the distribution of results that for house dust mite there is general consensus across the range of methods. However, for cat and for grass and tree pollen there is a bimodal distribution, with higher values obtained using the assay represented by the coloured columns. Whether these higher results reflect enhanced analytical sensitivity or false positivity is unknown. It is likely that differences in the composition of allergen extracts between manufacturers are a significant factor.

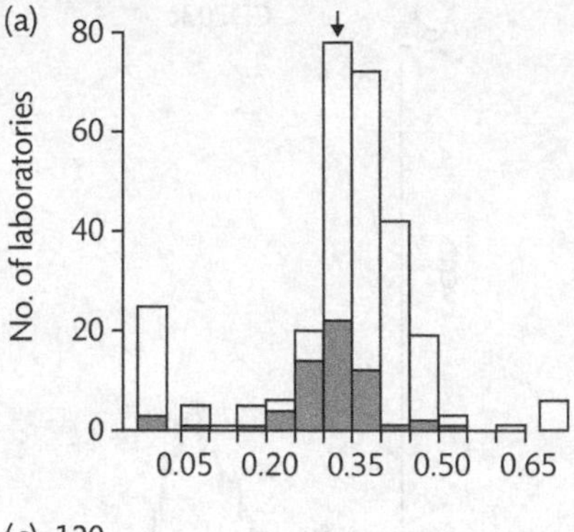

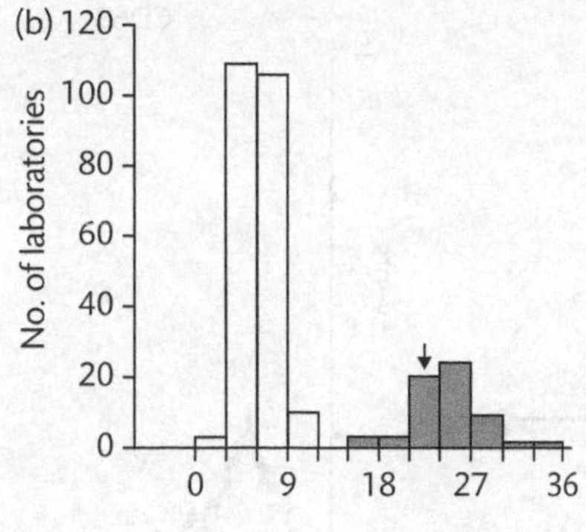

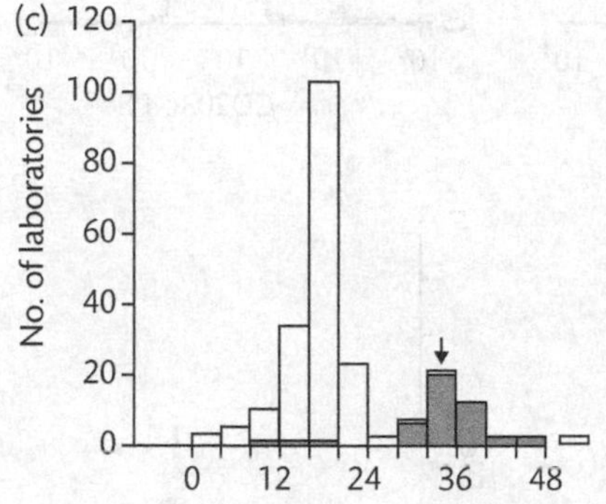

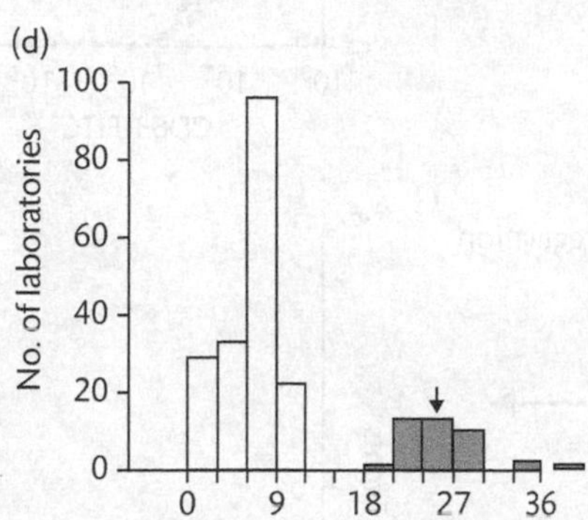

FIGURE 3.6

Cumulative results from a UK NEQAS specific IgE distribution which tested for reactivity to four allergens: (a) house dust mite; (b) cat; (c) grass pollen; (d) birch pollen. Coloured columns indicate values reported by laboratories using the same assay, all columns represent the distribution of values reported using different analytical platforms. x axis: kUA/L; y axis: number of participating laboratories. Reproduced with permission from UK NEQAS.

3.13 Flow cytometric basophil activation test

A novel approach to the laboratory diagnosis of allergy is offered by the analysis of allergen-induced basophil activation by flow cytometry. The basis of the test is the demonstration of an altered membrane phenotype on activated peripheral blood basophils. Basophil activation is used rather than mast cell activation as they circulate in blood and are relatively easy to measure, whereas mast cells reside in tissues.

Interaction of allergen with membrane bound IgE results in cross-linking of the IgE molecules and subsequent basophil activation. As well as secretion of bioactive mediators, upregulation of cell surface activation markers occurs, most notably CD63 and CD203c. The general characteristics of these molecules are summarized in Table 3.6 and Figure 3.7.

TABLE 3.6 Surface membrane characteristics of CD63 and CD203c on unstimulated and stimulated basophils.

	CD63	CD203c
Unstimulated	Barely detectable	Constitutively present
Stimulated	Upregulation within 10 mins	Upregulation within 5 mins
	Expressed at high density	Expressed at lower density than CD63

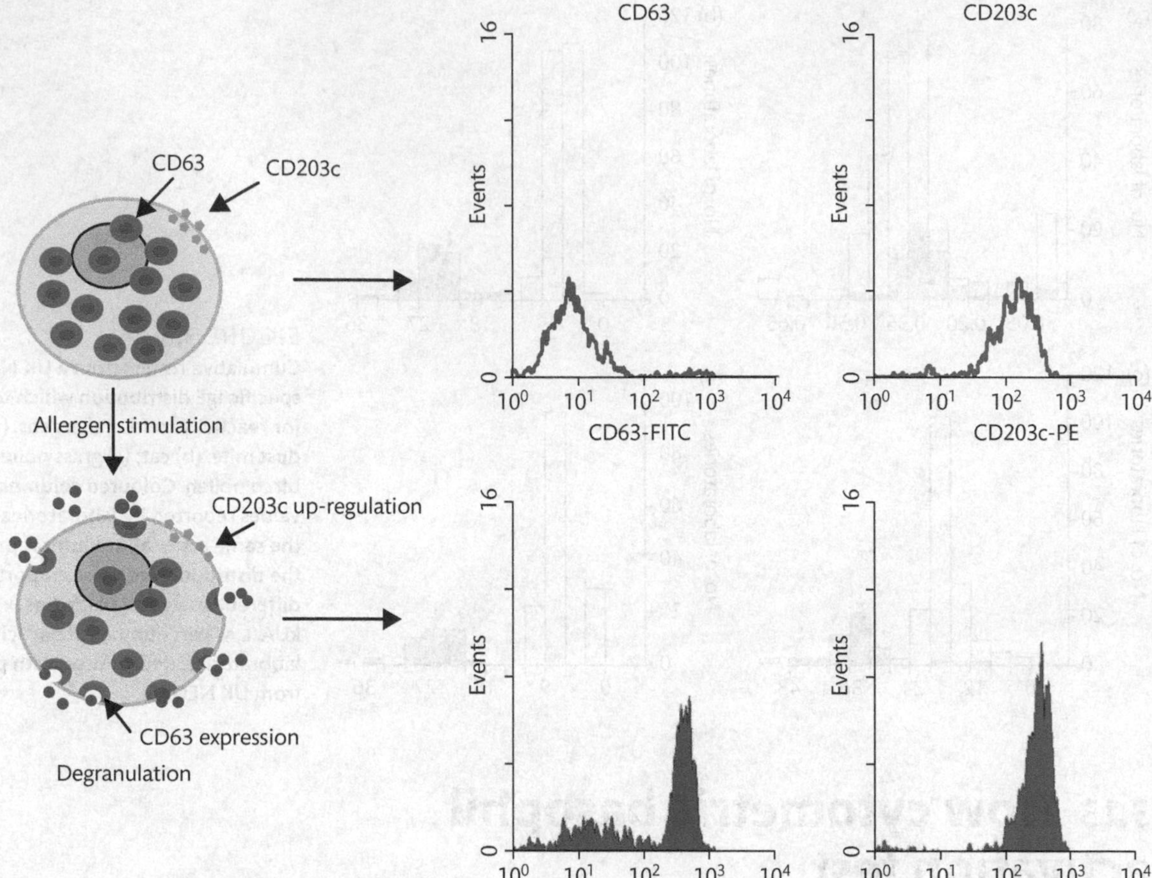

FIGURE 3.7

In resting basophils CD63 is located in intracellular granules. On activation the granules fuse with the surface membrane and CD63 is expressed on the cell surface. This change in CD63 expression can be detected by flow cytometry. Upper left quadrant (red) shows the background resting signal. The lower left quadrant (red) shows increased CD63 expression–positive signal. CD203c is constitutively expressed on the surface membrane of resting basophils and becomes upregulated following activation. This can be detected by flow cytometry. Upper right quadrant (blue) shows low level resting signal. The lower right quadrant (blue) shows positive CD203c signal. x axis: fluorescence intensity; y axis: number of events. Adapted, with permission, from Ebo et al. (2006) *Allergy*, 61, 1028. Copyright © 2006, John Wiley and Sons.

The attraction of this methodology is that it may more accurately mimic the *in vivo* situation of allergen challenge rather than, as with sIgE testing, indicate previous exposure to the allergen. The technique may be particularly applicable in the following situations:

- where sIgE tests are unavailable
- where skin test and/or specific IgE tests provide results that do not match the clinical presentation (see Case Study 3.4 for an example of this)
- when sIgE tests have poor diagnostic sensitivity or specificity, for example, in drug allergy.

The assays, however, are labour intensive and unlikely to replace sIgE testing in most cases. They are only currently available in specialist referral centres.

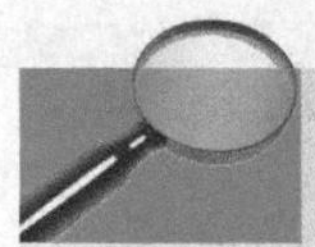

CASE STUDY 3.4 Venom allergy

Patient history

- 45-year-old male. Stung on the hand whilst at work. Thought that it was a wasp.
- Within minutes he had generalized itch all over the body, felt hot and sweaty, and began to have trouble breathing.
- His colleagues called for an ambulance and paramedics treated him with adrenaline, antihistamines, and steroids prior to taking him to hospital.
- When seen by an expert in allergy he gave a history of previously being stung at age 19 years by a bee and had no reaction.
- He is a keen gardener, therefore it is important to correctly identify the insect that caused the reaction as it is likely to be encountered again whilst in the garden.

Results (1)

- Skin prick tests were positive to both bee and wasp.
- Specific IgE to bee was 16.9 kUA/L and wasp was 1.3 kUA/L.

Significance of results (1)

- The results of the skin prick tests and specific IgE tests show that the patient was positive for bee and wasp. These results are not consistent with the clinical presentation. It was decided to carry out intradermal tests and request bee and wasp specific IgE components.
- Specific IgE to bromelain was tested to check for CCD cross-reactivity.
- Basophil activation tests to bee and wasp were also requested.

Results (2)

- Intradermal test to wasp was positive, negative to bee.
- Wasp-specific IgE components (Ves v 5, Pol d 5, and Ves v 1) all positive.
- Bee-specific IgE component (Api m 1) negative.
- Bromelain-specific IgE positive (15.7 kUA/L).
- Basophil activation test (BAT) positive to wasp (look at Figure 3.8 to see this), negative to bee.

Significance of results (2)

- Intradermal tests, component resolved diagnostics tests, and basophil activation test results led to a diagnosis of wasp venom allergy.
- CCD cross-reactivity is a common cause of dual positive venom-specific IgE results.

In cases where there are unexpected positive results, it is important to follow them up with other investigations, in order to clarify what the causative agent is. In this particular case it was important as the patient is a gardener, therefore is more likely to be stung. He now carries an adrenaline auto-injector and antihistamines. He has started to have wasp venom desensitization.

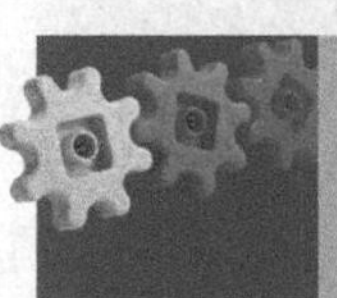

METHOD 3.3 Basophil activation test (BAT)

- Basophils in a whole blood sample are incubated with allergen extract at a range of concentrations.
- Positive controls (FcεRI stimulant and FMLP) and negative controls (dilution buffer) are included.
- **Fluorochrome** conjugated monoclonal antibodies–C-C Chemokine receptor type 3 (CCR3)(to aid in the identification of basophils) and anti-CD63 and/or CD203c (activation markers)–are added.

Fluorochrome
A fluorescent chemical that emits a specific colour when illuminated by light.

- Samples are incubated with allergen and labelled monoclonal antibodies, typically for 15 minutes.
- Red cells are removed by lysing the sample prior to analysis on the flow cytometer.
- On the flow cytometer, basophils are identified on the basis of side scatter laser light and CCR3 expression.
- The percentage of CD63 and/or CD203c expressed by the basophils is determined (see Figure 3.8 for an example).
- A sample from a healthy volunteer is usually set up at the same time as the patient as another form of quality controlling the assay.

Evaluative studies have reported good correlation with clinical diagnoses for inhalant allergy (e.g. pollens and house dust mite), hymenoptera venom allergy, and latex allergy. A representative series of flow cytometric plots following the basophil activation test on a blood sample from the patient described in Case Study 3.4 with wasp venom allergy is shown in Figure 3.8. The diagnostic sensitivity of the test is lower for drugs, probably reflecting the weaker allergenicity of these molecules. Nonetheless the technique has potential diagnostic utility in the investigation of reactions caused by neuromuscular blocking agents and β-lactam antibiotics.

Key Points

- Basophil activation tests can provide useful diagnostic information, particularly when specific IgE tests are unavailable or have poor diagnostic sensitivity or specificity, e.g. drug allergy.
- Allergen-induced basophil activation is assessed by flow cytometric analysis of CD63 and/or CD203c expression.

Cross reference

You can read more about flow cytometry in Chapter 11.

BOX 3.3 Quality control of basophil activation tests

- Internal Quality Control (IQC) for the basophil activation test relies on concurrent analysis of a blood sample from a healthy individual that does not react to the allergen being tested. This is of use to show if the allergen acts as an irritant causing non-IgE-mediated basophil activation.
- Positive and negative controls, as described in Method 3.3, show whether the method is capable of detecting basophil activation in that particular patient and also what the background level of stimulation is.
- It is important to check that the positive control has worked as up to 10% of patients may be non-responders. In these cases the results cannot be reported.

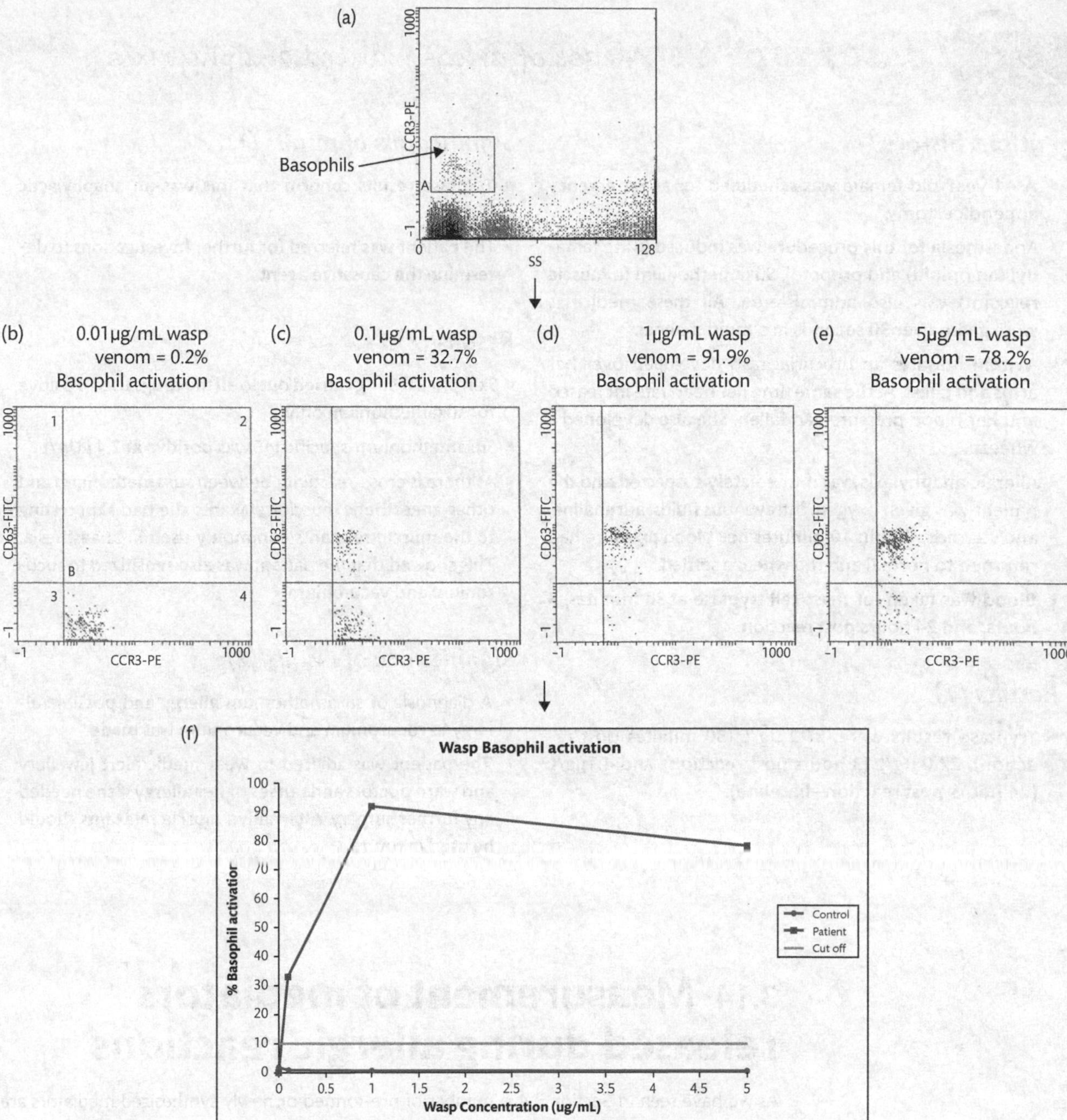

FIGURE 3.8

Flow cytometric dot plots demonstrating basophil activation and CD63 positivity in a patient with wasp venom allergy. (a) The basophils are initially gated based on laser side scatter (ss) and phycoerythrin (PE) labelled CCR3. (b, c, d, & e) Fluorescein isothiocyanate (FITC) labelled anti-CD63 is used to determine the percentage of activated basophils over a series of concentrations of wasp venom. Activated basophils are present in quadrant B2. (f) When plotted on a graph it can be seen that the patient gives a positive result (pink line) when compared to the venom cut-off of 10% activation (yellow line) and healthy control (blue line).

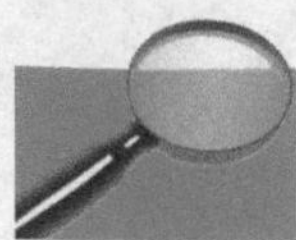

CASE STUDY 3.5 A case of drug-induced anaphylaxis

Patient history

- A 44-year-old female was scheduled for an emergency appendicectomy.
- Anaesthesia for this procedure was induced using fentanyl (an opioid) and propofol. Suxamethonium (a muscle relaxant) was also administered. All these medicines were given over 30 seconds in a rapid manner.
- Within minutes an urticarial rash developed over her arms and chest. At the same time her heart rate increased and her blood pressure had fallen. She also developed a wheeze.
- Allergic anaphylaxis was immediately suspected and the patient was given oxygen, intravenous fluids, adrenaline, and steroids. Within 10 minutes her blood pressure had returned to normal and the wheeze settled.
- Blood was taken for mast cell tryptase at 30 minutes, 3 hours, and 24 hours post reaction.

Results (1)

- Tryptase results were: 81.2 μg/L (30 minutes post reaction), 22.0 μg/L (3 hours post reaction), and 4.1μg/L (24 hours post reaction–baseline).

Significance of results (1)

- Tryptase results confirm that this was an anaphylactic reaction.
- The patient was referred for further investigations to determine the causative agent.

Results (2)

- Skin prick testing carried out to all the drugs used. Positive for suxamethonium only.
- Suxamethonium-specific IgE was positive at 2.4 kUA/L.
- As there is cross-reactivity between suxamethonium and other anaesthetic muscle relaxants she had skin testing to the muscle relaxants commonly used in anaesthesia. This showed that the patient was also sensitized to rocuronium and vecuronium.

Significance of results (2)

- A diagnosis of suxamethonium allergy and possible allergy to rocuronium and vecuronium was made.
- The patient was advised to wear medic alert jewellery and warn doctors and nurses of her allergy if she needed any further surgery. Alternative muscle relaxants should be used in future.

3.14 Measurement of mediators released during allergic reactions

As we have seen in Section 3.4, a number of pre-formed or newly synthesized mediators are released during an allergic reaction. However, very few of these molecules are measured in the routine diagnostic laboratory. This is due to difficulties of detection, either because the molecules have short half-lives, or because standardized assays are unavailable.

3.14.1 Mast cell tryptase

Mast cell tryptase exists in two major forms: α-tryptase and β-tryptase. Both forms of the enzyme are synthesized and secreted as precursors: pro-α-tryptase and pro-β-tryptase, respectively. Together, pro-α-tryptase and pro-β-tryptase comprise the baseline levels of mast cell tryptase detected in the circulation. As these enzymes are virtually unique to mast cells, blood levels typically reflect the body's mast cell content; i.e., the higher the level, the greater the number of mast cells present.

As well as being directly secreted, β-tryptase is stored in mast cell granules, where it is the principal pre-formed mediator within these structures. Activation of mast cells (by IgE- and non-IgE-mediated mechanisms) results in degranulation and release of β-tryptase along with other pre-formed mediators. Thus, detection of elevated levels of β-tryptase in the circulation is an indication of mast cell activation.

Following mast cell degranulation, blood tryptase levels peak within 1 hour, with a return to normal levels within 24 hours. The half-life of tryptase is approximately 2–3 hours. This contrasts with the mediator histamine, also released during mast cell activation, where maximal blood levels are observed within 5 minutes of degranulation, with a return to baseline within 30 minutes. Given this short time frame, collection of blood samples for histamine analyses can pose problems. Hence, measurement of mast cell tryptase is the preferred assay for clinical laboratories assessing mast cell activation in, for example, anaphylaxis.

Serum or plasma mast cell tryptase may be measured by fluorescence immunoassay. The capture antibody employed in the assay identifies both α-and β-tryptase and so detects total tryptase. The normal range in serum/plasma is 2–14 μg/L, the majority of which is α-tryptase. Following mast cell degranulation the predominant form which is measured is β-tryptase.

Measurement of mast cell tryptase in post-mortem blood samples can be measured to provide supportive evidence for suspected anaphylactic deaths. The upper limit of normal range (0–50μg/L) for post-mortem tryptase results is higher as tryptase may be released during the tissue breakdown that occurs after death.

CLINICAL CORRELATION 3.4

Causes of raised tryptase results

- **Anaphylaxis. Mast cell tryptase levels are elevated in the majority of cases of anaphylaxis. The timing of sample collection is critical for detection of anaphylaxis-induced tryptase release. It is recommended that three tryptase samples are taken:**
    1. **At the time of reaction (within 1 hour)**
    2. **3 hours post reaction**
    3. **24 hours post reaction (level should have returned to baseline normal for that patient).**

Time of venepuncture in relation to the reaction should be clearly indicated on the request forms as well as clinical history, including information about potential allergens. This allows for a proper interpretation of results to be made.

- **Systemic and cutaneous (urticaria pigmentosa) mastocytosis. Mastocytosis is a disease characterized by proliferation of mast cells in various tissues (bone marrow, skin, liver, spleen, and the gastrointestinal mucosa). Skin rashes, itching, and hives are generally observed in the cutaneous form. Systemic mastocytosis symptoms involve the whole body and include: skin involvement, anaphylaxis, gastrointestinal upset, and fainting. Clinical manifestations are caused by mast cell infiltration into tissues and release of bioactive mediators acting locally or at distant sites.**

Microscopic analysis of tissue biopsy, in which increased numbers of mast cells are detected, is a key laboratory test. However, measurement of mast cell tryptase is also helpful in that increased levels, usually >20μg/L are found. Monitoring mast cell tryptase levels during therapy may be helpful as decreasing levels may reflect a reduction in mast cell burden.

- **Mast cell activation syndromes. Normal numbers of mast cells in tissues but they rapidly degranulate. Similar symptoms to those of mastocytosis.**
- **Haematological neoplasms. For example; acute myeloid leukaemia and chronic myeloid leukaemia.**
- **Idiopathic. Some patients have unexpected, unexplained borderline raised tryptase. Causes such as mastocytosis have been excluded in these cases.**
- **Assay interference. Human anti-mouse antibodies and raised rheumatoid factor (RF) have been documented as causes of unexplained raised tryptase levels.**

SELF-CHECK 3.6

Why is it important to know the time of blood sampling in relation to an anaphylactic reaction when interpreting mast cell tryptase levels?

3.14.2 Urine methylhistamine

Methylhistamine is a relatively stable metabolite of histamine that is excreted by the kidneys. Therefore, an increase in histamine levels after anaphylaxis or during mastocytosis leads to increased levels of urinary methylhistamine. In some patients methylhistamine levels may remain within the normal range during anaphylaxis or mastocytosis. Care must be taken when interpreting the results and the clinical history must be taken into account.

The test can be performed by Enzyme Linked Immunosorbent Assay (ELISA) on acylated urine samples, or by liquid chromatography–mass spectrometry. There is no international reference preparation available for methylhistamine, therefore the units used and normal range can differ between methods.

The test can provide additional evidence of anaphylaxis. It can be useful to obtain a urine sample for methylhistamine quantitation at the same time as a tryptase sample is taken.

3.14.3 Eosinophil cationic protein

Eosinophil cationic protein (ECP) is a single chain, zinc-containing protein which is stored in the secretory granules of eosinophils. Activation of eosinophils results in release of ECP. Within the airways, ECP may contribute to epithelia damage and increased hypersensitivity leading to chronic inflammatory airways disease. Consequently, ECP has been investigated as a potential biomarker of airway inflammation, particularly in asthmatic patients.

ECP can be measured by fluorescence immunoassay. The assay is straightforward but standardization of sample collection and handling is critical for assay reproducibility. This is because of *in vitro* release of ECP which occurs during the clotting process. Consequently, serum ECP measurement combines the physiological level with that released by *in vitro* activation. The latter element reflects the propensity of activated eosinophils to release granule proteins. As 'primed' eosinophils are a feature of airway inflammation, ECP is more readily released from these cells than from 'unprimed' eosinophils. Thus, discrimination between the levels observed as a consequence of airway inflammation compared with those detected in health is enhanced. Serum measurements are regarded, therefore, as being superior when assessing and monitoring airway inflammation. Values of >15 μg/mL are considered to be elevated for both adults and children (>2 years).

BOX 3.4 Steps to reduce in vitro ECP release

- **Use of blood collection tubes with gel barriers to decrease cell transfer to the serum phase.**
- **Standardization of clotting times (60–120 minutes) and temperature (20–24°C).**
- **Transfer of serum into a fresh tube within 1 hour of separation.**

In asthmatic patients, ECP levels in blood (and bronchoalveolar lavage and sputum) reflect airway inflammatory status. Monitoring ECP during anti-inflammatory therapy (e.g. with corticosteroids) may be helpful in assessing compliance and/or efficacy of treatment.

CLINICAL CORRELATION 3.5

Allergy treatments

- **The most effective way of treating allergy is to avoid the allergen. This is not always practical as it is difficult to avoid allergens such as pollen and cross-contamination of food products cannot always be avoided.**
- **The use of antihistamines is commonly advised to reduce the daily symptoms of allergies such as rhinitis. Regular corticosteroids may also be prescribed to minimize symptoms.**
- **Injectable adrenaline can be administered in anaphylactic situations to quickly reduce symptoms of the allergic reaction. Patients with life-threatening allergies such as those to peanut or venom are usually prescribed, and trained how to use, adrenaline auto-injectors. These should be carried with them at all times.**
- **Desensitization or specific immunotherapy can be offered in some cases. Treatment starts by giving the patients small amounts of allergen. Then increasing amounts are given as treatment progresses. It may take months to desensitize a patient. The aim is to produce tolerance to the allergen by changing the response from IgE-mediated to IgG-mediated. Desensitization is not effective in all patients. Component resolved diagnostics may help to decide if a patient is suitable for desensitization. If they are sensitized to a component in the desensitization treatment they are suitable for the treatment. If the allergen that they are sensitized to is not in the treatment then it will have no effect if given.**

3.15 IgG antibodies in hypersensitivity

Allergen specific IgG antibodies may be detected in patients with type III hypersensitivity. The clinical value of measuring allergen specific IgG antibodies (often termed 'precipitating antibodies') is limited to a relatively small number of conditions in which chronic exposure to inhaled allergens gives rise to elevated levels of these antibodies.

BOX 3.5 Quality control of allergen-specific IgG tests

- **Appropriate IQC should be tested and checked prior to reporting patient results.**
- **As with specific IgE, it may be difficult to obtain IQC for each of the specific IgG tests. In practice, an IQC targeted at monitoring a clinically relevant specific IgG test can be used to represent the performance of all the tests.**
- **An EQA scheme is available for monitoring test performance of specific IgG tests in suspected cases of farmer's lung, bird fancier's lung, and *Aspergillus fumigatus*.**

3.15.1 Precipitating IgG antibodies (precipitins)

Chronic exposure to organic dusts containing, for example, moulds or bird droppings can result in hypersensitivity reactions involving lung interstitium and terminal bronchioles. Specific IgG antibodies can be detected in pulmonary diseases such as:

- Farmer's lung: IgG antibodies to *Micropolyspora faeni; Thermoactinomyces vulgaris.*
- Extrinsic allergic alveolitis and allergic bronchopulmonary alveolitis: IgG antibodies to *Aspergillus fumigatus.*
- Bird fancier's lung: IgG antibodies to avian serum/faecal extracts.

Traditionally these antibodies are detected by the Ouchterlony plate double diffusion technique whereby the antigen–antibody reaction is visualized as a precipitin line. Hence the terminology: precipitating IgG antibodies or precipitins. Specific IgG immunoassays, similar to IgE immunoassays, are now more commonly employed.

The presence of specific IgG in the serum indicates exposure to the antigen and hence the antibodies can be detected in both symptomatic and asymptomatic subjects. However, a high level of antigen-specific IgG in a symptomatic individual would be supportive of the diagnosis.

3.15.2 Immunotherapy

It has been proposed that desensitization or specific immunotherapy may work, in part, by promoting a change in immune response from IgE production via T_H2 cells to IgG production via a T_H1 response. This has led to the suggestion that specific IgG could be used to monitor immunotherapy. However, specific IgG levels do not necessarily correlate with control of clinical symptoms, meaning that monitoring of specific antibodies has not entered mainstream clinical practice. An exception appears to be wasp and bee venom desensitization where quantifying venom-specific antibodies can be used to guide dosing schedules.

Cross reference

You can read more about immunotherapy in Clinical correlation 3.5.

3.15.3 Food allergy

Determination of food-specific IgG has no clinical relevance in the investigation of food allergy. IgG antibodies to dietary antigens can be detected in healthy individuals and food-specific IgG antibody levels do not correlate with the results of oral food challenges.

SELF-CHECK 3.7

Can you identify the conditions in which allergen-specific IgG antibody testing provides useful diagnostic information?

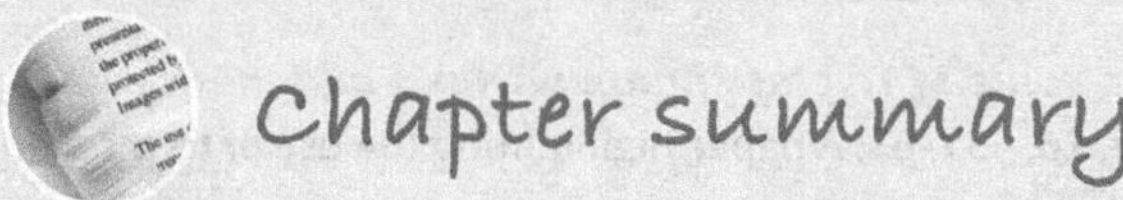

Chapter summary

- The incidence of allergic disease is increasing.
- Allergy is a type I hypersensitivity reaction. IgE antibodies initiate a two-stage reaction: induction/sensitization and reactive phases.
- Allergy is a systemic disease. Patients can present with single or multiple symptoms.
- Allergy diagnosis is based on clinical assessment supplemented by laboratory investigations. Taking an accurate clinical history, skin testing, and appropriate selection of allergen-specific IgE tests are the primary diagnostic tools used to diagnosis allergic disease.
- Allergens are heterogeneous and IgE antibody cross-reactivity can occur. It is important to bear this in mind when looking at test results.
- Component resolved diagnostics (CRD) can be used to define disease eliciting components and aid in decision making for avoidance advice and whether the patient is suitable for desensitization.
- Quality assurance for allergy testing can be problematic. There are no reference standards available for any allergen preparation. Consequently, assessment of results should be made with a peer group using a comparable assay platform.
- Determination of *in vitro* induced basophil activation by flow cytometry has a role in the investigation of certain allergic reactions, for example in suspected drug allergy.
- Circulating levels of mast cell tryptase are raised during anaphylaxis. Detection of elevated levels in serum would support a diagnosis of anaphylaxis provided the blood sample has been taken within 3 hours of a suspected reaction.
- Allergen-specific IgG antibody testing can aid in the diagnosis of respiratory conditions caused by chronic exposure to inhaled allergens. This is not immediate type I hypersensitivity. Food-specific IgG antibody testing is not useful in the investigation of food allergy.

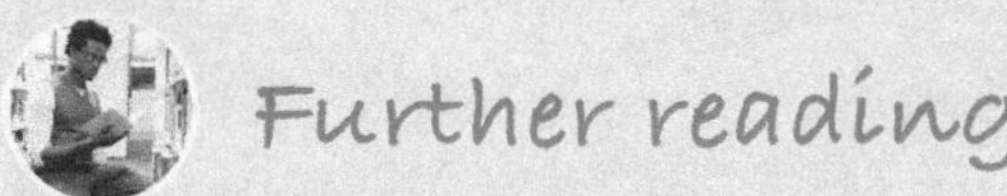

Further reading

- **Bernstein IL, Li JT, Bernstein DI, *et al.* (2008). *Allergy diagnostic testing: An updated practice parameter*. *Annals of Allergy, Asthma and Immunology*, 100, S1-148. A comprehensive review detailing clinical and laboratory investigations for allergy diagnosis.**

- Ferrer M, Sanz ML, Sastre J, *et al.* (2009). *Molecular diagnosis in Allergology: Application of the microarray technique*. *J Investig Allergol Clin Immunol*, **19**, 19–24. Discussion of the principles and performance of allergen microarrays.
- Murphy K (2014). *Janeway's Immunobiology*. 8th Edition, Garland Science. Chapter 14 provides a major reference source describing the different mechanisms of the four types of hypersensitivity, key examples, methods of detection, and available treatments.
- Sanz ML, Ganboa PM, De Weck AL (2007). *In vitro tests: Basophil activation tests*. In: Pichler WJ, *Drug Hypersensitivity*, pp. 391–402. Karger, Basel. Overview of the theory of basophil activation tests and their application in allergy testing.
- Schwartz LB (2006). *Diagnostic value of tryptase in anaphylaxis and mastocytosis*. *Immunol Allergy Clin North Am*, **26**, 451–63. A paper highlighting the use of tryptase in anaphylaxis.
- Williams P, Sewell WA, Bunn C, *et al.* (2008). *Clinical immunology review series: an approach to the use of immunology laboratory in the diagnosis of clinical allergy*. *Clinical and Experimental Immunology*, **153**, 10–18. A paper that explains the role of the diagnostic laboratory in the assessment of patients with allergic disease.

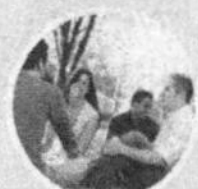

Discussion questions

3.1 What are the relative advantages and disadvantages of using natural allergen extracts and individual components as diagnostic tools?

3.2 How should quality assessment be undertaken in a laboratory performing allergy tests?

3.3 What is the role of flow cytometry in allergy diagnosis?

Answers to self-check questions are provided in the book's Online Resource Centre.

 Visit www.oxfordtextbooks.co.uk/orc/hall2e

4

Complement

Learning objectives

After studying this chapter you should be able to:

- outline the common features of the complement pathways
- outline the assays and techniques used to test for complement
- discuss the limitations of these techniques
- explain the effects of complement deficiencies
- explain the clinical features of hereditary and acquired angioedema
- outline the treatment of hereditary and acquired angioedema.

Introduction

The complement system consists of a group of soluble plasma and membrane-bound proteins which interact with one another in three distinct enzymatic activation cascades and a final common terminal pathway:

- the classical pathway (CP)
- the alternative pathway (AP)
- the lectin pathway (LP)
- the non-enzymatic assembly of a cytolytic complex (the membrane attack pathway).

The naming of the classical and alternative pathways is historical, as the classical pathway was described first. However, in evolutionary terms the alternative pathway is likely to have arisen first. The names are potentially confusing; it should be remembered that the alternative pathway is not an alternative to the other pathways, but a pathway in its own right, an activation loop with its own role in immune defence. The more recently described lectin pathway represents an antibody-independent route for classical pathway activation. Complement plays a central role in innate immune defence, providing a system for the rapid destruction of a wide range of invading micro-organisms. The control of complement activation is essential to prevent rapid consumption of complement *in vivo*. Control is provided by ten or more plasma and

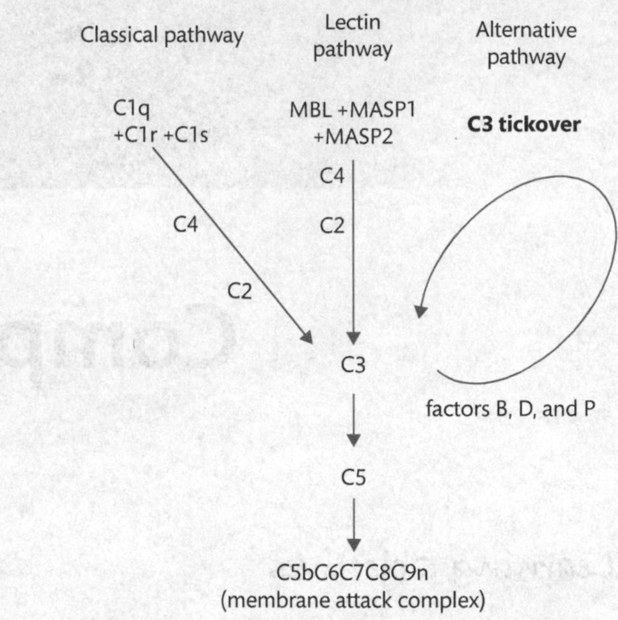

FIGURE 4.1
Overview of the complement system.

membrane-bound inhibitory proteins acting at multiple stages of the system. The major source of most of the complement components and soluble control proteins is the liver. Other tissues and cells may synthesize specific proteins and local synthesis by macrophages and other cells at sites of inflammation may be of importance in maintaining local concentrations in the tissues during activation. Figure 4.1 shows an overview of the complement system.

> **Key Point**
>
> **The classical and alternative pathways are so named for historical reasons. Each is an important pathway in its own right.**

4.1 Actions of complement

> **Opsonization**
> **The binding of complement and antibodies to the surface of a pathogen or foreign substance to aid phagocytosis.**

Complement, through its different components, is important in three main areas: first, *host defence against infection* (**opsonization**, chemotaxis and activation of leukocytes, and lysis of bacteria and cells); second, *interface between innate and adaptive immunity* (augmenting the antibody response and enhancing immunological memory); and third, *disposal of waste* (clearance of immune complexes and apoptotic cells).

The different pathways of complement are triggered in different ways. The alterative and lectin pathways are triggered by microbial cell surfaces and the classical pathway is triggered by antibody/antigen complexes. During complement activation, the components are cleaved into active forms. These are labelled 'a' for the small fragment and 'b' for the large fragment. For example, C5 is cleaved into C5a and C5b. C5a binds to the C5a receptor present on a number of cell types including endothelial cells and phagocytes and mediates an inflammatory response. C5b binds to C6 and C7 and initiates assembly of the membrane attack complex which punches holes in cell membranes. Look at Table 4.1 for a list of complement components and their actions.

TABLE 4.1 Complement components and their functions.

Pathway	Component	Action
Classical	C1q	Binds to Fc portion of antibodies (IgM and IgG in particular) leading to activation of C1r.
	C1r	Cleaves and activates C1s.
	C1s	Cleaves C4 and C2.
	C4	C4b binds to C2 which is then cleaved by C1s. (C4a is a weak inflammatory mediator probably inactive.)
	C2	As part of C4bC2a cleaves C3 and forms C4b2a3b which cleaves C5.
Lectin	MBL	Binds to sugars present on bacterial cell walls and activates MASP2.
	MASP1 and 2	Cleaves C4 and C2 leading to the formation of C4b2a3b as above.
Alternative	C3	Spontaneously hydrolyses (tickover) forming C3a and C3(H2O). C3(H2O) is stabilized if bacterial cell wall is present.
	Factor B	Binds to C3b on bacterial cell wall and is then cleaved by factor D. The resultant C3bBb cleaves C5.
	Factor D	Cleaves factor B into Ba and Bb.
	Properdin	Stabilizes the C3bBb complex.
Common	C3	Activated as above. C3a mediates inflammation. Bb in the C3bBbC3b complex cleaves C5. C3b binds C5 and presents it for cleavage by Bb.
Membrane attack complex	C5	C5a is a potent inflammatory mediator. C5b initiates formation of the membrane attack complex.
	C6 and C7	Bind to C5b forming C5b67. C5b67 inserts into the target cell membrane.
	C8	Binds to C5b67 and anchors the complex more tightly to the cell wall.
	C9	Multiple C9 molecules bind to C5b-8 and polymerize forming an open pore in the cell membrane.

4.1.1 Classical pathway

The **classical pathway** is triggered by antibody bound to particulate antigen. Many other substances including components of damaged cells, bacterial lipopolysaccharide, and nucleic acids can also trigger the classical pathway in an antibody-independent manner.

The first step in the classical pathway involves binding of C1 to surface or immune complex bound IgG or IgM antibody. C1 is a large multicomponent complex with a molecular weight of approximately 800 kDa. It consists of a single molecule of C1q and two molecules each of C1r and C1s. Binding of multiple heads of the six-headed C1q molecule by aggregated IgG or IgM triggers activation of the other components of the C1 complex. C1r and C1s are homologous single chain molecules with a molecular weight of 80 kDa, which associate with one another and with C1q in a calcium-dependent complex (Reid 1986, Reid and Day 1989). Conformational

Classical pathway

The complement pathway that is triggered by antibody bound to particulate antigen. Many other substances including components of damaged cells, bacterial lipopolysaccharide, and nucleic acids can also trigger the classical pathway in an antibody-independent manner.

changes in C1q trigger the auto-activation of the pro-enzyme C1r, and activated C1r in turn activates C1s in the complex. C1s in the activated C1 complex will cleave and activate the next component of the classical pathway, C4.

C4 is a large (200 kDa) plasma protein containing three disulphide-bonded chains (α, β, and γ) (Schreiber and Muller-Eberhard 1974, Janatova and Tack 1981). C1s cleaves plasma C4 at a single site near the amino-terminus of the α chain, releasing a small fragment, C4a (Mw ~ 9kDa) and exposing a labile, reactive thioester group in the α chain of the large fragment, C4b. Once exposed in C4b the thioester forms covalent amide or ester bonds with exposed amino or hydroxyl groups respectively on the activating surface, locking the molecule to the activating surface. Membrane-bound C4b provides a receptor for the next component of the classical pathway, C2.

C2 is a single chain plasma protein of molecular weight 102 kDa. In the presence of Mg^{2+} ions, C2 binds membrane-bound C4b and is cleaved by C1s in an adjacent C1 complex. The carboxy-terminal fragment, C2a, remains attached to C4b to form the C4b2a complex, the next enzyme in the classical pathway.

C3, a 185 kDa heterodimeric molecule, is the most abundant of the complement components (1–2 g/L in serum) and is essential for activity of both the classical and alternative pathways (Lambris 1988). C3 binds the C4b2a complex and is cleaved by the C2a enzyme, releasing a small fragment, C3a (9kDa), from the amino-terminus of the α chain and exposing in the large fragment, C3b, a labile thioester group. C3b binds via the thioester either to the activating C4b2a complex or to the adjacent membrane (Kozono et al., 1990, Ebanks et al. 1992). C3b bound to the activating C4b2a complex constitutes a new enzyme, C4b2a3b, the C5 cleaving enzyme (convertase) of the classical pathway.

C5 is a heterodimeric protein of 190 kDa molecular weight that is structurally related to C3 and C4 but lacks a thioester. C5 binds to C3b in the C4b2a3b convertase and is cleaved by C2a in the complex. A small fragment, C5a (~10 kDa), is released from the amino terminus of the α chain, whilst the large fragment, C5b, remains attached to the convertase.

4.1.2 Alternative pathway

Alternative pathway
The complement pathway that provides a rapid, antibody-independent route for activation and amplification of complement on foreign surfaces. C3 is the key component of the alternative pathway but three other proteins, factor B (fB), factor D (fD), and properdin, are also required.

The **alternative pathway** provides a rapid, antibody-independent route for activation and amplification of complement on foreign surfaces. C3 is the key component of the alternative pathway but three other proteins, factor B (fB), factor D (fD), and properdin, are also required. Factor B, a single-chain protein closely related to C2, binds C3b in a Mg^{2+}-dependent manner. This renders factor B susceptible to cleavage by factor D, a 26 kDa serine protease present in plasma in its active form. Cleavage releases the smaller Ba fragment and exposes a serine protease domain in the large (60 kDa) fragment, Bb (Gotze 1986). The C3bBb complex can then cleave more C3 to generate C3b. Properdin binds and stabilizes the C3bBb complex.

Initiation of the alternative pathway occurs spontaneously, a phenomenon known as 'tickover'. C3 in plasma is hydrolysed to form a metastable $C3(H_2O)$ molecule which binds factor B in solution and renders it susceptible to cleavage by factor D to form a fluid phase C3 convertase (Lachmann and Hughes-Jones 1984, Law and Dodds 1990). The surface features of many micro-organisms and foreign cells favour amplification of the alternative pathway and rapidly become coated with C3b molecules.

Binding of a second C3b molecule to the C3bBb complex generates the C5-cleaving enzyme of the alternative pathway, C3bBbC3b. C5 is cleaved by Bb in a manner identical to that described in Section 4.1.1 for cleavage in the classical pathway, in which the large fragment C5b remains attached to the convertase.

4.1.3 Lectin pathway

The more recently described **lectin pathway** provides a second antibody-independent means of activation of complement on bacterial and other micro-organism surfaces. It is highly analogous to the classical pathway with which it shares C2, C3, and C4. Mannan binding lectin (MBL) is a high molecular weight serum lectin made up of multiple copies of a single 32 kDa chain that binds mannose and N-acetyl glucosamine residues in bacterial cell walls (Reid and Turner 1994, Holmskov et al. 1994). The structure of MBL resembles that of C1q and it too is associated with serine proteases, in this case MBL-associated serine proteases (MASPs). The MBL-MASP complex activates C4 in a manner identical to that described in Section 4.1.1 for the activated C1 complex.

Lectin pathway
The complement pathway that provides a second antibody-independent means of activation of complement on bacterial and other micro-organism surfaces. It is highly analogous to the classical pathway and shares C2, C3, and C4 with it.

4.1.4 Membrane attack pathway

The **membrane attack pathway** involves the non-covalent association of C5b with the four terminal complement components to form an amphipathic membrane-inserted complex, the **membrane attack complex (MAC)**. C5b, while attached to the C5 convertase, binds C6, a large single chain plasma protein. The C5b6 complex then binds C7, a single chain protein homologous to C6, which triggers the release of the complex from the convertase. The C5b67 complex binds tightly to the surface membrane of the micro-organism through its labile hydrophobic binding site. C8 is a heterotrimeric protein and binds C7 in C5b67, causing the complex to insert deeper in the membrane. Finally, multiple copies of C9 bind the C5b-8 complex to form a large transmembrane pore (MAC) which can cause lysis of the target cell by allowing free diffusion of molecules in and out of the cell.

Membrane attack complex (MAC)
A large transmembrane pore formed from the terminal complement components which can cause lysis of the target cell by allowing free diffusion of molecules in and out of the cell.

Key Point

All three complement pathways result in the formation of C5 convertase, leading to the formation of the membrane attack complex (MAC), which can result in the lysis of target cells.

SELF-CHECK 4.1

Can you name the three complement activation pathways and describe what triggers each pathway?

4.2 Regulation of complement

The complement system is tightly controlled at multiple stages in the pathway by regulatory proteins present in plasma and on cell membranes (Morgan and Harris 1999).

The first step of the classical pathway is regulated by C1-inhibitor (C1inh), a serine protease inhibitor which binds activated C1 and removes C1r and C1s from the complex (Davis 1988, Davis 1989). C1inh is the only plasma inhibitor of activated C1, and as a serine protease is also the most potent regulator of the bradykinin pathway. Even partial deficiency can result in uncontrolled activation of the contact kinin pathway, with increased capillary permeability resulting in angioedema at sites including the airway, gut, and skin–the condition is known as **hereditary angioedema (HAE)**.

Hereditary angioedema (HAE)
Genetic mutations resulting in reduced levels of C1 esterase inhibitor in serum are found in approximately 85% of patients (type I). The remaining 15% of patients have normal or elevated serum concentrations, but the protein produced by one allele is dysfunctional (type II). In either case, this clinically results in angioedema.

TABLE 4.2 Complement control proteins.

	Control Protein	Mechanism of Action
Liquid phase	C1 inhibitor (C1inh)	Binds and deactivates C1qrs complex.
	Factor I (FI)	Cleaves C3b and C4b.
	C4 binding protein (C4bp)	Accelerates decay of C4bC2b and acts as a cofactor for fI cleavage of C4b.
	Factor H (fH)	Accelerates decay of C3bBb and acts as a cofactor for fI cleavage of C3b.
Membrane bound	Complement receptor 1(CR1)	Accelerates decay of both C4b2a and C3bBb. Acts as a cofactor for fI cleavage of C3b and C4b.
	Decay accelerating factor (DAF)	Accelerates decay of C4b2a and C3bBb.
	Membrane cofactor protein (MCP)	Cofactor for fI cleavage of C3b and C4b.
	CD59	Prevents formation of the membrane attack complex (blocks incorporation of C9).

Control of the C3 and C5 convertases is provided by factor I (fI), a plasma serine protease which, in the presence of essential cofactors, cleaves C3b and C4b to inactivate the convertases. In plasma, two proteins act as cofactors for factor I; factor H (fH) in the alternative pathway and C4bp in the classical pathway. Both factor H and C4bp also inhibit the pathways by accelerating the decay (breaking up) of the convertases. On the membrane, decay accelerating factor (DAF) acts to accelerate the decay of convertases whereas membrane cofactor protein (MCP) acts as cofactor for the cleavage of C4b and C3b by factor I, irreversibly inactivating the enzyme. Complement receptor 1 (CR1) is a large transmembrane protein which has both decay accelerating and cofactor activities.

The membrane attack pathway is also regulated by inhibitors present in the fluid phase and on membranes. The fluid-phase C5b-7 complex is the target of S-protein (vitronectin) and clusterin, abundant serum proteins which, among their many roles, help regulate complement activation by binding to the hydrophobic site in C5b-7. On the membrane, CD59 binds to C8 in the C5b-8 complex and blocks incorporation of C9 and assembly of the MAC (Lachmann 1991).

Table 4.2 summarizes the complement control proteins.

SELF-CHECK 4.2

Name five proteins involved in the regulation of complement. For each protein, describe its method of action.

4.3 Complement deficiencies

Deficiencies of almost every complement protein and regulator have been described and more detailed accounts of the various complement deficiencies can be found in several reviews (Morgan and Walport 1991, Colten and Rosen 1992, Figueroa et al. 1993). Several of the assays to be described in this chapter are useful in screening for complement deficiency; however, an understanding of the clinical presentations associated with deficiencies of different components is essential for selecting the most appropriate tests.

Deficiencies of components of the classical pathway (C1, C4, or C2) are associated with an increased susceptibility to immune complex disease, a consequence of the failure of immune complex solubilization. The frequency and severity of disease is greatest with deficiencies of one of the subunits of C1 (C1q, C1r, or C1s), closely followed by total C4 deficiency, each giving rise to severe immune complex disease and often secondary systemic lupus erythematosus (SLE). Deficiency of C2 is the most common homozygous complement deficiency in Caucasoids but is often without consequence and causes much less severe disease. Inherited or acquired deficiency of C1 inhibitor causes uncontrolled activation of the classical pathway (and other proteolytic cascades) that can lead to episodes of swelling of skin and mucosa–angioedema due to the action of bradykinins on vascular smooth muscle.

Cross references

Look at Section 4.5 for more information on C1 inhibitor deficiency.

You can read in more detail about SLE in Chapter 5.

C3 is an essential component of all activation pathways and is vital for efficient opsonization of bacteria. C3 deficiency is associated with a marked susceptibility to bacterial infections. Acquired C3 deficiency due to a nephritic factor (C3 nef) is associated with **membranoproliferative glomerulonephritis type II (MPGN II)**. Deficiencies of the regulators factor I and factor H cause a secondary deficiency of C3 and also present with recurrent bacterial infections. Furthermore, a deficiency or mutations in either factor H or factor I can lead to susceptibility to **atypical haemolytic uraemic syndrome (aHUS)** which consists of the triad of thrombocytopenia, Coombs negative microangiopathic haemolytic anaemia, and acute renal failure. aHUS is caused by mutations of the *CFH* (complement factor H) gene in 30% of cases. HUS is the commonest cause of renal failure in children, although the large majority of cases are secondary to a severe diarrhoeal illness caused by infection with specific types of *E. coli* bacteria and not due to the CFH mutations.

Membranoproliferative glomerulonephritis (MPGN)

A disorder of the kidney caused by immune complex deposition in the glomerular basement membrane. Complement activation results in inflammation of the glomeruli, causing disrupted kidney function and can progress to chronic renal failure.

Haemolytic uraemic syndrome (HUS)

A syndrome consisting of the triad of thrombocytopenia, Coombs negative microangiopathic haemolytic anaemia, and acute renal failure; deficiency of or mutations in factor H and factor I can lead to a susceptibility in HUS.

Deficiencies of the alternative pathway components are rare. A few individuals deficient in factor D have been described, all of whom have presented with recurrent *Neisseria* infections, usually meningococcal meningitis. Deficiency of the positive regulator properdin is the commonest disorder of the alternative pathway and is also associated with meningococcal infection. Properdin deficiency is X-linked and so is exclusively seen in males; infections usually occur in infancy or childhood (the average age of presentation being 12–14 years) and can be catastrophic.

Deficiencies of terminal pathway components (C5, C6, C7, C8, or C9) also cause susceptibility to infection with organisms of the genus *Neisseria*—often presenting as recurrent meningococcal meningitis or systemic infection with meningococcus.

4.3.1 Use of deficient and depleted sera to characterize complement deficiencies

Sera deficient in or depleted of individual components can be used to identify the specific component that is missing in complement deficient individuals. Table 4.3 lists the complement components, their structure, and normal plasma concentration. If a particular patient serum fails to restore haemolysis when mixed with a particular deficient or depleted test serum then the patient and test sera must be missing the same component. Human and animal sera deficient in many individual components are now widely available from many suppliers but they are expensive and of variable quality. It may be easier to generate in-house depleted sera for use in these assays. Sera may be depleted of individual complement components by 'classical' or immunochemical methods. 'Classical' methods for depletion are summarized in Method 4.1.

TABLE 4.3 The component proteins of the complement system. The proteins which constitute the classical, alternative, and membrane attack pathways are listed.

Component	Structure	Plasma Conc. (mg/L)
Classical pathway:		
C1	Complicated molecule, composed of 3 subunits, C1q (460kDa), C1r (80kDa), C1s (80kDa) in a complex (C1qr2s2)	180
C4	3 chains: α, 97kDa; β, 75kDa; γ, 33kDa; from a single precursor	600
C2	single chain, 102kDa	20
Alternative pathway:		
fB	single chain, 93kDa	210
fD	single chain, 24 kDa	2
Properdin	oligomers of identical 53kDa chains	5
Common:		
C3	2 chains: α,110kDa; β,75kDa	1300
Terminal pathway:		
C5	2 chains: 115kDa, 75kDa	70
C6	single chain, 120kDa	65
C7	single chain, 110kDa	55
C8	3 chains: α, 65kDa; β, 65kDa; γ, 22kDa	55
C9	single chain, 69kDa	60

Modified from Morgan BP and Harris CL (1999) *Complement Regulatory Proteins*. Academic Press, London.

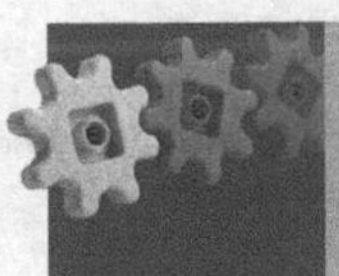

METHOD 4.1 Depletion of sera of individual complement components

Complement C1

C1 is a euglobulin and can be removed from serum by dialysis against low ionic strength buffer. Dialyse fresh serum (5ml) overnight at 4 °C against 2L of 10mM barbitone buffer pH7.4 containing $CaCl_2$ (5mM) and NPGB [nitrophenylguanidinobenzoate] (0.1mM). Centrifuge at 5000g for 15min at 4 °C. Store C1-depleted serum (R1) in aliquots at −70 °C.

Complement C4

The thioester group in C4 (and C3) is inactivated by treatment of serum with ammonia. To 8.5ml of serum (guinea pig serum is most commonly used) add 1.5ml NH_4OH diluted to 150mM in H_2O. Incubate for 45min at 37 °C; adjust pH to 7.4 with dilute HCl. Store C4-depleted serum (R4) in aliquots at −70 °C.

Complement C2

C2 and factor B are the most heat labile of the complement components. Place fresh serum (1ml) in a glass tube preheated in a 56 °C water bath and incubate at 56 °C for precisely 6 min with constant shaking. C2-depleted serum (R2) generated in this manner should be stored on ice and used immediately.

Complement C3

Incubation of serum with zymosan efficiently depletes C3 and partially depletes C5 and the terminal components. Zymosan depletion of C3 works better in guinea pig serum than in human serum. Incubate 1mg boiled zymosan (Sigma) in 10ml serum at 37 °C for 60 min; centrifuge (1000g for 5 min) to pellet zymosan. Store supernatant (R3) in aliquots at −70 °C.

Complement Factor B

Place fresh serum (1-2 ml) in a glass tube preheated to 50 °C in a water bath. Incubate for 20 min with continuous shaking. Factor B-depleted serum generated in this manner should be stored on ice and used immediately.

Complement Factor D

Factor D can be selectively depleted from serum by virtue of its small size. Apply fresh serum (1ml) to a Sephadex G-75 gel filtration column (0.5 × 30cm) equilibrated in veronal buffered saline (VBS). Factor D is significantly retarded on this column. Develop the column in VBS and pool the void volume fractions, containing the bulk of the serum proteins minus factor D. Store in aliquots at −70 °C.

Mannose Binding Lectin

Mannose binding lectin can be depleted from serum by utilizing its affinity for specific carbohydrates.

With the increasing availability of monoclonal antibodies against the complement components, immunoaffinity methods are now widely used to generate depleted sera. The general principle involves immobilizing the appropriate monoclonal antibody on sepharose and applying fresh serum to the column at 4 °C. The completeness of the depletion can be easily assessed in haemolytic assays. Orren and colleagues have described a simple and sensitive haemolysis-in-gel assay utilizing known complement-deficient sera to simultaneously screen patient serum for deficiencies of each of the terminal complement components (Orren et al. 1994). Although with the increasing availability of the essential reagents, assays of this sort could easily be established in most Clinical Immunology laboratories, we do not advise this course of action. Artefacts induced in sample handling and the influence of *in vivo* complement activation can make interpretation of results difficult. Laboratories experienced in complement assays will be better equipped to recognize and correct these problems.

Key Point

Sera deficient in or depleted of individual components can be used to identify the specific component that is missing in complement deficient individuals.

4.3.2 Complement in pathology

Activation of complement occurs in a large number of inflammatory diseases and is likely to be an important contributor to tissue damage in these diseases. Complement deposition can be detected in the tissues and products of complement activation are found in the plasma. Assays for individual complement components may be of help in identifying complement activation and measurement of complement activation products can provide additional information.

The development of a monoclonal antibody that inhibits C5 cleavage (Eculizumab™, Alexion Pharma UK Ltd) provides a means by which the generation of C5a and activation of the membrane attack pathway can be inhibited. This drug is currently licensed for the treatment of

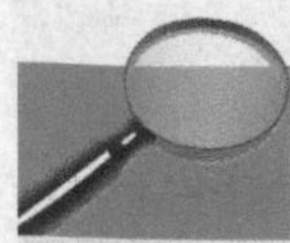

CASE STUDY 4.1 Complement C7 deficiency

Patient history

- 37-year-old female.
- Admitted to hospital with suspected septicaemia.
- Previous meningococcal meningitis at age 16 and 35.

Results

- Group C meningococci isolated from blood culture.
- CT scan showed no cranial bony abnormality.
- C3 1.31 g/L (0.75–1.65).
- C4 0.18 g/L (0.14–0.54).
- Classical pathway CH50 174 (1000–2000).
- Alternative pathway AP50 0 (80–200).
- Immunochemical measurement of individual complement components revealed complete deficiency of C7.

Significance of results

- Two previous episodes of meningococcal infection.
- Normal C3 and C4.
- Low CH50 and absent AP50 suggest a possible terminal complement component deficiency.
- Measurement of C5, C6, C7, C8, and C9 confirmed C7 deficiency.
- Family members were screened using CH50 and AP50.
- Her daughter and 3 siblings had CH50 values within the normal range.
- One brother had low CH50 with normal AP50.

The patient recovered fully after treatment and upon discharge was started on life-long Penicillin V 250 mg once daily. She was immunized with the tetravalent meningococcal vaccine that contains relevant immunogens of the A, C, Y, and W135 meningococcal groups, as patients with terminal pathway deficiencies are at risk of infection with all of these strains (Morgan and Orren 1998). This vaccine is different from the usual commercially available bivalent vaccine which contains immunogens from groups A and C only, but is not suitable for children (as a true polysaccharide they often don't respond). Newer vaccines are available for meningococcus B and C which are the most prevalent strains in the UK and are conjugated, so useful in children.

paroxysmal nocturnal haemoglobinuria and atypical haemolytic uremic syndrome, though is in clinical trials in several further conditions where the complement cascade is involved in pathogenesis of the disease. Given the mechanism of action, Eculizumab increases patient susceptibility to infection, in particular to meningococcal infection and possibly to other encapsulated bacteria. Patients should receive vaccination against meningococcal serotypes A, C, Y, and W135 prior to commencing treatment and should be instructed to seek prompt medical advice if they develop symptoms suggestive of meningococcal infection (fever > 39 °C, headache accompanied with fever and/or stiff neck or sensitivity to light).

Cross reference

Section 4.4 provides more detail about the assays available for measuring complement activity.

4.4 Measurement of complement activity

4.4.1 Sample handling for measurement of complement components

The majority of the complement proteins are heat-labile and so correct handling of samples is essential if reliable, meaningful results of complement assays are to be obtained. Improper handling of samples may result in incorrect or uninterpretable results. This applies especially to assays of complement haemolytic activity and complement activation products. Serum is used for measurement of C3 and C4 and for measuring the haemolytic activity of the classical and alternative pathways (CH_{50} and AP_{50} assays). Clotted blood taken for these assays (2–4ml) should reach the laboratory on the day of venesection where sera should be assayed directly or separated, aliquotted and frozen (at −20 °C for up to one month, −70 °C for longer periods). Repeated freezing and thawing of specimens should be avoided as it can lead to loss of activity. For assays of complement activation products, EDTA plasma is used. By chelating Ca^{2+} and Mg^{2+}, EDTA inhibits *in vitro* activation through the classical and alternative pathways. Again, plasma should be obtained fresh and either assayed immediately or stored frozen as described above. Some commercial additives have been developed specifically to inhibit activation *in vitro* of complement. The advantages of these agents over EDTA are minor.

Key Point

The handling of samples for complement analysis is critical to ensure that reliable results are achieved in the laboratory.

4.4.2 Assays of complement haemolytic activity

Assay of the serum complement haemolytic activity (CH_{50}) involves measuring the ability of all the complement protein molecules involved to lyse target cells. This measures the functional activity of the whole system from initiation through to end-point. The main indication for measuring CH_{50} is when a deficiency of a complement component protein is suspected. In addition CH_{50} is being used to monitor the effect of biological therapies such as Eculizumab. There is rarely any reason to assay CH_{50} in any fluid other than serum. Patients who have complement deficiencies present typically in one of three ways clinically, these being:

- Severe and/or recurrent infection with *Neisseria meningitidis*, the causal organism of meningococcal meningitis and meningococcal septicaemia (which can coexist). Any patient who has two or more infections with this organism should have the CH_{50} assayed. It is debatable whether this should be assayed after the first episode of meningococcal infection, although infections with atypical meningococcal serotypes (X, Y, Z, W135, or 29E), or family history, should heighten suspicion.
- Failure to clear immune complexes, giving a clinical picture resembling systemic lupus erythematosus (SLE).
- Recurrent infections, usually bacterial.

Figure 4.2 outlines the assays to assess complement activity.

Classical pathway activity CH_{50}

The classical pathway CH_{50} measures the amount of a serum sample required to lyse 50% of a standardized suspension of sheep erythrocytes (Esh) coated with optimal amounts of rabbit anti-Esh antibody (EshA; made by pre-incubation with antibody and subsequent washing). The assay assesses activity from C1 activation through to cell lysis by the membrane attack pathway. Different dilutions of a standard and the test sera are incubated with EshA in different wells of a 96-well microtitre plate and the degree of haemolysis in each well is measured. This enables calculation of the amount of classical pathway haemolytic activity per ml of test serum. The

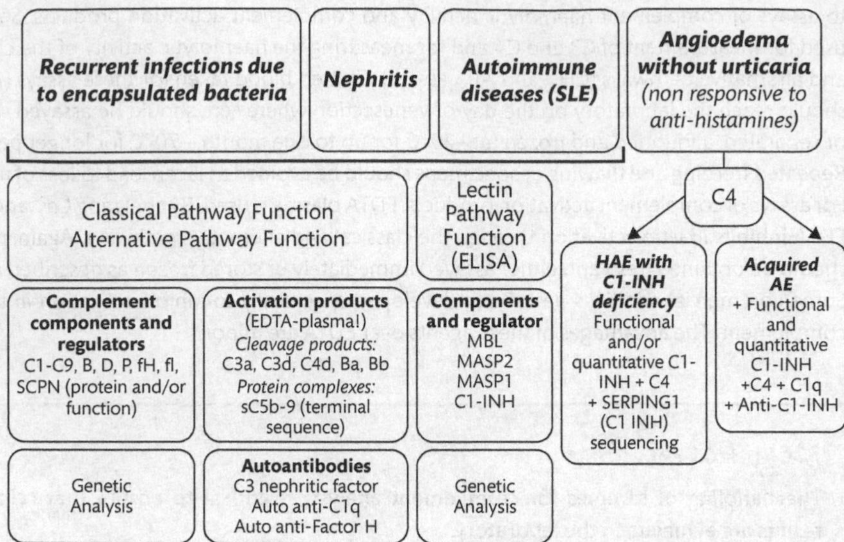

FIGURE 4.2
Tests associated with specific complement mediated disorders.

measured CH_{50} will be dependent on the concentration of EshA in the system, the relative concentrations of reactants, ionic strength, and many other variables, and so it is important to standardize the assay conditions.

Alternative pathway activity CH_{50}

The alternative pathway CH_{50} measures the activity of the alternative pathway from initiation of C3 activation through to lysis. Washed rabbit erythrocytes (Erb) without any antibody bound to their surface are used as the target cells because Erb are extremely susceptible to non-antibody dependent haemolysis by human complement (i.e. haemolysis via the alternative pathway). The reagents and conditions used are similarly standardized. Selectivity for the alternative pathway is ensured by using the chelating agent ethylene glycol tetra-acetic acid (EGTA) with excess magnesium ions, the former eliminating the calcium-dependent function of C1 and the presence of the latter permitting the assembly of the magnesium-dependent C3bBb complex.

Cross reference

Other technologies in use for measuring CH_{50} activity are detailed later in this section.

Key Point

You must find out which technology is used by your local laboratory and what considerations are taken for the quality control, technical aspects, and interpretation of the results provided by the test system in place.

Standardization and quality control

The classical pathway assay is standardized against a commercially available freeze-dried standard material purchased from Sigma (human complement serum, product no S-1764). Each lot of material has an ascribed value for the classical pathway CH_{50}. This material is also included in every alternative pathway assay, although no value for the alternative pathway CH_{50} has been ascribed to it by the manufacturers.

Internal quality control is achieved by running an aliquot of a standard normal human serum in every assay run. This material is obtained from a single normal donor, aliquotted, and frozen at −70 °C, and a fresh aliquot used for each assay. There is currently no external Quality Assurance Scheme available for complement haemolytic activity assays, although the International Complement Society is preparing such a standard.

Expression of results in CH_{50} units/ml from activity in X_{50} µl

The classical pathway CH_{50} results are expressed in arbitrary units using the following calculation, on the basis that the amount of complement haemolytic activity is inversely proportional to the amount of serum required to produce 50% haemolysis of the erythrocyte.

$$CH_{50} = \frac{1}{X_{50}} \times 2000$$

The alternative pathway CH_{50} results are expressed similarly. For historical reasons a different multiplication factor is used to generate a different range of values for results.

$$CH_{50} = \frac{1}{X_{50}} \times 200$$

Normal ranges for these assays should be calculated locally. The normal ranges for the classical pathway and alternative pathway CH_{50} were calculated in our laboratory by measuring a number of normal sera. This provided a range of 1000–2000 units/ml for the classical pathway and 80–200 units/ml for the alternative pathway. Some laboratories report the haemolytic activity as a percentage of normal; >50% activity when compared with a normal serum is considered to be normal activity.

Inter-run correction factor

As this is a bioassay, a significant amount of variation may occur from one assay run to another. This has the potential of producing results that may be significantly influenced by variables such as the laboratory temperature or extraneous influences upon the susceptibility of the erythrocytes to haemolysis. In order to compensate for these variables it is recommended to modify the calculated CH_{50} values obtained.

The necessary modification is made by multiplying every measured test CH_{50} value by a correction factor, as follows:

$$\text{Corrected serum } CH_{50} = \text{Measured serum } CH_{50} \times \frac{^{*}\text{Standard material mean } CH_{50}}{\text{Standard material measured } CH_{50}}$$

(* = the running mean of many serial measurements of the standard material CH_{50}).

Acceptability of results

In order to measure the CH_{50} values of the test sera accurately, the absorbance of the samples and the standard are measured at three-minute intervals. This provides multiple calculations of the CH_{50} at different incubation times. As the standard material has an expected value (from experience ±15% from its target value), the incubation time that gives a CH_{50} standard value nearest to the target value is chosen, and it is at this time that the patient's CH_{50} values are reported.

When a patient serum gives a low CH_{50} result, it is recommended to perform a repeat assay without a prior dilution step. This will attempt to quantify low levels of haemolytic complement.

Interpretation of results

High or low normal values of CH_{50} activity do not have any clinical significance.

Low values of CH_{50} most often result from complement consumption. The serum concentrations of C3 and C4 may or may not be low and so clinical details are required to clarify such situations. Low values of alternative pathway CH_{50} activity are frequently seen in infants; these values usually rise into the normal range after a few months. In such cases, repeat assays after a suitable interval are recommended, with prophylactic antibiotics being recommended in the interim if clinically indicated.

Key Points

- **When interpreting functional complement assay results, the levels of complement C3 and C4 must be taken into account.**
- **Clinical details are required to interpret the results of complement assays.**

Alternative assays for measuring CH_{50}

Several assays have been described which have sought to establish a simplified system for measurement of CH_{50} levels, removing the requirement for erythrocytes as indicator cells.

Numerous liposome-based assays have been reported (Canova-Davis et al. 1986, Bowden et al. 1986, Yamamoto et al. 1995). A commercially available kit (Autokit CH50; Wako Ltd, Osaka, Japan) utilizes liposomes loaded with the enzyme glucose-6-phosphate dehydrogenase (G6PD). The antibody-sensitized liposomes are incubated with the test and control sera and released enzyme is quantified in the supernatant by monitoring the conversion of NAD in the substrate buffer to NADH (increased absorbance at 340nm). The kit is simple, sensitive, and correlates well with assays utilizing $E_{sh}A$ as an indicator.

Recently, several protocols have been described for measurement of CH_{50} which eliminate altogether the need for an indicator cell or liposome. Enzyme immunoassay (ELISA) methods measure the appearance of complement activation products and generate results which can be expressed in CH_{50} equivalent units (Goldberg et al. 1997, Zwirner et al. 1998). A commercially available kit (CH50 Eq EIA Kit; Quidel Inc., San Diego, CA) measures the generation of the terminal complement complex (TCC). These assays have also been shown to correlate well with 'classical' CH_{50} techniques.

The Binding Site Total Haemolytic Complement assay is an adaptation of a traditional radial immunodiffusion assay. It uses the principle that sheep erythrocytes coated with anti-sheep erythrocyte antibody (haemolysin) will activate the classical pathway in the presence of normal serum. Erythrocytes coated with haemolysin are incorporated into an agarose gel. Serum is added to wells in the plate and incubated to allow diffusion of complement components. Activation of the classical pathway results in a clear zone of haemolysis around the well and the diameter of this zone will be proportional to the haemolytic activity of the sample

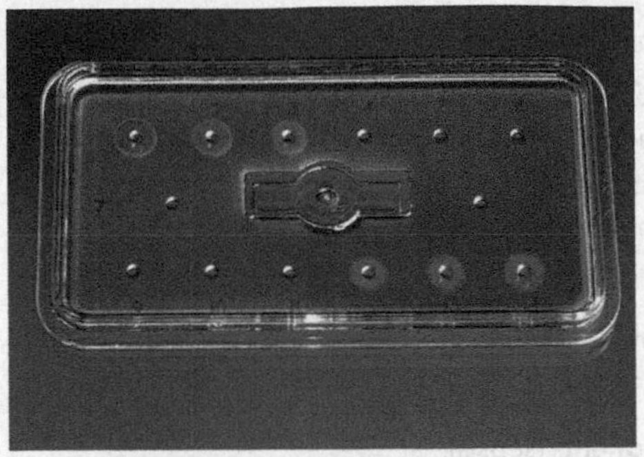

FIGURE 4.3
Haemolysis of sheep erythrocytes coated with anti-sheep erythrocyte antibody by complement. Courtesy of The Binding Site.

FIGURE 4.4
Measurement of complement component protein by RID. Courtesy of The Binding Site.

(see Figure 4.3). A similar assay is available for the alternative pathway. This uses the principle that chicken erythrocytes will activate the alternative pathway, resulting in haemolysis of the erythrocytes.

SELF-CHECK 4.3

Why is sample handling for CH_{50} important?

4.4.3 Immunochemical measurement of individual components

The complement proteins C3, C4, and C1 inhibitor (C1inh) are present in serum at sufficient concentrations and antisera of uniformly good quality are commercially available so as to allow them to be reliably assayed by nephelometry or turbidimetry. Other complement proteins (C1, C2, C5 to C9) may be assayed immunochemically by radial immunodiffusion (see Figure 4.4). They have alternatively been assayed by rocket electrophoresis but this is a cumbersome method that is now infrequently used. ELISAs for the majority of complement proteins are now available and are increasingly replacing gel-based assays.

Online Resource Centre

To see an online video demonstrating the immunochemical measurement of complement components, log on to www.oxfordtextbooks.co.uk/orc/fbs

Standardization and quality control

Most of the immunochemical assays have been standardized using an international reference preparation for plasma proteins provided by the International Federation of Clinical Chemistry (IFCC).

Internal quality control is achieved by running an aliquot of a standard normal human serum in every assay run. This material is obtained from a single normal donor, aliquotted, and frozen at −70 °C, and a fresh aliquot used for each assay. UK NEQAS offer external quality control schemes for complement C3, C4, and C1 inhibitor (both antigenic and functional activity).

Interpretation of results

You need to understand the complement pathways and the relationship of the different components in order to interpret the immunochemical results.

- An increase in the plasma concentrations of C3 and C4:
  - commonly seen during inflammation. C3 and C4 are acute phase proteins and can be seen together with an increase in CRP and ESR (erythrocyte sedimentation rate). As C3 and C4 increase as acute phase proteins, levels can sometimes appear normal even when the proteins are being rapidly consumed.
- A decrease in both C3 and C4:
  - commonly seen when the classical pathway is activated
  - immune complex mediated diseases such as SLE
  - consumption of the complement components (sepsis).
- C3 is decreased and C4 is normal:
  - commonly seen when the alternative pathway is predominantly activated (Gram-negative sepsis)
  - post-streptococcal glomerulonephritis
  - C3 nephritic factor.
- C3 is normal and C4 is decreased:
  - Type II cryoglobulinaemia associated with hepatitis C infection
  - C1 inhibitor deficiency (discussed in more detail in Section 4.5)
  - active SLE
  - genetic deficiency (C4 null alleles).

Cross reference

You can read in more detail about nephelometry, turbidimetry, and radial immunodiffusion in the *Biomedical Science Practice* textbook of this series.

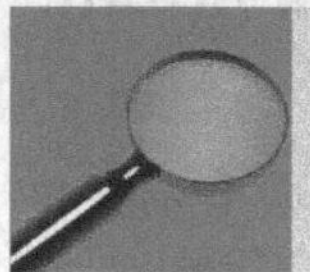

CASE STUDY 4.2 Complement deficiency

Patient history

- **Male child age 11 weeks presented with a group B meningococcal meningitis.**
- **No siblings.**
- **Non-consanguinous parents.**
- **Born by vaginal delivery at 36 weeks gestation.**
- **Developed pneumonia soon after birth.**
- **Again at 5 weeks.**
- **No organisms isolated.**
- **RSV bronchiolitis at 7 weeks.**

Results

- **Whilst ill, 5 weeks after birth:**
- **C3 0.66g/L** **(0.75–1.65)**
- **C4 0.14 g/L** **(0.14–0.54)**
- **Classical pathway CH_{50} 1106** **(1000–2000 units)**

- **Alternative pathway AP_{50} 0 (80–200 units)**
- **When well, aged 12 weeks:**
- **C3 0.90 g/L (0.75–1.65)**
- **C4 0.14 g/L (0.14–0.54)**
- **Classical pathway CH50 2139 (1000–2000 units)**
- **Alternative pathway AP50 70 (80–200 units)**

Significance of results

- **A primary complement deficiency or alternatively a combination of complement consumption due to pneumonia and delayed acquisition of adult serum levels were considered as possibilities. He was thus started on prophylactic broad spectrum antibiotic treatment.**
- **This case illustrates firstly that age-specific ranges for relevant complement values still require definition, particularly for neonates (despite there being a higher incidence of meningitis in childhood than in adulthood) and secondly that prophylactic antibiotic treatment may need to be started empirically and later withdrawn when complement values normalize.**

4.4.4 Measurement of activation fragments and complexes

Assay of fragments and/or complexes generated during complement activation provide an accurate and dynamic picture of the complement activation status at the time of sampling. The small fragments C4a, C3a, C5a, and Bb, the large fragments iC3b and C4d, and the complexes C1r, C1s/C1inh, C3bBbP, and SC5b-9 (TCC) all represent potential targets for assay (Wurzner et al. 1997). Judicious choice of assays can yield information on the pathway by which complement is activated as well as the degree of activation. Of the fragments, C3a has been most used as an index of complement activation. C3a is rapidly inactivated in serum by removal of a single Arg residue from its carboxy-terminus and all available assays measure both C3a and its metabolite C3adesArg. Radioimmunoassays for C3a(desArg) are commercially available from GE Healthcare (Amersham, UK) and have been widely used in research and diagnosis. ELISA assays for C3a(desArg) have more recently become available. A comprehensive panel of ELISA assays for complement activation products is available from Quidel and several other manufacturers. The majority of these assays measure the generation of neoantigens not expressed by native complement components thus providing specificity for the activation product. Measurement of complement activation products may yield clinically useful information, when interpreted appropriately within the clinical context.

4.5 C1 inhibitor deficiency

C1 inhibitor functions as an essential regulator of the complement, coagulation, and contact (kinin-forming) systems. It is a serine protease inhibitor and acts as a suicide inhibitor in that it becomes consumed during its inhibition of complement C1r and C1s, the contact system Factor XII and kallikrein, and the coagulation Factor XI (Davis et al. 1993a; see Figure 4.5). Lack

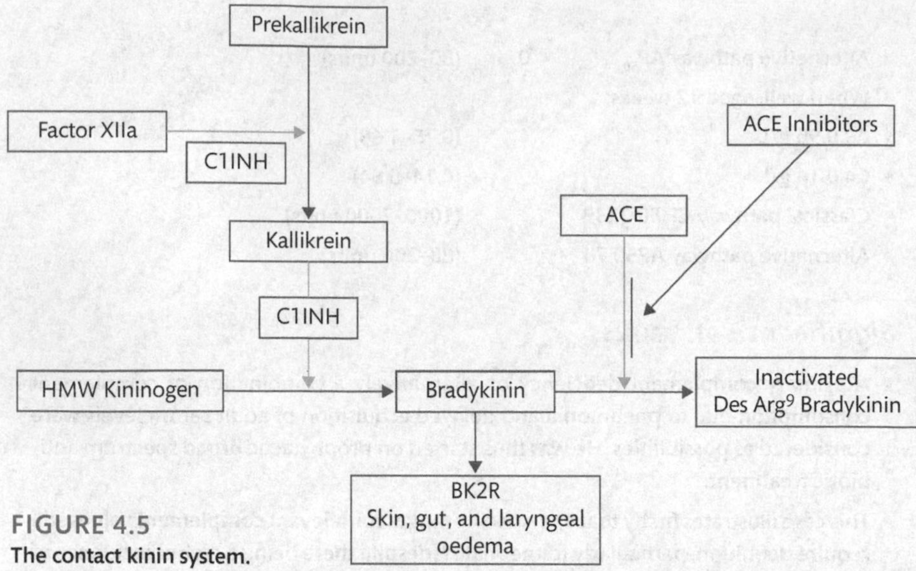

FIGURE 4.5
The contact kinin system.

of inhibition of these systems by C1 inhibitor leads to the formation of vasoactive peptides, the most important of which is bradykinin, predominantly via the bradykinin-2 receptor, which causes relaxation of vascular smooth muscle and capillary leak. C1inh is encoded at a single locus, and expression of adequately functioning paternal and maternal alleles is necessary to provide sufficient serum enzymatic activity for health. When one copy encodes a dysfunctional or non-expressed protein, clinical angioedema can result (homozygous deficiency is very rare). Subcutaneous swellings lasting from 1–5 days are important to control as they may be painful and disabling. Abdominal swellings can mimic an acute abdomen and upper airways swelling can cause life-threatening laryngeal oedema. Some patients have a family history of deaths from asphyxia and a recent study underlined the importance of diagnosis and appropriate treatment, as the mortality of HAE patients who had not been diagnosed was 29% compared to 3% in those who had been diagnosed (Bork et al. 2012).

Hereditary angioedema (HAE) has an autosomal dominant inheritance, but symptoms may sometimes first appear only in adulthood. Heterozygotes manifest the condition which affects about 1:50 000 people (Davis 1988). In more than 20% of patients with HAE the mutations are spontaneous and therefore there is no family history of disease (Agostoni and Circardi 1992). The majority of mutations result in the absence of a protein product of that allele in serum, and reduced immunochemical concentrations of C1 inhibitor are found in approximately 85% of patients (Type I HAE). The remaining 15% of patients have normal or elevated serum concentrations, but the protein produced by one allele is dysfunctional, usually due to point mutations causing amino acid substitutions at or near the enzyme's active site (Type II HAE) (Davis et al. 1993b). A recent study in the UK showed a smaller proportion of 6% of patients diagnosed with Type II HAE (Jolles et al. 2014).

Acquired angioedema (AAE) is rare and due to increased consumption rather than deficient production of C1 inhibitor. Autoantibodies to C1 inhibitor bind to the molecule in such a way as to allow it to become cleaved by other plasma proteases, or consumed and cleaved during its interaction with the C1r–C1s complex whilst preventing its inhibition of the complex's activity (Mandle et al. 1994). Serum assays thus show reduced C1 inhibitor function (due to consumption), but immunochemical levels as measured by nephelometry may be normal due to the presence of cleaved C1 inhibitor. The latter may be detected by staining a Western blot of the patient's serum with an anti-C1 inhibitor antibody, when two bands are seen that represent the normal and cleaved molecules respectively. In addition the serum concentrations of C1, C4, and C2 are reduced as they are consumed. These auto-antibodies may occur in association with leukaemia, lymphoma, and rarely other tumours (Type 1 AAE) (Cicardi et al. 1996). They may alternatively occur in isolation or in relation to non-organ-specific autoimmune diseases such as rheumatoid arthritis and SLE (Type II AAE) although this is much less frequent.

4.5.1 Differential diagnosis of angioedema

A thorough drug history should be taken as some drugs such as angiotensin converting enzyme inhibitors can cause angioedema. Patients with C1 inhibitor deficiency usually have low plasma levels of C4 (which is the substrate of the C1r–C1s complex) in between attacks, and these fall significantly further during attacks. A normal 'resting' C4 concentration virtually excludes the diagnosis, though it may be normal in HAE patients when taking prophylactic attenuated androgens. When assessing new patients it is expedient to assay serum immunochemical concentrations of C3, C4, and C1 inhibitor at the same venesection. Low serum C4 indicates C1 inhibitor deficiency. If this is not confirmed by immunochemical assay then C1 inhibitor function should be assayed. If this is normal, then assay of C1 and investigations for causes of Types I and II AAE should be performed. There is a further cause of HAE previously known as Type III HAE (now renamed HAE with normal C1inh) due in some cases to mutations in Factor XII (FXII) (Bork et al. 2000; Zuraw et al. 2012). Most frequently, all laboratory results are normal and no cause for the angioedema is found and many patients end up with a label of 'idiopathic angioedema'. Subdivisions into 'histaminergic idiopathic angioedema' and 'non-histaminergic idiopathic angioedema' can be made depending on the clinical response to anti-histamines.

4.5.2 Laboratory diagnosis—C1 inhibitor functional assay

C1 inhibitor function may be measured in assays that have haemolytic or esterolytic end-points. The latter involves incubating appropriate dilutions of normal and test sera and a standard reference material with a substrate which yields a coloured product following hydrolysis by C1 inhibitor. Such assays should always be performed in specialist or reference laboratories. Many laboratories have used a chromogenic assay for C1 inhibitor activity marketed by Behringwerke (Berichrom C1-inactivator kit; Behringwerke AG, Marburg, Germany). This kit contains chromogenic substrate for C1s, substrate buffer, and freeze-dried purified C1s. ELISA-based assays for C1 inhibitor functional activity are also commercially available (C1 inhibitor EIA Kit; Quidel).

4.5.3 Treatment of C1 inhibitor deficiency

Hereditary angioedema

Treatment varies according to the patient's clinical phenotype. For patients with frequent attacks anabolic, attenuated androgenic steroids danazol or stanozolol (which increase transcription of many genes, including the normally functioning copy of C1 inhibitor) may be helpful (Frank et al. 1976, Waytes et al. 1996). They may have unacceptable androgenic adverse effects in women (especially if pregnancy is wanted) and they are contraindicated in pre-pubertal children as they limit growth. In these cases tranexamic acid may be tried, but is frequently less effective than attenuated androgens in HAE. Acute upper airway obstruction and significant peripheral swellings (including abdominal) require emergency treatment. In the UK, one of the C1 inhibitor concentrates (Berinert and Cinryze, both plasma derived), the bradykinin B2 receptor antagonist (Icatibant), or recombinant C1inh (Ruconest) may be used. In the United States the kallikrein inhibitor ecallantide is a further option. Fresh frozen plasma is a poor substitute for C1 inhibitor, but may be used when there is no other alternative. The existing preparations were also virus free and can also be used for prophylaxis. Adrenaline, while life-saving in allergic reactions (anaphylaxis), provides no benefit in the treatment of HAE.

Acquired angioedema

The treatment of AAE may involve a number of approaches, initially with tranexamic acid or attenuated androgens as a prophylactic agent, the dose of which may be temporarily increased to help manage milder attacks. Unlike HAE, tranexamic acid is the prophylaxis of choice in AAE. Plasma derived and recombinant C1inh may be used for more severe acute attacks though due to consumption much higher doses compared to HAE are sometimes needed. The bradykinin B2 receptor antagonist Icatibant is an attractive option as it acts at the final part of the pathway leading towards angioedema and is unaffected by factors leading to consumption of C1inh. Effective treatment of the underlying condition will also often improve the AAE.

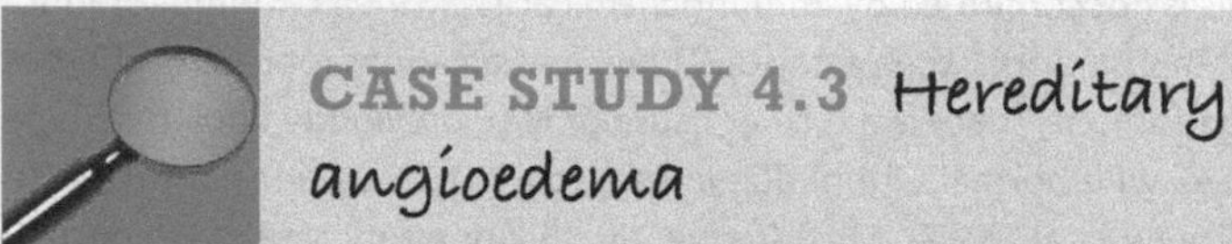

CASE STUDY 4.3 Hereditary angioedema

Patient history

- **18-year-old woman, previously well.**
- **Began taking oral contraceptive pill.**
- **One month later admitted to hospital with abdominal pain.**
- **Spontaneously resolved after 3 days allowing discharge from hospital.**
- **Began to have deep cutaneous swellings affecting her hands and arms.**
- **Elective dental treatment caused facial swelling requiring hospital admission.**
- **Over the following year she continued to have occasional swellings.**

Results

Whilst well:

- **C3 1.31 g/L (0.75–1.65),**
- **C4 0.07 g/L (0.14–0.54),**
- **C1 esterase inhibitor 0.09 g/L (0.15–0.35).**

Significance of results

- **Low serum C4 level with low C1 esterase level consistent with Type 1 hereditary angioedema.**
- **Symptoms not uncommonly first only appear in adulthood.**
- **Frequency of attacks may be increased by oral contraceptives and pregnancy.**
- **Can be life threatening if the airway is obstructed.**
- **May result in unnecessary laparotomies for abdominal pain.**

The combined oral contraceptive pill was stopped and, due to reluctance to take androgens, tranexamic acid 1-1.5g TDS was started. However, attacks remained frequent. Daily danazol treatment started and resulted in satisfactory management with four minor swellings only in the following 2 years. At this point the patient wished to become pregnant, the danazol was stopped, and attacks returned frequently. C1 inhibitor prophylaxis was then successfully used to manage the pregnancy and after breastfeeding the patient elected to use high dose progestogens as an effective alternative.

SELF-CHECK 4.4

Which laboratory tests should be performed in the investigation of hereditary angioedema?

4.6 Auto-antibodies against complement components and complexes

Numerous auto-antibodies directed against complement components have been described; so far all are directed against neoepitopes on activated or conformationally altered molecules. The reasons why some individuals develop an antibody response against these neoepitopes is not known.

Auto-antibodies to the collagen-like region (CLR) of C1q (anti-C1qCLR) have been detected in numerous individuals (Wener et al. 1989, Strife et al. 1989). These antibodies only bind solid-phase C1q.

ELISA systems in which C1q or its CLR are immobilized on the plate have been developed and have demonstrated the presence of anti-C1qCLR antibodies in SLE, membranous glomerulo nephritis, rheumatoid vasculitis, hypocomplementaemic urticarial vasculitis (HUVS), and other diseases. The presence of anti-C1q CLR antibodies correlates strongly with the severity of renal disease in SLE. Virtually all patients with HUVS have anti-C1q CLR antibodies; the presence of these antibodies has been used as a diagnostic aid for this syndrome (Wisnieski and Naff 1989, Wisnieski et al. 1995).

Auto-antibodies against C1 inhibitor have been demonstrated by ELISA in some patients with acquired angioedema (AAE). It has been suggested that the auto-antibody binds at a site close to the reactive centre of C1inh and thus blocks function (Mandle et al. 1994). The frequency of such antibodies in AAE is still not certain.

Auto-antibodies to the C3 convertase complexes are termed nephritic factors. C3 nephritic factor (C3 NeF) is an IgG auto-antibody that stabilizes the C3bBb convertase, promoting the continued activation of C3 and profound hypocomplementaemia. C3NeF has been found in association with membranoproliferative glomerulonephritis (MPGN) and partial **lipodystrophy**. Published assays for C3NeF measure the capacity of the test serum to enhance complement activation through the alternative pathway in a fluid-phase activation assay. The products of complement activation (usually C3 breakdown products) are measured after a defined incubation by two-dimensional electrophoresis, ELISA, or other appropriate method. Testing for C3NeF should be considered in patients with a low C3 and the presence of glomerulonephritis and/or partial lipodystrophy.

Lipodystrophy

The progressive loss of fat. Lipodystrophy may be congenital or acquired, and can affect all of the body (generalized lipodystrophy) or just parts of the body (partial lipodystrophy).

C4 nephritic factor (C4NeF), an IgG auto-antibody which stabilizes the C3 convertase of the classical pathway C4b2a, has been reported in patients with SLE and glomerulonephritis (Daha et al. 1976). The measurement of C4NeF is not performed routinely.

SELF-CHECK 4.5

What is C3 nephritic factor? When would you measure it?

4.7 Complement allotyping

Polymorphism
Variations in a gene locus at a frequency greater than 1% (adj. **polymorphic**).

Allotypes
Allelic polymorphisms in a gene that can be determined using specific antibodies for the gene product.

Genotyping
The process of defining the genotype of an individual using laboratory techniques such as DNA sequencing and PCR. This is useful in determining if an individual has disease-associated genes.

It is apparent that most complement components, receptors, and regulators are **polymorphic**, some with several tens of different **allotypes**. Analysis of polymorphisms in complement proteins can provide information of relevance for genetic studies and insights into function of the different allotypes. Analysis can be undertaken at the phenotypic and genotypic levels. Most of the complement polymorphic variants can now be easily **genotyped**. Phenotypic analyses involve methods such as SDS-PAGE analysis and isoelectric focusing, separating different allotypes on the basis of altered size or charge of the protein. In recent years, allotype-specific monoclonal antibodies have been developed for several of the complement components, including C4, C6, C7, and factor H. These provide a very easy and rapid way of assessing the relative frequencies of different complement component allotypes (Wurzner et al. 1997).

ELISAs specific for the two isotypes of C7 have been used in numerous research studies but have not found a place in clinical practice. Indeed, although of considerable academic interest, it is debatable whether allotyping of complement components has any place in the clinical laboratory. Where allotyping might be of use, is in the determination of null alleles in a patient with chronically low C4 level–could this be due to consumption (e.g. immune complexes in SLE) or reflection of a genetic deficiency? This could help with the clinical conundrum of chicken or egg with severe refractory lupus and low C4. A low gene copy number of C4 is seen as a risk factor for SLE, whereas a high copy number of C4 is protective

Cross references

For more information on polygenic variations of C4, you can read Yang et al. (2003).

For more information on the involvement of C4 allotypes in the pathogenesis of human diseases, you can read Samano et al. (2004).

4.8 Molecular testing for complement deficiencies

Molecular testing for many of the complement components is now available in specialist laboratories. If a clear diagnosis has been made, by measurement of protein and/or function, molecular testing may not be required; however, there are certain circumstances when knowledge of the genetic mutation may be helpful. If a diagnosis is required in young children below the age of one year then functional assays may be difficult to interpret and molecular analysis or the identification of a family mutation may allow definitive diagnosis and a management plan to be put in place. Sometimes there is ambiguity in the protein and functional assays and clarification may be achieved by molecular testing. A defined molecular defect will also allow informed genetic counselling and appropriate testing of family members. Given the stability of DNA samples, they may be posted to the testing centre following appropriate consent. There may also be merit in knowledge of a molecular defect to support the use of potentially costly long-term treatments. In some instances it is important to rule out defects in a particular gene to allow investigations to explore other avenues (e.g. C1inh, the gene for which is SERPING1) or to allow genetic diagnosis in offspring from cord blood.

Some complement defects such as properdin are described in three forms; type I where there is complete lack of protein; type II designating residual levels (1–10%); and type III having normal concentration of dysfunctional protein (Fijen et al. 1999).

Protein assays will detect only types I and II and either functional assays or molecular testing would be needed to detect type III properdin deficiency. If there is limited availability of protein assays then again sequencing to identify a mutation may be helpful, particularly as the costs of sequencing continue to come down. It is likely that with next generation sequencing it will be possible to efficiently sequence all of the components of the complement pathway in one step, further speeding up identification of molecular defects.

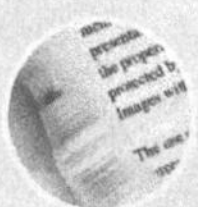

Chapter summary

- Complement is an important part of the immune system. There are three pathways which initiate complement activation, the classical, lectin, and alternative pathways. All the pathways result in the cleavage of C3 forming C3a and C3b, the cleavage of C5 forming C5a and C5b, and the formation of the membrane attack complex.
- Complement activation results in opsonization of targets, clearance of antigen–antibody complexes, inflammation, phagocyte recruitment, and formation of the membrane attack complex which can result in cell lysis.
- Deficiency of complement components leads to susceptibility to infection. Deficiency of components of the classical pathway can increase the risk of SLE due to a lack of clearance of immune complexes.
- There are many regulatory proteins which normally hold the activation of complement under tight control. Deficiency of these can lead to disease, hereditary angioedema being one example.
- The assessment of complement in the laboratory requires samples which have been handled appropriately. Laboratory tests can assess both the concentration of complement components, and their function.

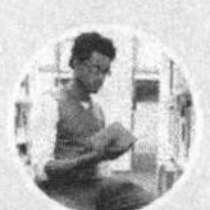

Further reading

- **Botto M, Kirschfink M, Macor P, *et al.* (2009) *Complement in human diseases: lessons from complement deficiencies*. *Mol Immunol*, 46, 2774–83.**
- **Pettigrew HD, Teuber SS, Gershwin ME (2009) *Clinical significance of complement deficiencies*. *Ann N Y Acad Sci*, 1173, 108–23.**
- **Samano EST, *et al.* (2004) *Involvement of C4 allotypes in the pathogenesis of human diseases*. *Rev Hosp Clin Fac Med Sao Paolo*, 59, 138–44.**

• **Yang Y, Chung EK, Zhou B, *et al.* (2003)** ***Diversity in intrinsic strengths of the human complement system: serum C4 protein concentrations correlate with C4 gene size and polygenic variations, hemolytic activities and body mass index. J Immunol*, 171, 2734–45.**

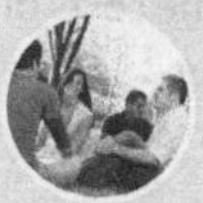

Discussion questions

4.1 Name the ways in which the complement system protects against infection.

4.2 HAE results from a deficiency of which complement regulator and what is the inheritance? What symptoms might a patient with HAE suffer from? What treatments are available?

4.3 Compare and contrast the classical and lectin pathways.

Answers to self-check questions are provided in the book's Online Resource Centre.

Visit www.oxfordtextbooks.co.uk/orc/hall2e

5

Autoimmune rheumatological disease

Learning Objectives

After studying this chapter you should be able to:

- outline the clinical presentation of the autoimmune rheumatological diseases seen in the Immunology laboratory
- outline the assays and techniques used to test for auto-antibodies seen in autoimmune rheumatological diseases
- understand the performance characteristics of these tests
- describe the auto-antibodies tested in the clinical immunology laboratory to aid diagnosis of autoimmune rheumatological diseases
- describe common patterns of immunofluorescence routinely seen on HEp-2 slides.

Introduction

The laboratory plays an increasing role in the diagnosis and clinical management of patients with rheumatic diseases. It is therefore essential that the results of laboratory tests are both accurate and reliable, and give clinicians correct information. It is also important to keep clinicians informed of the changes occurring in the rapidly evolving field of investigation of auto-antibodies.

In rheumatology the detection of auto-antibodies is useful in diagnosis, prognosis, and monitoring disease activity. The first two are firmly established, while with certain exceptions, such as the quantitation of anti-double stranded DNA, the value of the third is still not fully assessed.

This chapter focuses on the rheumatic diseases seen in the clinical laboratory and the tests used to aid the clinical diagnosis.

5.1 Systemic lupus erythematosus (SLE)

SLE is a disease that most commonly affects women of the age group 20–45. Cases do occur in men but it is approximately nine times as common in females. It can occur in children and there is no sex bias before the onset of puberty. SLE is a **multisystem disease** capable of affecting many different organs in the body. In reality it is probably not one disease but a group of closely related diseases which share common features. As a result of this the symptoms of SLE vary greatly from person to person. For some patients with SLE it represents little more than a mild nuisance condition, but for some the disease is very troublesome, even life-threatening resulting from major organ failure. This heterogeneity is reflected in the 11 criteria laid out for the diagnosis of the disease, from which each patient only requires four to fulfil the diagnosis, thus giving many possible combinations. Thus there is no typical clinical presentation and diagnosis can often be delayed whilst other diseases are excluded.

Multisystem disease
A disease affecting more than one component of the body.

From the American College of Rheumatology 1997 update of the 1983 revised criteria for classification (Hochberg 1997), the eleven diagnostic criteria are:

1. Malar rash
2. Discoid rash
3. Photosensitivity
4. Oral ulcers
5. Nonerosive arthritis
   - Involving > 2 peripheral joints
6. Pleuritis **or** pericarditis
7. Renal disorder
   - Persistent proteinuria **or** cellular casts
8. Neurological disorder
   - Seizures **or** psychosis in the absence of drugs or known metabolic disorders
9. Haematologic disorder
   - Haemolytic anaemia **or** leukopenia **or** lymphopenia **or** thrombocytopenia
10. Immunologic disorder
    - Antibodies to dsDNA **or** Sm **or** positive finding of antiphospholipid antibodies (anticardiolipin, lupus anticoagulant or a false positive syphilis test)
11. Positive antinuclear antibodies.

Cross reference
More information on the criteria for diagnosing SLE and other rheumatological diseases can be found at www.rheumatology.org.

There is a strong genetic background to SLE. It is associated with null alleles within the complement region of chromosome 6 and with genes within the HLA region (DR2 in African-Caribbeans and DR3 in Caucasians).

The **aetiology** of this disease remains unclear. There are strong indications from human and mouse studies that deficiencies in **apoptosis**, the clearance of apoptotic material, and the removal from the circulation of **immune complexes** may all play a role in the induction of antibodies to self antigens which are the characteristic hallmark of this disease. These defects result

Aetiology
The cause or origin of disease.

Apoptosis
Programmed cell death.

Immune complexes
Antigen and antibody complexes which can be soluble or insoluble. This depends on the size of the complex and the presence of complement.

in a failure of the body to clear potentially antigenic material from the circulation, thus allowing it to be processed by the immune system. However it remains debatable what role, if any, auto-antibodies play in the **pathogenesis** of this disease. Complement levels (C3 or C4) may be decreased as a result of increased breakdown and may be used to monitor disease activity.

Pathogenesis
The origination and development of a disease.

Environmental factors such as stress and UV light may play a part in triggering disease flares in patients but there is little evidence linking them to its induction.

Cross reference
Look at Chapter 4 for more information on complement.

Key Point

SLE is a mimic disease and may present in a number of different ways. This is a clinical problem in which auto-antibody serology can be helpful in diagnosis.

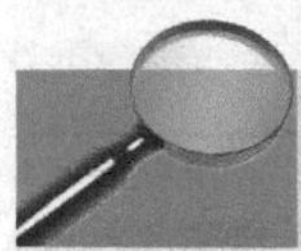

CASE STUDY 5.1 Suspected SLE

Patient history

- **23-year-old female**
- **Presents to general practitioner with increasing lethargy and a facial rash which becomes more pronounced following sunbathing.**
- **Significant associated hair fall.**

Results

- **FBC–Hb–130 g/L [Reference range 115–160]**
- **WCC 5 × 10^9/L [Reference range 4–11]**
- **Platelets 90 × 10^9/L [Reference range 150–400]**
- **U&E/LFT normal**
- **Urine dipstick NAD**
- **Antinuclear antibody positive 1/640 Speckled**
- **ENA–Ro60 positive**
- **dsDNA Ab negative.**

Significance of results

- **Facial rash suggestive of cutaneous lupus.**
- **UV light exacerbates Ro antibody associated skin symptoms.**
- **FBC demonstrates thrombocytopenia.**
- **No renal involvement on bloods or urine testing.**
- **ENA consistent with SLE or Sjögren's.**
- **dsDNA Ab negative, which is consistent with the ANA pattern and suggests lower risk of renal involvement.**

The patient had a biopsy of a patch of skin affected on the forearm and this demonstrated a leukocytoclastic vasculitis. This is not specific to, but consistent with, SLE. The patient was advised to cover sun exposed skin with high factor sun block and started on hydroxychloroquine and their symptoms improved.

This patient fulfils the ACR diagnostic criteria (Hochberg 1997) for SLE by having four distinct features; a typical malar skin rash, photosensitivity, haematologic disorder (thrombocytopenia), and ANA positivity.

Ro antibody positive disease may be cutaneous only or associated with systemic symptoms (such as thrombocytopenia), as in this case. Purely cutaneous disease rarely progresses to involve other organs, but all patients should be tested for other involvement at baseline.

SELF-CHECK 5.1

What specificities of ANA are found predominantly in SLE?

SELF-CHECK 5.2

Why is it important to test for all relevant auto-antibodies when investigating patients with suspected SLE?

5.2 Rheumatoid arthritis (RA)

Rheumatoid arthritis is a multisystem disease, which can affect almost all organs within the body. The principal site of inflammation is found within the joint but the consequences of this process can cause symptoms in many other tissues, e.g. lungs, kidneys, and blood vessels, leading to the manifestations referred to as extra-articular disease, that is disease occurring outside of the joints.

Synovial membrane
The thin membrane that lines the inside of a joint. Its function is to lubricate the joint and produce synovial fluid.

Within the joint there is a proliferation of cells within the **synovial membrane**. These cells set up an inflammatory process which causes the further influx of immune cells into the joint space and the dysregulation of the bone remodelling processes. This results in an excess of bone loss over bone regeneration, leading to small cavities being formed in the bone called erosions, and over time these erosions merge and weaken the bone causing severe damage to the structure. Look at Figure 5.1 which shows an erosive joint by plain radiography.

Within this process there is evidence for an active role of T cells, macrophages, and endothelial cells. There are large amounts of biologically active substances like pro-inflammatory cytokines and chemokines found within the fluid of the joint. These potent immunoregulatory molecules ensure continued activation of cells and the recruitment of additional immunologically active cells into the joint. Look at Figure 5.2 to see the difference between a normal joint and a rheumatoid arthritis joint.

Citrullinated proteins
Citrullination is the post-translational modification of arginine within a protein to citrulline by enzymes called PADs (peptidylarginine deiminases) to form citrullinated proteins.

The increased levels of these immunological mediators are also found within the circulation, and presumably reflect both a leakage from the joint space and some systemic production. In addition a number of different auto-antibodies have been detected in the circulation of patients with RA and these include rheumatoid factor and antibodies to **citrullinated proteins**. Although these are useful in the diagnosis of RA, it is still unclear whether they play any role in the aetiology or pathogenesis of the disease. Other serological manifestations may include the presence of cryoglobulins and the increase of proteins associated with an acute phase response

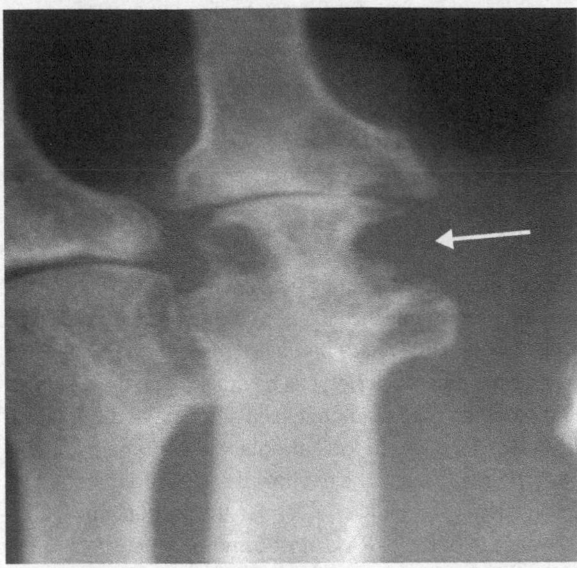

FIGURE 5.1
Erosive arthritis illustrated by plain radiography. Reproduced by kind permission of Professor Peter Taylor, Imperial College London.

such as fibrinogen and C-reactive protein. Complement levels (C3 or C4) may appear normal or even raised due to excess production as part of the acute phase response. However, measurement of complement breakdown products (C3d or C4d) indicates that these patients often have increased levels of complement consumption as well.

Clinically the patient will often present with symptoms such as early morning stiffness and fatigue together with joint swelling and pain. In more advanced cases there may also be symptoms in the lungs, kidneys, blood vessels, spleen, muscles, or neurological system. The onset may be slow and symptoms will develop over a period of months and years. However in about 20% of patients this process is accelerated and the damage occurs more rapidly. In addition a further 20% may always have a mild disease which does not progress over time.

Cross references

You can read more about cryoglobulins in Chapter 2.

You can read more about complement in Chapter 4.

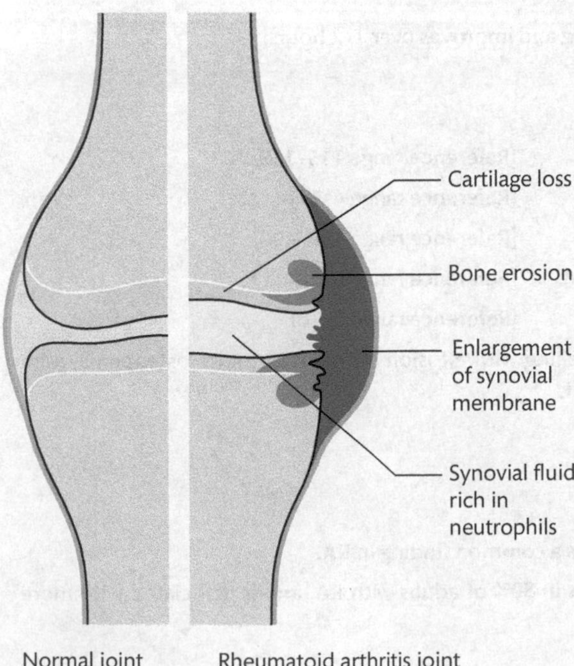

FIGURE 5.2
Pathogenesis of rheumatoid arthritis.

The aetiology of RA is unknown. There is a well described genetic link within the histocompatibility region (HLA) with a number of DRβ genes which code for a similar epitope on the HLA DR molecule and this is referred to as the shared epitope. Frequencies of shared epitope are much higher in patients with RA than in the normal population. It has been calculated that possession of HLA DR containing the shared epitope has approximately twice the risk of any person developing RA. In addition to the shared epitope a number of other genetic variants have been described in association with RA (e.g. PTPN22) but the contribution to the risk and the strength of the association is much lower than in RA.

There are also indications of the effect of environmental triggers associated with the disease. There has been a long history of searching for an infective agent and prospective candidates have included EBV, *Mycobacterium tuberculosis*, and *Proteus mirabilis.* However the evidence is not strong and further work is required before any conclusion can be drawn from these studies. Work from Sweden (Stolt et al. 2003) has suggested a link between smoking and RA, which has opened the discussion on environmental triggers to look at potential airborne pollutants as potential initiators of the immune response. It is still unclear how these environmental triggers would, in an appropriate genetically susceptible individual, lead to the production of autoantibodies and the onset of disease. The age of onset for RA is most commonly between 40 and 50 and there are four times as many cases in females than in males. However it is important to remember that cases can occur at any time in life. There are a separate, but related group of diseases which occur in children and these may first present from the early months of life.

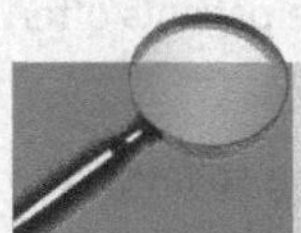

CASE STUDY 5.2 Suspected RA

Patient history

- **67-year-old man**
- **Presents to general practitioner with joint stiffness and pain, mainly affecting the small joints of both hands.**
- **Stiffness worst in the morning and improves over 1-2 hours.**

Results

- **FBC–Hb–100 g/L [Reference range 115-160]**
- **WCC 7 × 10^9/L [Reference range 4-11]**
- **Plts 110 × 10^9/L [Reference range 150-400]**
- **Rheumatoid Factor 400 IU/mL [Reference range 0-20]**
- **CCP–250 IU/ml [Reference range 0-10]**
- **Joint X-ray–periarticular swelling with effusion of the MCP joints, osteopenia, joint space narrowing, and erosions**
- **CXR–NAD.**

Significance of results

- **Anaemia of chronic disease is a common finding in RA.**
- **Rheumatoid factor is present in 80% of adults with RA, and is associated with more aggressive disease.**

- **CCP is highly specific for RA and positivity frequently predates diagnosis, sometimes by years.**
- **Plain radiography remains the key diagnostic test and this patient has the classical features.**
- **RhF is associated with skin and lung nodules—the CXR is normal in this patient.**

The patient was commenced on methotrexate and had a clinical and radiological remission.

The diagnosis of rheumatoid arthritis is clinical, with radiology an essential component (Aletaha 2010). Symptoms of joint involvement should be present for at least 6 weeks without another explanation. The presence of high RhF, CCP, and elevated ESR and CRP all add to the probability of a definite diagnosis. Early treatment can prevent joint damage and significant morbidity.

SELF-CHECK 5.3

What is the primary site of inflammation in rheumatoid arthritis?

5.3 Scleroderma

Systemic sclerosis is a disease in which an abnormal fibrotic process brings about changes in the structure of the skin, which leads to a decrease in permeability and flexibility. These processes may also occur in other organs of the body, which may lead to damage to kidney, lung, or digestive tract tissues.

Women are affected three to four times more often than men. The disease usually starts between the ages of 25 and 50, but occasionally it begins in children or in the elderly.

There are a number of variants of scleroderma but the two commonest are

1. Limited cutaneous systemic sclerosis (sometimes called 'CREST').

   In this syndrome the patient has a combination of

   - **Calcinosis** (calcium deposits).
   - **Raynaud's phenomenon** (a vascular defect).
   - **Esophageal (Oesophageal) dysmotility**—problems with swallowing.
   - **Sclerodactyly** or enlarged swollen fingers.
   - **Telangectasia**, a defect with surface blood vessels in the skin.

2. Diffuse cutaneous systemic sclerosis.

This combines the presence of sclerodermatous changes in the skin with those in other organs of the body. These might include blood vessels, the digestive system, the lungs, and the kidneys. These changes may lead to a decrease in the functioning of these organs.

The aetiology and pathogenesis of scleroderma are unknown. The connective tissue cells of patients with scleroderma can produce too much collagen. Collagen is an essential building block of the body's tissues, but if present in excess, then inflexibility of the tissue results and this may lead to an abnormal structure and consequent altered function.

Calcinosis
The formation of tiny deposits of calcium in the skin.

Raynaud's phenomenon
Spasm of the tiny artery vessels supplying the blood to the extremities during periods of low ambient temperature.

Oesophageal dysmotility
Involvement of the oesophagus in scleroderma.

Sclerodactyly
Localized thickening and tightness of the skin of the fingers or toes.

Telangiectasias
Dilated capillaries that form tiny red areas, frequently on the face.

Cross reference

The auto-antibodies seen in autoimmune rheumatic diseases are discussed in Section 5.8.

These diseases are characterized by the production of specific auto-antibodies that correlate well with the different disease sub-types. However it remains unclear what role these auto-antibodies play in the disease process.

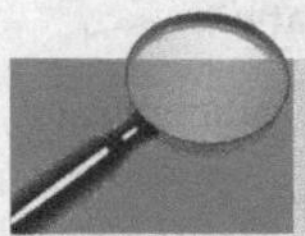

CASE STUDY 5.3 Suspected scleroderma

Patient history

- **42-year-old female**
- **Complains of fingers undergoing colour change—white followed by blue. This is painful. Fingers become red when rewarmed.**
- **Also complains of increasing breathlessness which is becoming more pronounced with very little exertion.**

Results

- **FBC–Hb–100 g/L [Reference range 115-160]**
- **WCC 7 × 10^9/L [Reference range 4-11]**
- **Plts 110 × 10^9/L [Reference range 150-400]**
- **U&E -**
  - **Na–140 [Reference range 135-145]**
  - **K–3.8 [Reference range 3.5-5.0]**
  - **Cr 150 [Reference range 70-130]**
  - **Urea 3.5 [Reference range 3-7]**
- **Chest X-ray–Interstitial shadowing**
- **ANA–Positive 1/640 Nucleolar/Homogeneous**
- **ENA–SCL-70 on ENA Characterization.**

Significance of results

- **Anaemia of chronic disease is a common finding in systemic sclerosis.**
- **The elevated Cr needs follow-up investigation and suggested renal involvement.**
- **The chest X-ray is suggestive of pulmonary involvement—a CT chest would be needed to confirm and stage this further.**
- **The ANA is consistent with systemic sclerosis and the U3-RNP (fibrillarin) is typically associated with renal involvement.**

The patient was treated with pulsed methylprednisolone and then started on oral immune suppression.

Systemic sclerosis may be limited or systemic. SCL-70 is typically associated with pulmonary fibrosis and renal involvement in systemic sclerosis.

The presence of Raynaud's, and lung and renal involvement should alert the clinician to the possible diagnosis and ensure that rapid referral for review is made.

SELF-CHECK 5.4

What are the two most common types of scleroderma and what ANA specificities are most commonly associated with them?

5.4 Sjögren's syndrome

Sjögren's syndrome is an autoimmune disease in which there is lymphocytic infiltration of the glands of the exocrine system (e.g. salivary glands and tear glands) which leads to dysfunction of the production of secretions. Other tissues of the body that may be affected include the lungs, kidneys, skin, and the nervous system. It occurs mostly in women between the ages of 40 and 60. It is much less common in men than in women (1 in 10 of those with Sjögren's syndrome are men), and occurs only rarely in childhood. It affects all races.

There is a well-documented genetic link with genes in the HLA region. There has been much research into looking for an environmental trigger in this disease, but although a number of viruses have been proposed as candidates the story is still unclear.

SELF-CHECK 5.5

Which autoimmune rheumatic disease is associated with the dysfunction of the exocrine gland system, e.g. salivary glands or tear glands?

5.5 Polymyositis and dermatomyositis

Polymyositis is an autoimmune disease that affects mainly the large muscles of the body, such as those around the shoulders, hips, and thighs. Dermatomyositis is a related condition, which affects the skin in addition to the muscles. Polymyositis and dermatomyositis are rare diseases, affecting only 6–8 people out of every 100 000 of the population.

The disease processes that lead to the development of polymyositis and dermatomyositis are not well understood. If muscle biopsies from people with polymyositis and dermatomyositis are examined histologically, infiltrating inflammatory cells can be seen. In addition muscle fibres can show an up-regulation of HLA molecules and the presence of deposited complement indicating an active immune process. In the case of dermatomyositis there are also pathological changes in the skin and the small blood vessels leading to the muscles.

Polymyositis and dermatomyositis are frequently associated with the presence of disease-specific auto-antibodies which can be helpful in differentiating myositic disease caused by autoimmunity from those found in cancer or in metabolic diseases. Recently an up-regulation of auto-antigen in affected tissues has been documented, although it is unclear whether this is a precursor of disease or as a response to inflammation (Suber et al. 2008; Casciola-Rosen et al. 2005).

Genetic influences are seen in some variants of myositis, mostly with genes in the HLA region. There has been much research looking for potential environmental triggers in these diseases, but so far this has failed to reveal any strong associations.

5.6 Antiphospholipid syndrome (APS)

APS is a disorder in which the blood has a tendency to clot too easily. This can affect any vein or artery in the body. There are two main problems caused by APS. They are, firstly, blood clotting in inappropriate blood vessels (**thrombosis**) and secondly, a tendency to miscarriage during

Thrombosis
The formation of a blood clot (thrombus) within the blood vessels.

pregnancy. Symptoms may include headaches, memory loss, forgetfulness and fatigue, visual disturbances, and seizures or fits. It is estimated that as many as 1 in 5 people under 40 years who suffer from strokes may have APS. Deep vein thrombosis (DVT) of the leg is the commonest type of venous thrombosis, but patients with APS may also have arterial complications. There are two main areas of the heart that can be affected: the heart valves and the coronary arteries that supply blood to the heart muscle. The heart valves may become thickened and fail to work properly. The coronary arteries may also become thicker, leading to angina. In addition, other organs such as the kidneys and lungs may also be affected.

All age groups can be affected, from infants to the elderly. However, the majority of people with APS are aged between 20 and 50 years. It seems to affect the health of women more than men because of its effect on pregnancy.

Like many of the autoimmune rheumatic diseases APS may have both genetic and environmental triggers. It is characterized by the presence of circulating antibodies to phospholipids and phospholipid co-factors, but the role of the auto-antibodies has yet to be fully elucidated. It can be shown experimentally that the antibodies are capable of interfering with the functioning of the clotting and fibrinolytic cascades and thus present a potential mechanism for a pathogenic role in the disease process. They may also be capable of interacting with endothelial cells and platelets to encourage conditions promoting the formation of blood clots.

Cross reference

You can read the classification criteria for definitive antiphospholipid syndrome in more detail in Mikyakis et al. (2006).

In 2006 revised guidelines for the diagnostic criteria for antiphospholipid syndrome were published. These guidelines break the criteria down into two areas.

1. Clinical criteria
   - Vascular thrombosis
   - Pregnancy morbidity
2. Laboratory criteria
   - Lupus anticoagulant
   - Anti-cardiolipin antibody
   - Beta-2-glycoprotein antibody (β2GP1).

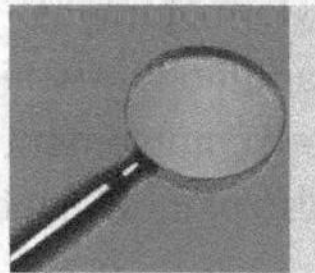

CASE STUDY 5.4 Antiphospholipid syndrome

Patient history

- **33-year-old female.**
- **Has suffered spontaneous miscarriages in the second trimester of pregnancy.**
- **Had an unexplained painful calf swelling which lasted for 2 months after a long-haul plane flight.**

Results

- **FBC–Hb–130 g/L** **[Reference range 115–160]**
- **WCC 5 x 10^9/L** **[Reference range 4–11]**
- **Plts 160 x 10^9/L** **[Reference range 150–400]**
- **U&E/LFT normal**

- ANA–Positive 1/160 Homogenous
- dsDNA and ENA Ab negative
- IgG ACL–180 GPLU/ml [Reference range 0-10]
- IgG B2GP–70 U/ml [Reference range 0-10]
- Clotting screen APTT 40 seconds [Reference range 20-33]
- Lupus anticoagulant–positive.

Significance of results

- ANA is a non-specific finding in this setting.
- The ACL and B2GP are both positive, and if consistent when repeated at a three-month interval would be part of the diagnostic criterion for APS.
- The prolonged APTT is consistent with the presence of a lupus anticoagulant, which has much greater specificity for the diagnosis of APS.

The patient was put on low dose aspirin and heparin and had a further pregnancy with a healthy baby born at term.

APS is a clinical diagnosis and the presence of unexplained recurrent foetal loss as in this case should raise suspicion of the diagnosis. The leg swelling may also have been a venous thromboembolism.

Management depends on the clinical scenario; caution is needed in pregnancy, travel, and for elective surgery.

SELF-CHECK 5.6

Which autoimmune rheumatic disease most commonly presents as either thrombosis or recurrent foetal loss?

5.7 Overlapping connective tissue diseases

Overlapping connective tissue diseases are syndromes where patients may exhibit clinical and serological features from more than one autoimmune rheumatic disease. The most common of these is mixed connective tissue disease (MCTD) in which patients exhibit symptoms of SLE, polymyositis, and scleroderma. In addition to this, there are also well described overlap syndromes between:

- Limited cutaneous systemic sclerosis (CREST), primary biliary cirrhosis, and Sjögren's syndrome.
- Polymyositis and scleroderma.
- SLE and rheumatoid arthritis.
- SLE and scleroderma.

In some cases the auto-antibody profiles of these diseases may reflect one or other of the diseases or in some cases both diseases. In some however the auto-antibody profile is associated

Cross reference

You can read more about primary biliary cirrhosis in Chapter 9.

with the overlap syndrome and not with the diseases in isolation (e.g. anti-PM/Scl antibodies in polymyositis–scleroderma overlap syndrome).

Key Point

Patients with overlap syndromes may appear to have different rheumatic diseases at different times, e.g. a patient with SLE/scleroderma overlap may present as SLE but develop more sclerodermatous features as the disease develops due to the acute versus chronic nature of the two diseases.

5.8 Auto-antibodies

Cross reference

The clinical and technical specificity and sensitivity is described in Method 5.1.

This section aims to describe the auto-antibodies that are tested in the clinical immunology laboratory to aid the diagnosis of autoimmune rheumatological diseases. In order to interpret the results of these tests an understanding of the performance characteristics of the test is essential. This applies to any of the assays performed in the Clinical Immunology laboratory and must considered when interpreting any result.

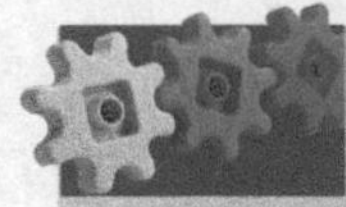

METHOD 5.1 Specificity and sensitivity of the test

Sensitivity is defined as the percentage of patients within a defined disease group who have the antibody, whereas specificity is defined as the percentage of positive results which are contained within the target disease group.

An ideal diagnostic assay is highly specific for the disease and occurs in the majority of patients with that disorder (high sensitivity). It must be borne in mind that diagnostic sensitivity may increase with frequent blood sampling since the level of auto-antibody (e.g. rheumatoid factor) may correlate with the activity and stage of the disease and may be affected by the drugs that are being used to treat the disease. Sensitivity may also reflect genetic heterogeneity and ethnic origins of populations under study, a notable example being the frequency of anti-Sm in SLE, which is 60% in African-Caribbean populations but only 5% in Caucasoid populations. Sensitivity and specificity may also depend on the method. Thus enzyme-linked immunosorbent assays (ELISA) are more sensitive than gel precipitation techniques. However, increased sensitivity often goes hand in hand with a decrease in specificity as increasingly small amounts of antibody are detected; thus an assay with very high sensitivity may be of little use diagnostically assay due to very low specificity. The specificity of an assay may also be affected by the material used as the antigenic source, by its purity, and the nature and conformation of the peptides and epitopes presented in the assay.

Specificity is usually measured in relation to a population of healthy subjects, but suitable age-matched control populations should be used, since some auto-antibodies occur in healthy elderly people. It is often of greater relevance to compare the test population with others displaying clinical features which are likely to be confused (e.g. rheumatoid arthritis and SLE), or that are part of a differential diagnosis.

5.8.1 Anti-nuclear antibodies

Anti-nuclear antibodies (ANA) are auto-antibodies directed against cellular components. The term 'ANA' is something of a misnomer as some of these antigens are actually cytoplasmic in location. Chromosomal antigens include single- and double-stranded deoxyribonucleic acid (DNA), deoxyribonucleoprotein (DNP), and histones. Antibodies have also been described against the centromeric proteins and various nucleolar proteins. Soluble nuclear or cytoplasmic antigens which are readily extracted in phosphate-buffered saline (pH 7.2) have been termed 'extractable nuclear antigens' (ENA) or 'soluble cellular antigens'. Some of these antigens are named according to their biochemical nature (e.g. ribonucleoproteins: RNP) or according to the diseases in which they occur (e.g. Sjögren's syndrome: SS-A). ANA are usually initially tested by indirect immunofluorescence on HEp-2 cells or historically on cryostat sections of rodent tissues. In addition to the strength of reaction, either as intensity or titre, the pattern of staining should be recorded as this may indicate certain specificities, such as the centromeric antigen, and those located in the nucleolus. Look at Figure 5.3 for some commonly recognized ANA patterns seen on immunofluorescence and their antigen associations.

Online Resource Centre

To see an online video demonstrating immunofluorescence, log on to www.oxfordtextbooks.co.uk/orc/fbs

Other screening methods, including ELISAs and multiplex bead-based assays using purified antigens or cell homogenates, are also gaining in popularity. These have become more popular as they do not demand the same level of expert practice as indirect immunofluorescence in their interpretation. Whilst such screening techniques give an indication as to the presence or absence of antibodies, it is the specificity of the antibody which is important in determining disease associations. It should be remembered that not all antigens are nuclear in cellular location and that for certain antibodies (e.g. anti-Ro or anti-Jo-1) the ANA is not a useful test for their presence as they may not be detected on ANA immunofluorescence.

The specificity of the antibody is determined by techniques such as radioimmunoassay, gel diffusion, ELISA, or immunoblotting. ANA with high specificity are termed 'disease markers'. These antibodies are rarely found other than associated with their designated diseases. Look at Table 5.1 for a list of these antibodies. Certain specificities are also associated with specific clinical features and may point to future clinical developments. Look at Table 5.2 for a list of these antibodies.

5.8.2 Anti-dsDNA

Antibodies to deoxyribonucleic acid (DNA) in SLE are directed to the double-stranded variant. These antibodies occur almost exclusively in SLE and are present in 60–70% of patients with active disease. Increasing levels may predict increasing disease activity; this rise in antibody levels is often coupled with a decrease in complement C3 and C4 levels, indicating complement consumption. Patients in remission or with inactive disease may also have very high levels

TABLE 5.1 **Marker auto-antibodies in autoimmune rheumatic diseases.**

Disease	Auto-antibody	Sensitivity	Specificity
SLE	dsDNA	Medium	High
	Sm	Low	High
Sjögren's syndrome	La	Medium	High
Neonatal lupus erythematosus	Ro	High	High
Diffuse systemic sclerosis	Scl-70	High	High
Limited systemic sclerosis	Centromere	High	High
Polymyositis	Jo-1	Low	High
Dermatomyositis	Mi-2	Medium	High
Rheumatoid arthritis	CCP	High	High

	Pattern on Hep 2 cells	Target	Disease association
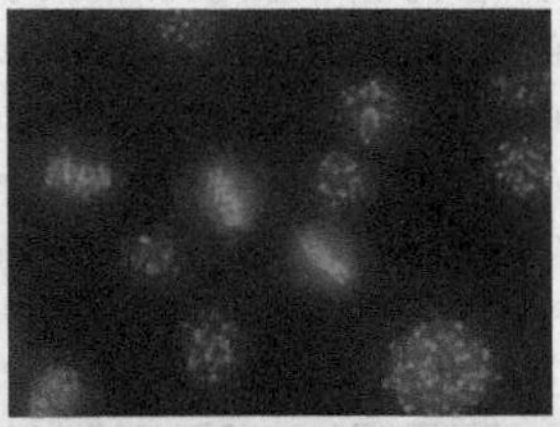	Centromere	Cenp A, B, C	Limited scleroderma / CREST (60%) Raynaud's phenomenon
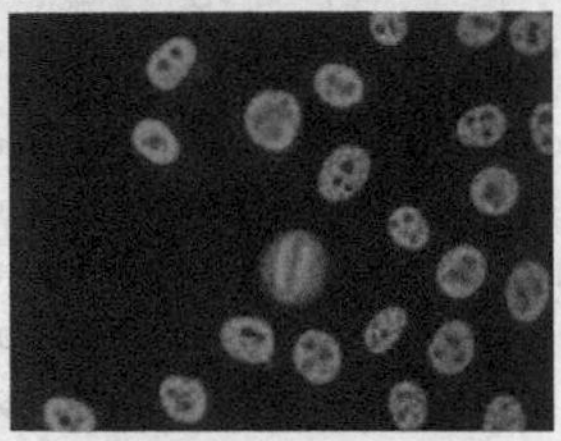	Coarse speckled	U1RNP, Sm	SLE
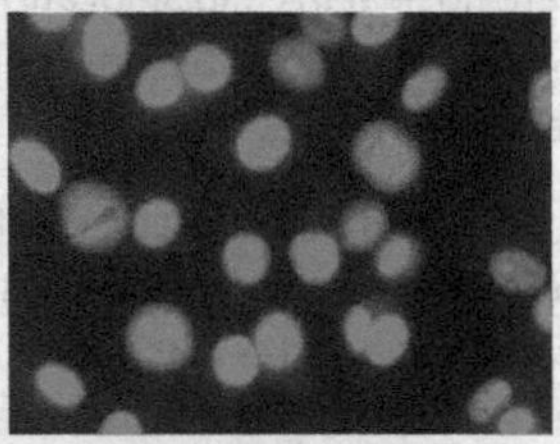	Fine speckled	Ro (SS-A), La (SS-B)	Sjögrens' syndrome (95%) SLE (40%) Scleroderma (5%)
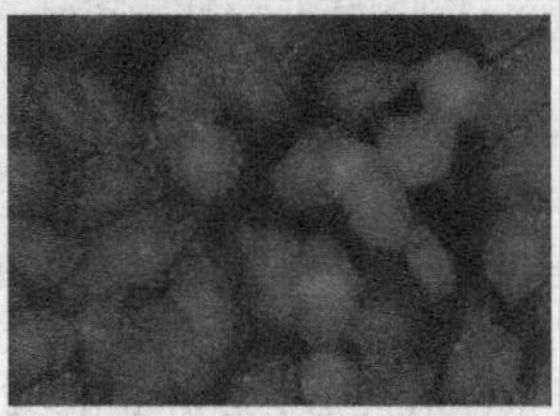	Cytoplasmic speckled	Jo-1	Polymyositis
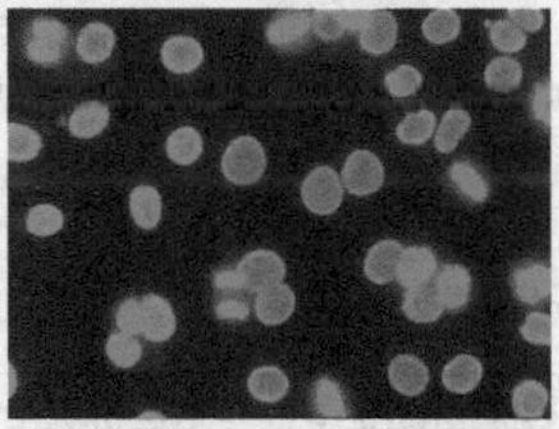	Homogenous	dsDNA, Histones	SLE (95%) Discoid lupus
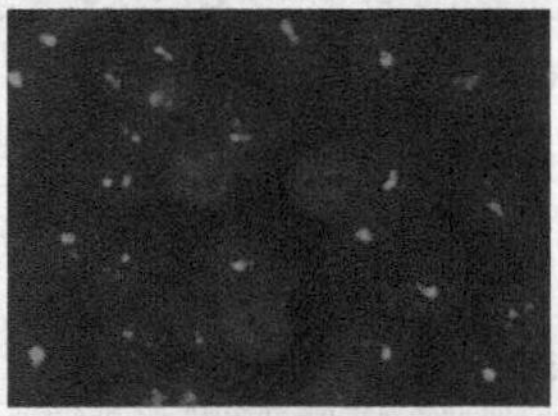	Nuclear homogenous	Pm-Scl	Scleroderma (30%) Polymyositis / Scleroderma overlap
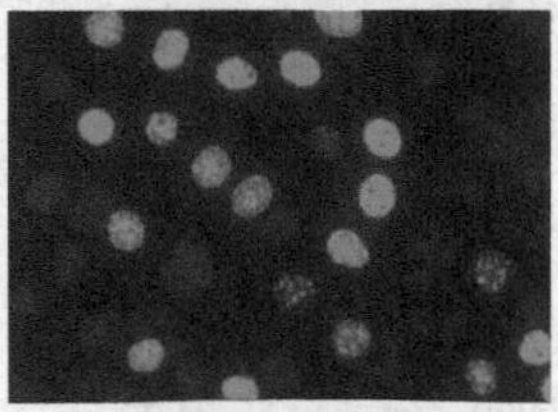	Pleiomorphic (PCNA)	Cyclin	SLE (1–3%)

FIGURE 5.3
Commonly recognized ANA patterns and their antigen associations.

TABLE 5.2 Associations of auto-antibodies with clinico-pathological features.

Clinico-pathological feature	Auto-antibody	Comment
Diffuse glomerulonephritis	dsDNA	SLE with kidney disease
Membranous glomerulonephritis	Sm, Ro	SLE with kidney disease
Neonatal heart block	Ro	Maternal antibody
Raynaud's phenomenon	U1-RNP	As part of overlap syndromes
Fibrosing alveolitis	Jo-1	In polymyositis
	U1-RNP	As part of overlap syndromes
Erosive joint damage	CCP	In RA and overlap syndromes

of antibodies and this has led to the suggestion that it is change in antibody level rather than absolute antibody level that may equate with changes in disease activity.

Anti-dsDNA antibodies are associated with the development of kidney failure in SLE and are associated with a specific lesion that can be seen on kidney biopsy (diffuse proliferative glomerulonephritis).

It should be noted that there are a number of different methodologies for the detection of anti-dsDNA and that each of these may detect a different sub-population of antibodies. The Farr radioimmunoassay, once regarded as the gold standard assay for antibodies in SLE, detects only high avidity binding antibodies and has a strong association with both renal and active systemic disease. The ***Crithidia lucillae*** immunofluorescent test also has a high specificity for SLE but is less sensitive than the Farr assay. However the *Crithidia* test is semi-quantitative and so is not useful in monitoring patients. Look at Figure 5.4 to see how dsDNA antibodies appear on *Crithidia* substrate. Generally speaking ELISA assays for anti-dsDNA have a high sensitivity but a lower specificity, and thus some people have suggested that they have a greater role in monitoring patients' disease activity than in diagnosis.

Crithidia lucillae

A micro-organism with a kinetoplast that contains only double-stranded DNA. Commercial preparations of this organism are available for test purposes.

Anti-dsDNA may be found occasionally in diseases other than SLE. Most commonly this is connected to the patient being on certain medication such as sulphasalazine or TNF-blockers. The occurrence of these antibodies may be accompanied by lupus-like symptoms, and this is

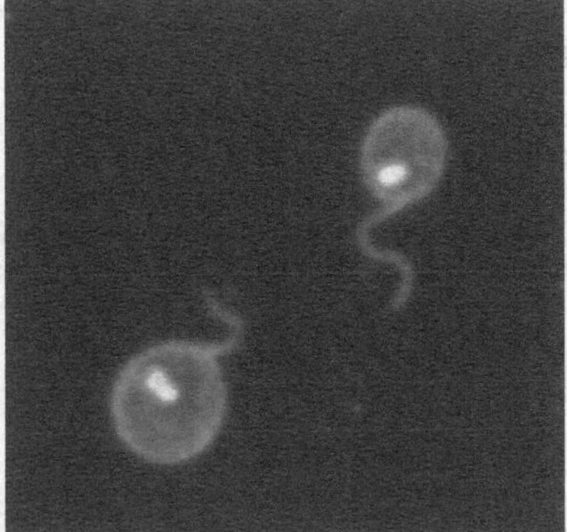

FIGURE 5.4

dsDNA antibodies on *Crithidia* substrate. Note the staining of the kinetoplast, a bundle of pure DNA.

referred to as 'drug-induced lupus'. However it is important to note that the incidence of anti-dsDNA antibodies in these patients is far higher, 10 to 100 fold, than the incidence of clinical symptoms of SLE in these patients. This indicates that the presence of auto-antibody alone is probably insufficient to cause disease, and that maybe other factors, such as a suitable genetic or environmental background, are also necessary for the clinical expression of the disease.

5.8.3 Anti-Ro

Antibodies to Ro are directed to two different antigens which are usually termed Ro52 and Ro60 based on the molecular weight of the respective antigens. Anti-Ro60 is detected in about 60–80% of patients with primary Sjögren's syndrome and 40% of patients with SLE. Anti-Ro52 is also found in a higher frequency in patients with SLE and Sjögren's syndrome, but in addition it is also found in systemic sclerosis, polymyositis, and overlap connective tissue disease and has little diagnostic value. Anti-Ro has also been detected in a small group of healthy adult controls.

Anti-Ro60 in all these groups may be associated with foetal congenital heart block. This condition is found in 5% of pregnant women who have circulating anti-Ro60, and rises to 25% in women who have previously had one or more affected babies. These findings suggest that the damage may be caused by a subgroup of antibodies to Ro60, probably directed against a particular epitope. Maternal Anti-Ro60 is also associated with neonatal lupus, a condition in which maternal antibodies cross the placenta and cause a cutaneous disease, which regresses following birth as the maternal antibody is cleared from the baby's circulation. It is interesting to note that neonatal lupus and congenital heart block, although both associated with antibodies to Ro60, are very rarely seen occurring together in the same baby, although cases have been described where both have occurred to different babies born to the same mother.

Anti-Ro60 is also associated with a number of subsets of SLE, including the so-called ANA negative SLE syndrome, subcutaneous lupus erythematosus, and the lupus-like syndrome associated with homozygous complement C2 and C4 deficiency.

5.8.4 Anti-La

Antibodies to La are found in approximately 50% of patients with primary Sjögren's syndrome. In the absence of SLE associated antibodies, anti-La is a diagnostic marker for primary Sjögren's syndrome, particularly in patients with extraglandular features of the syndrome. In general, patients with lupus and anti-La have a later age of onset and a lower incidence of nephritis than other SLE patients.

5.8.5 Anti-U1RNP and anti-Sm

This group of antibodies is directed to a group of uridine-rich ribonucleic acids and their associated proteins The U1 RNP antigens are located exclusively on the U1 RNA particle, whereas the antigenic targets for anti-Sm are found on the U2, U4, U5, and U6 ribonucleoproteins. Antibodies to U1 RNP react with the 71kd, A, and C peptides, whereas anti-Sm react with the B, B1, and D peptides. The E, F, and G proteins are rarely targets for antibodies in the autoimmune diseases.

5.8.6 Anti-Sm

Anti-Sm is found almost exclusively in SLE. Antibodies to Sm show a marked variation in frequency. In Caucasoid populations it occurs in less than 5% of SLE patients, but the reported prevalence rises to 40–60% in African-Caribbean populations. Anti-Sm and anti-U1 RNP antibodies are often found in combination, although rarely monospecific anti-Sm antibodies can occur.

5.8.7 Anti-U1 RNP

Anti-U1 RNP is found in 80% of patients with mixed connective tissue disease (MCTD), one of the overlap syndromes, and in 10% of patients with SLE or scleroderma. The presence of this antibody is associated with Raynaud's phenomenon and fibrosing lung disease.

5.8.8 Anti-Jo-1

Antibodies to Jo-1 (histidyl tRNA synthetase) are present in 20% of patients with primary polymyositis, especially in those with pulmonary fibrosis and arthritis. Antibodies to five other tRNA synthetases have also been described: thryonyl (PL-7), alanyl (PL-12), isoleucyl (OJ), glycyl (EJ), and lysyl. All appear to be associated with a clinical syndrome similar to Jo-1, but are rare, each occurring in less than 4% of polymyositis patients.

5.8.9 Anti-Scl-70

Antibodies to Scl-70 are directed against the enzyme DNA topoisomerase 1 and are found in 30% of patients with systemic sclerosis. They are most commonly found in patients with the diffuse variant and are much less frequently seen in patients with limited disease. Their presence in patients with Raynaud's phenomenon or limited scleroderma may indicate that the disease is becoming more aggressive.

5.8.10 Anti-centromere

This antibody gives a characteristic pattern visualized in an immunofluorescent test using cells in **mitosis**. Antibodies are directed against the A, B, and C proteins of the centromeric complex. It appears that the B protein is the immunodominant epitope and antibodies to this are found in >95% of sera containing anti-centromere antibodies. However, occasional patients are seen whose antibodies will react with only the A or C proteins. The antibody is found in approximately 30% of patients with systemic sclerosis, and in 80–90% of patients with the limited cutaneous variant. Occasionally, anti-centromere antibodies may also be present in other autoimmune diseases such as primary biliary cirrhosis or SLE, where it may identify patients who will subsequently develop features of scleroderma.

Mitosis
Division of a somatic cell to form two genetically identical daughter cells.

5.8.11 Anti-phospholipid

Antibodies directed against negatively charged phospholipids occur in SLE and other connective tissue diseases. They are responsible for false positive syphilis serology and for the **lupus anticoagulant** reaction. In patients with SLE, anti-phospholipid antibodies (APL) have been associated with vascular thrombosis, recurrent foetal loss, and thrombocytopenia. In some patients with a similar clinical syndrome, the only serological abnormalities are the presence of anti-phospholipid antibodies and occasionally a weak ANA. This syndrome has been termed 'anti-phospholipid syndrome'. Anti-phospholipid antibodies have also been detected in infections and other diseases and may reflect part of the immune response to phospholipid antigens within the membranes and cell walls of infective agents. However, the association with thrombosis, foetal loss, and thrombocytopenia has frequently not been found in these groups. It has been suggested that the lupus anticoagulant test, a functional measure of coagulation activity, is a more reliable predictor of risk for foetal loss, thrombosis, and thrombocytopenia.

Lupus anticoagulant
An auto-antibody which interferes with blood coagulation, as well as *in vitro* tests of clotting function, causing elevation in the partial thromboplastin time.

Some assays for APL give variable results and may give false positive reactions due to non-specific binding. Co-factors may be required for the binding of anti-cardiolipin to its antigen, such as β2GP1, and it is important that these are included in assay systems. Due to these variations it is difficult to compare the many studies of APL in different diseases.

5.8.12 Rheumatoid factor

The association of IgM rheumatoid factor and the diagnosis of RA is well known, but rheumatoid factors are also found in other immunoglobulin classes. IgA rheumatoid factor levels correlate with cartilage loss and bone erosion in RA, and correlate well with disease activity. IgG rheumatoid factors have been associated with vasculitis, but have not, so far, found a useful role in diagnosis and management.

IgM rheumatoid factor is not specific for RA and is also found in high levels in Sjögren's syndrome, and in ANCA related vasculitis. Lower levels may also be found in SLE, systemic sclerosis, polymyositis, and in patients with infections. The diagnostic specificity of IgM rheumatoid factor is therefore quite low, and when the appropriate control groups are tested may only be about 50%.

5.8.13 Anti-CCP

Anti-CCP (cyclic citrullinated peptide) antibodies were first described in 1998. Second and third generation CCP antibody assays use a synthetically formed cyclic citrullinated peptide which shows no homology to tissue proteins, and was generated using RA sera to screen citrullinated peptide libraries. The benefit of synthetic peptide production and purification is that it is cheap and reproducible, with homogeneous citrullination of the peptides.

The anti-CCP assay has been reported with a sensitivity as high as 81% and specificity of 91%. It has been found to identify IgM rheumatoid factor negative (so called sero-negative) patients and offer prognostic value. However, while IgM RF concentrations have been found to decrease with treatment, anti-CCP antibody concentrations do not appear to change, limiting the use of anti-CCP as a marker of disease activity or as an indicator of response to treatment. There is increasing evidence that anti-CCP antibodies are also detected in patients with other connective tissue diseases, including Sjögren's syndrome, systemic lupus erythematosus, systemic sclerosis, mixed connective tissue disease, and idiopathic inflammatory myositis, and may be linked to the occurrence of joint erosions in these conditions. Several studies have observed the detection of anti-CCP antibodies many years prior to disease onset (Nielen et al. 2004, Rantapää-Dahlqvist et al. 2003).

Overall, anti-CCP antibodies are a useful marker for aiding the diagnosis of early RA, especially in sero-negative patients, and aid the identification of patients needing aggressive treatment for future erosive disease.

5.8.14 Other auto-antibodies

Antibodies to ribosomal RNP (rRNP) or ribosomal P protein are present in approximately 15% of patients with SLE. They were originally described as a marker for neuropsychiatric SLE, but more recent studies suggest that they are more likely to be a marker for active generalized disease.

Anti-nucleolar antibodies react with diverse antigens located within the nucleolar region of the cell. These include anti 6-7S RNA, RNA polymerase-I, fibrillarin, and U3 RNA, which are all present in low frequencies in scleroderma. Another nucleolar specific antibody, PM-I or PM/Scl, is found in patients with overlapping features of polymyositis and scleroderma. Anti-nucleolar antibodies in low titre are occasionally seen in other connective tissue diseases.

Antibodies to Ku are found in patients with SLE, MCTD, Sjögren's syndrome, scleroderma, and myositis.

Anti-proliferating cell nuclear antigen (PCNA) antibodies are a specific marker for SLE, and are found in approx. 5% of patients. There is no known association with clinical features.

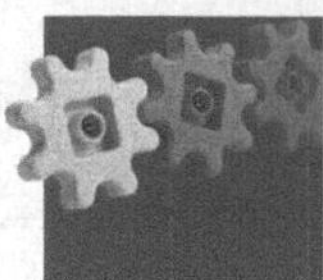

METHOD 5.2 Methods used in detecting auto-antibodies in rheumatic diseases

Antinuclear antibodies (ANA)

- Indirect immunofluorescence using cultured cells e.g. HEp-2.
- Indirect immunofluorescence using rodent tissue sections e.g. rat liver.
- ELISA using mixtures of purified or recombinant antigens.
- ELISA using cell homogenates.

Traditionally ANA screening has been performed using indirect immunofluorescence. However, many laboratories have switched in recent years to using ELISA-based assays as these require less interpretative skill and produce objective results rather than a subjective opinion.

Anti dsDNA

- ELISA using biochemically pure mammalian DNA.
- FPIA using biochemically pure mammalian DNA.
- Radioimmunoassay using biochemically pure mammalian DNA.
- Indirect immunofluorescence using *Crithidia lucillae*. (The kinetoplast of this flagellate contains only dsDNA.)

Radioimmunoassay and *Crithidia* indirect immunofluorescence tend to have a lower sensitivity and a higher specificity than ELISA-based assays. Quantitative results obtained from ELISA and radioimmunoassay are useful in monitoring disease activity in patients following diagnosis.

Anti ENA (e.g. Ro, La, U1-RNP, Sm, Jo-1, Scl-70)

- ELISA using purified or recombinant antigens.
- FPIA using purified or recombinant antigens.
- Immunodiffusion using purified or recombinant antigens.
- Dot or line blotting using purified or recombinant antigens.
- Western blotting using cell homogenates.
- Addressable bead immunoassay using purified or recombinant antigens.

The many different techniques that are available for the detection and identification of antibodies to ENA can be confusing. The variations in technology and in the antigen sources can lead to discrepancies in the results obtained between different technologies. Some laboratories operate a system whereby a serum must be positive in two different technologies before the antibody is assigned to a patient. This avoids the problems of both false positive and false negative results, which may arise due to the technological variations.

Anti-phospholipid

- ELISA using biochemically purified cardiolipin or other phospholipids.

IgM rheumatoid factor

- Particle agglutination using beads coated with IgG.
- Nephelometry.
- ELISA.
- Addressable bead immunoassay.

Anti-CCP

- ELISA.
- FPIA.

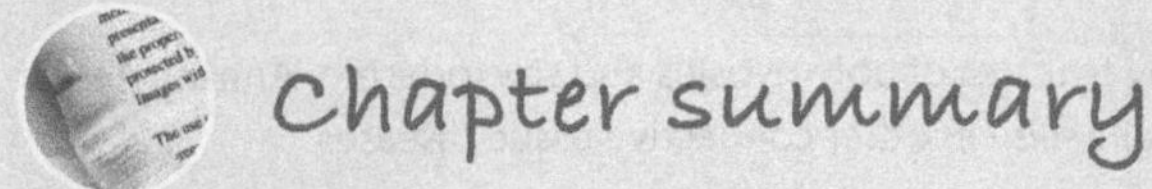

Chapter summary

- Auto-antibodies are useful tools in the diagnosis and management of autoimmune rheumatic diseases.
- SLE is a systemic autoimmune disease which may affect many organs within the body.
- Rheumatoid arthritis is an inflammatory disease of the joints, which may have systemic features.
- Scleroderma (systemic sclerosis) is a disease in which an abnormal fibrotic process causes changes in the structure of the skin and other organs.
- Sjögren's syndrome is an autoimmune disease which results in a dysfunction of the exocrine glands (e.g. salivary and tear glands).
- Polymyositis is an autoimmune disease which results in tissue destruction and weakness.
- Anti-phospholipid syndrome is a disease which is characterized by an increase in thrombosis and recurrent foetal loss.
- Overlapping connective tissue diseases are syndromes in which patients show the features of more than one autoimmune rheumatic disease.
- Anti-dsDNA antibodies occur in 60–70% of patients with SLE and levels are commonly correlated to disease activity.
- Anti-Ro antibodies are detected in SLE and Sjögren's syndrome.
- Anti-La antibodies are detected in SLE and Sjögren's syndrome.
- Anti-Sm antibodies are detected in SLE.
- Anti-U1 RNP is detected in 80% with mixed connective tissue disease.
- Anti Jo-1 is detected in patients with polymyositis.
- Anti-Scl-70 is detected in patients with diffuse systemic sclerosis.
- Anti-centromere is detected in patients with limited systemic sclerosis.
- Anti-CCP is a specific and sensitive marker for the diagnosis of rheumatoid arthritis.

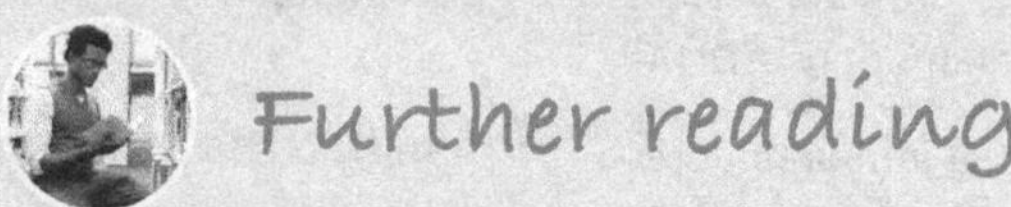

Further reading

- **Mikaykis S *et al.* (2006) *International consensus statement on an update of the classification criteria for definite antiphospholipid syndrome (APS)*. *J Thromb Haemost*, 4(2), 295–306.**
- **Wilson WA, Gharavi AE, Koike T, *et al.* (1999) *International consensus statement on preliminary classification criteria for definite antiphospholipid syndrome*. *Arthritis Rheum*, 42, 1309–11.**

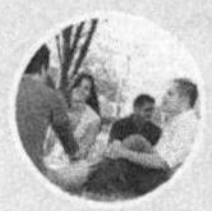

Discussion questions

5.1 Describe the symptoms and laboratory findings included in the ACR diagnostic criteria for SLE. How many need to be present for a diagnosis to be made?

5.2 Describe the methods for detection of ANA and comment on their relative advantages and disadvantages.

5.3 Discuss the immunological mechanisms which may play a part in the pathogenesis of rheumatoid arthritis.

Answers to self-check questions are provided in the book's Online Resource Centre.

Visit www.oxfordtextbooks.co.uk/orc/hall2e

6

Autoimmune kidney disease

Learning objectives

After studying this chapter you should be able to:

- outline the common features of autoimmune kidney disease
- explain the clinical features of granulomatosis with polyangiitis, microscopic polyangiitis, and eosinophilic granulomatosis with polyangiitis
- explain the clinical features of anti-GBM (Goodpasture's) disease
- explain the clinical features of membranous nephropathy
- outline the treatment and monitoring of these diseases
- describe the laboratory techniques used to test for anti-neutrophil cytoplasmic antibodies (ANCA)
- describe the laboratory techniques used to test for antibodies to myeloperoxidase (MPO) and proteinase 3 (PR3)
- describe the laboratory techniques used to test for glomerular basement membrane (GBM) antibodies
- describe the laboratory techniques used to test for antibodies to phospholipase A2 receptor (PLA2R)
- discuss the advantages and limitations of these techniques
- describe the quality assurance of these techniques in the clinical laboratory.

Introduction

Autoimmune kidney diseases can be broken into two major disease groups. The diseases associated with antibodies to anti-neutrophil cytoplasmic antibodies (ANCA) and those associated with antibodies to the glomerular basement membrane (GBM). In addition, this chapter will also introduce the novel antibodies to Phospholipase A2 Receptors (PLA2R) and their association with Membranous Nephropathy. Whilst these represent distinct syndromes it must also be recognized that there is some commonality in symptoms, which means that in an acute presentation of a patient in renal failure, it is not easy to distinguish them.

In all these diseases there is strong evidence that the degree of kidney damage at the time of onset of treatment is the biggest factor in determining long-term kidney survival emphasizing the need for early recognition, diagnosis, and treatment. The Immunology laboratory has an important role to play in this but this is not in isolation. As well as the autoimmune status of the patient, clinicians rely on the Clinical Biochemistry laboratory to determine the extent of the kidney involvement.

Cross reference

You can read more on the use of the glomerular filtration rate (GFR) and creatinine levels in determining kidney function in Chapter 3 of the *Clinical Biochemistry* textbook of this series.

In terms of the kidney pathology, these syndromes all can present as a rapidly progressive **glomerulonephritis**. However, it is also important to realize that, although the renal symptoms may represent the major immediate threat to recovery, these syndromes may also form part of a systemic inflammation of vascular organs (**vasculitis**) throughout the body.

Glomerulonephritis

Inflammation of the glomeruli of the kidney.

Vasculitis

Inflammation of the blood vessels.

6.1 Vasculitis and classification

Vasculitis, the inflammation and cellular infiltration of the blood vessels, may result in local inflammation as seen in glomerulonephritis, vessel wall damage leading to aneurism and haemorrhage or vessel occlusion, causing ischaemia and infarction. The clinical manifestations will depend on the size and location of the affected vessels. Vasculitis can be classified as either primary or secondary, according to the vessel size and whether this is due to ANCA-associated vasculitides.

Cross reference

For more information on the classification of vasculitides see Jennette et al. (2013).

6.1.1 Primary or secondary

Primary vasculitis often has an unknown cause, but is almost always an autoimmune mechanism of disease. A vasculitis is termed secondary when it is associated with infections such as endocarditis and hepatitis, secondary to malignancies such as lymphoma, or drug-induced following the use of anti-thyroid and anti-hypertensive medications such as propylthiouracil or hydralazine.

6.1.2 Vessel size

The Chapel and Hill consensus of nomenclature for vasculitis divides the vessels into large, medium, or small in size. Large vessels are the aorta and its major branches and the analogous veins. Medium vessels are the main visceral arteries and veins and their initial branches. Small vessels are intraparenchymal arteries. The kidney is an example of an organ with both medium and small vessels. Look at Figure 6.1 to see a diagrammatic representation of the vessels and their disease associations.

Small vessel vasculitis can further be broken down into a number of disease associations. Those that will be discussed in this chapter are the ANCA-associated small vessel vasculitides (AAV), anti-GBM disease, and membranous nephropathy. Since 2012 the AAV have been renamed as microscopic polyangiitis, granulomatosis with polyangiitis (formerly known as Wegener's granulomatosis) and eosinophilic granulomatosis with polyangiitis (formerly known as Churg-Strauss). As this is a relatively recent update, the old terminology remains a widely used nomenclature and still appears in many texts.

The AAV are rare, affecting approximately 20 per million people in Europe. Males and females are affected equally, with an increasing incidence with increasing age, the majority of cases occurring between 55 and 70 years of age. The diseases follow a relapsing-remitting course and can present with diverse clinical manifestations. Look at Table 6.1 to see the diversity of organs affected and the clinical presentations.

TABLE 6.1 The diversity of organs affected by ANCA-associated vasculitides and their clinical presentations.

Organ involved	Presentation	Investigations
Kidney	Asymptomatic urinary abnormalities (e.g. haematuria and proteinuria on dipstick) ranging from abnormal renal function through to rapidly progressive glomerulonephritis (RPGN) May be dialysis dependent at diagnosis	Kidney biopsy required Histologically: • Segmental fibrinoid necrosis • Established cellular crescent
Lungs	Cough Dyspnoea (shortness of breath) Haemoptysis–pulmonary haemorrhage Disproportionate anaemia Lung nodules and cavitation	Chest X-ray CT scan Lung function tests including transfer factor
Ear, Nose, and Throat	Sinusitis (nasal stuffiness, congestion) Nasal discharge Epistaxis (nosebleeds) Oral or nasal ulcers Otitis media (deafness) Cartilaginous involvement Collapse of nasal bridge Tracheal stenosis	
Neurological	Mononeuritis multiplex presenting as peripheral neuropathy Central nervous system disease	
Eyes	Conjunctivitis Scleritis (inflammation of the white of the eye) Uveitis (inflammation of the middle layer of the eye) Proptosis/Exopthalmus (bulging of the eye)	
Skin	Rash Ulcers Necrosis	

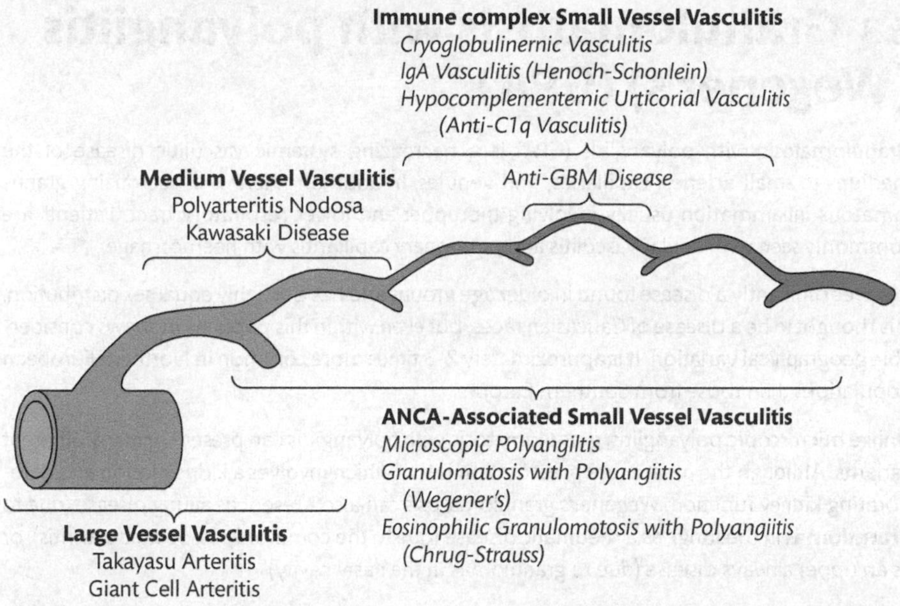

Immune complex Small Vessel Vasculitis
Cryoglobulinernic Vasculitis
IgA Vasculitis (Henoch-Schonlein)
Hypocomplementemic Urticorial Vasculitis
(Anti-C1q Vasculitis)

Medium Vessel Vasculitis
Polyarteritis Nodosa
Kawasaki Disease

Anti-GBM Disease

ANCA-Associated Small Vessel Vasculitis
Microscopic Polyangiltis
Granulomatosis with Polyangiitis
(Wegener's)
Eosinophilic Granulomotosis with Polyangiitis
(Chrug-Strauss)

Large Vessel Vasculitis
Takayasu Arteritis
Giant Cell Arteritis

FIGURE 6.1
Diagrammatic representation of the vessels and their disease associations. The diagram depicts (from left to right) aorta, large artery, medium artery, small artery/arteriole, capillary, venule, and vein. Anti-GBM = anti-glomerular basement membrane; ANCA = anti-neutrophil cytoplasmic antibody.

6.2 Microscopic polyangiitis (MPA)

Microscopic polyangiitis (MPA) is a necrotizing systemic vasculitic disease of the small arteries and capillaries. Histologically, there are few or no immune deposits seen. It is predominantly a disease found in older age groups and has a roughly equal sex distribution. It has a wider ethnic distribution than other ANCA-associated vasculitic diseases and is found commonly in both Caucasian and Oriental races. Within the Caucasian population its prevalence shows considerable geographical variation. It is approximately 3–4 times less common in Northern European populations than those found in Southern Europe. MPA is a rare disease with an incidence of approximately 2 cases per 100 000 persons in the United Kingdom.

Patients who have MPA often present with generalized symptoms (fatigue, fevers, loss of weight). They may also have shortness of breath or **haematemesis**. In addition they may also show rashes, and muscle and joint pain. The kidney disease may not always be evident until there is a significant deterioration in renal function.

Haematemesis
Vomiting blood.

In MPA, there is no granulomatous disease in the ear, nose, throat, or lungs. Inflammation is limited to the walls of the vessels. Patients are less likely to relapse following successful treatment.

Look at Section 6.8 for more information on the laboratory investigation of anti-neutrophil cytoplasmic antibodies (ANCA). Patients with MPA tend to have pANCA with specific antibodies to myeloperoxidase (MPO).

Key Points

- **The clinical features of Goodpasture's disease and the ANCA-associated vasculitic diseases can be similar and so all should be considered in a patient presenting with acute kidney failure.**
- **Evidence suggests that outcome, both in terms of kidney function and survival, is linked to early diagnosis and treatment**

6.3 Granulomatosis with polyangiitis (Wegener's) (GPA)

Granulomatosis with polyangiitis (GPA) is a necrotizing systemic vasculitic disease of the medium to small arteries, capillaries, and venules. In addition, there is a necrotizing granulomatous inflammation usually involving the upper and lower respiratory tract. Patients are commonly seen with ocular vasculitis and pulmonary capillaritis with haemorrhage.

It is predominantly a disease found in older age groups and has a roughly equal sex distribution. It is thought to be a disease of Caucasian races, but even within this population shows considerable geographical variation. It is approximately 2–3 times more common in Northern European populations than those from Southern Europe.

Unlike microscopic polyangiitis, granulomatosis with polyangiitis can present in many different variants. Although the most acute presentation is that which involves a kidney lesion and deteriorating kidney function, Wegener's granulomatosis can also present as a lung disease (due to **granulomas** in the lung), as a rheumatic disease (due to the commonly associated arthritis), or as an upper airways disease (due to granulomas in the nasal cavity).

Granuloma
A mass of immune cells (lymphocytes, macrophages) that accumulates at sites of inflammation, injury, or infection.

There does not appear to be an association between HLA genes and GPA; however there is some evidence that there may be a genetic component to disease susceptibility involving the genes governing diversity of the F_c gamma receptor on neutrophils and the intracellular enzyme PTPN22, although the exact role of these molecules in the disease remains unclear.

There is good evidence that antibodies to proteinase 3 (PR3) are pathogenic and play a direct role in the disease process. Antibody titres in many patients show a direct relationship to disease activity. They are capable of binding to primed neutrophils and initiate a respiratory burst, which leads to degranulation and the release of proteolytic enzymes, which are capable of causing damage to surrounding tissues. These antibodies may also bind directly to endothelial cells and thus render them susceptible to damage by cell-mediated or complement-mediated cytotoxicity.

Patients with GPA are more likely to relapse compared to the other AAV. The laboratory investigations tend to show a C-ANCA pattern on immunofluorescence and antibodies to proteinase 3.

SELF-CHECK 6.1

What are the three areas of the body most commonly associated with granulomatosis with polyangiitis (GPA)?

6.4 Eosinophilic granulomatosis with polyangiitis (Churg–Strauss) (EGPA)

Eosiniphilic granulomatosis with polyangiitis (EGPA) is an eosinophilic rich and necrotizing systemic vasculitic disease of the small and medium arteries and capillaries. There is involvement of the respiratory tract and patients usually are seen with nasal polyps. Patients have late onset allergic rhinitis, asthma, and eosinophilia. To have EGPA patients must have increased levels of eosinophils in the blood and tissues. The vasculitic involvement in EGPA can lead to presentation of skin nodules or purpura and mononeuritis multiplex where patients have numbness, tingling, or sudden loss of strength in the hands and feet. Cardiac involvement is also common.

Approximately 25% of patients without renal disease are ANCA positive and 75% of patients with renal disease are ANCA positive. Patients are more likely to have ANCA if renal involvement is glomerulonephritis (100% if documented necrotizing glomerulonephritis).

EGPA is a rare disease with an incidence of approximately 2 cases per million people in the United Kingdom. Similar to the other AAV, EGPA is found in older age groups with an average age of 50, although the disease can occur at any age, though very rarely in children. Again there is an equal sex distribution and it is found commonly in both Caucasian and Oriental races.

Generally in laboratory investigation patients have a P-ANCA on immunofluorescence with antibodies to myeloperoxidase (MPO).

6.5 Anti-GBM disease (Goodpasture's syndrome)

Anti-GBM disease is a vasculitic syndrome that affects either the glomerular capillaries of the kidney or the pulmonary capillaries of the lung or both. Goodpasture's syndrome is the term used when there is both renal and lung involvement. There is an immune complex formation, as autoantibodies bind to the α3 chain of type IV collagen.

It has two peaks of occurrence, one in the twenties and thirties and a second in patients over the age of sixty. Although there is some evidence of pre-presentation disease, it is usually seen as an acute presentation, more often than not when the patient has overt kidney failure.

There is a clear genetic association in that approximately 75% of patients are HLA-DR 2 positive (compared to 25% of the normal population). The disease rarely occurs before the onset of puberty and there does not seem to be a sex-bias in its distribution.

Although it has long been regarded as an autoantibody-mediated disease and the transfer of immunoglobulin from an affected individual can transfer disease in animal models, only a mild inflammation is seen. It requires the additional transfer of T cells or a T cell reactive peptide from the glomerular basement membrane to initiate a disease that resembles that seen in humans.

SELF-CHECK 6.2

What is another name for Goodpasture's syndrome?

6.6 Membranous nephropathy (MN)

Membranous nephropathy is a slow, progressive kidney disease in which there is an immune complex formation in the glomerulus, resulting in deposits in the glomerular basement membrane and complement activation. The disease affects mainly Caucasians between the age of 30 and 50, presenting with proteinuria, oedema, and with or without renal failure.

There are two types of MN—primary or idiopathic, and secondary. 85% of cases of MN are idiopathic, i.e. of unknown cause; however, recently in 75% of these cases antibodies to m-type phospholipase A2 receptor (PLA2R) have been described. MN can be secondary to autoimmune diseases (SLE), infections (Syphilis, Hepatitis B and C), drugs (NSAIDs) and tumours (lung and colon). There is a genetic association in primary MN to HLA DQA1 and PLA2R1 genes.

Recently, antibodies have been described to the m-type phospholipase A2 receptor (PLA2R) in 75% of cases of primary MN. Presence of these antibodies enables clinicians to differentiate between primary/idiopathic MN and secondary MN. Higher levels of antibodies to PLA2R are linked to active disease and patients are at a much increased risk of a decline in renal function. It is useful for clinicians to have confirmation that the MN is of primary type, as patients benefit from early treatment and may avoid unnecessary biopsy for type II.

6.7 Pathogenesis of renal related auto-antibodies

There are a number of in vitro and in vivo studies which strongly support the role of ANCA in the pathogenesis of ANCA-associated vasculitis. It is believed that ANCA are able to activate neutrophils and, together with the alternative components of complement, can lead to the lysis of the endothelium resulting in vasculitis. The successful treatment of the autoimmune vasculitides with Rituximab, successfully depleting B cells and removing ANCA from the circulation, demonstrates the importance of ANCA in the pathogenesis of these diseases.

There are well defined in vivo experiments to determine the role of MPO antibodies in GPA. Scientists immunized MPO-deficient mice with murine MPO, causing the mice to produce anti-murine MPO antibodies. Taking spleen cells or IgG from these mice and transferring these into immunocompromised or healthy mice leads to a pauci-immune necrotizing crescentic or focal crescentic glomerulonephritis respectively. The production of granulomas requires the presence of both neutrophils and alternative pathway complement components. Adding lipopolysaccharide (LPS) usually found in bacterial cell walls, as well as transferring IgG from these mice, enhances the response.

The association with *Staphylococcus aureus* and gram negative bacteria remains. It is thought that initial ANCA induction and disease expression is due to molecular mimicry; however, further study is required in this area.

There is a single case recorded of the passive transfer of anti-MPO antibodies from a mother with an MPO-associated vasculitis to her child resulting in a case of neonatal vasculitis.

There is not yet an animal model available for in vivo experiments of the role of PR3 ANCA, but in approximately 50% of cases of persisting GPA, ANCA is not detectable. This suggests that there are cellular mechanisms associated with disease activity. There is a strong association with $CD4^+$ T cells which produce IL-17, linked with granulomatous inflammation in the lesions. The role of the cellular immune response is important, as ANCA are not always detectable in patients with active disease. Patients are monitored for the presence of MPO and PR3 and there does seem to be some relationship with an increase in PR3 antibodies and relapse.

There is strong evidence that both antibodies to GBM and PLA2R are pathogenic and there are links in both cases to antibody concentration and disease activity. The binding of antibodies to both the glomerular basement membrane and to phospholipase A2 receptors leads to neutrophil stimulation and complement activation.

Antibodies to PLA2R have been shown to be mainly of IgG4 subclass, which should not be able to activate complement; however, there is evidence of complement activation and presence of the membrane attack complex. Patients with Membranous nephropathy have undetectable levels of C1q—therefore, similarly to the pathogenesis of ANCA, it is thought that complement is activated through the alternative pathway. Cellular mechanisms are also thought to be required.

6.8 Treatment and prognosis of autoimmune renal disease

In all of the autoimmune vasculitides, prognosis is poor if the disease is left untreated, with one year mortality as high as 80–90%. With current treatments, the prognosis is much more positive, with a 90% survival rate at one year. Only 14% of the deaths in AAV are disease related, with approximately 60% of deaths linked to side-effects of treatment, particularly due to infection.

The British Society for Rheumatology (BSR) and British Health Professions in Rheumatology (BHPR) published guidelines in 2013 for the management of adults with ANCA-associated vasculitis which are based on the 2009 EULAR recommendations (see Table 6.2).

The treatment of AAV is divided into induction of remission and maintenance. Unfortunately the most effective therapy to reliably induce remission is cyclophosphamide. This is relatively contraindicated in younger individuals who have not completed their family, because of the impact on fertility. Other therapies, such as rituximab have recently been licensed and approved by NICE for such patients. This highlights the importance of both the antibody and autoreactive B cells in the pathogenesis of disease.

To treat GBM disease, the first step is plasma exchange to remove the pathogenic antibody. Usually there is an exchange of 60ml/kg (max 4L) for 14 days or until the anti-GBM antibodies are undetectable. Then to prevent further antibody production, the patient is then immunosuppressed with cyclophosphamide, 2mg/kg daily. The dosage may be reduced if the patient is elderly or on dialysis. This is usually discontinued after 3 months. Then for the next 6 months, prednisolone is given as 1mg/kg daily (max 60mg), tapering weekly in order to reduce any tissue inflammation.

Primary membranous nephropathy is similarly a steroid responsive disease (analogous to AAV). There is now good evidence that patients with high titre of PLA2Rc antibody at diagnosis have a potentially worse outcome than those with lower titre. Persistent positivity of autoantibody is associated with disease progression, therefore patients are usually treated with steroids and/or cyclophosphamide until they both clinically and immunologically remit. At this point immune suppression may be withdrawn, thus the surrogate test is extremely important in management.

In cases of secondary membranous nephropathy, the treatment is of the underlying cause.

TABLE 6.2 EULAR recommendations for therapy of vasculitis.

DISEASE CATEGORY	RECOMMENDED THERAPY
REMISSION INDUCTION	
Early systemic/localized	Methotrexate + steroids
Generalized	Cyclophosphamide + steroids
Severe systemic	Adjunct: plasma exchange
MAINTENANCE THERAPY	Low dose steroids
	+ azathioprine
	or leflunomide
	or methotrexate

6.9 Auto-antibodies in autoimmune kidney diseases

There are a number of autoantibodies that are measured in the Clinical Immunology laboratory. This is still an area that relies on technical expertise for reading and interpreting patterns of immunofluorescence when screening for ANCA, in addition to the more automated techniques for confirmation of specific antibodies. ANCA testing is one of the few areas in Clinical Immunology that is considered an urgent test and many laboratories still offer an ANCA on-call service for weekends and bank holidays in departments that are not yet integrated into a seven-day working pattern.

6.9.1 Anti-neutrophil cytoplasmic antibodies (ANCA)

The first described technique for the detection of anti-neutrophil cytoplasmic antibodies (ANCA) was indirect immunofluorescence (IIF) using alcohol-fixed human granulocytes as a substrate. This is still a commonly used methodology in clinical laboratories today. Using alcohol as a fixative, most positive sera give one of two patterns. These are termed c-ANCA (classical or cytoplasmic) and p-ANCA (perinuclear). If you look at Figures 6.2 and 6.3, you can see examples of these patterns on IIF.

The main antigenic target for c-ANCA is proteinase 3 (PR3) and for p-ANCA the antigenic target is myeloperoxidase (MPO). The differentiation between staining patterns is, in fact, an artefact of fixation since in vivo both myeloperoxidase (MPO) and proteinase 3 (PR3) are found in the cytoplasmic granules. If the cells are fixed with an alternative fixative such as formalin, then no difference in pattern is seen between anti-PR3 and anti-MPO.

Initially the reactive antigens were unknown and it was noted that c-ANCA was found more commonly in GPA (Wegener's granulomatosis) and that p-ANCA was more common in other forms of systemic vasculitis such as microscopic polyangiitis. In time it was reported that anti-PR3 corresponded to c-ANCA and that anti-MPO corresponded with p ANCA. However,

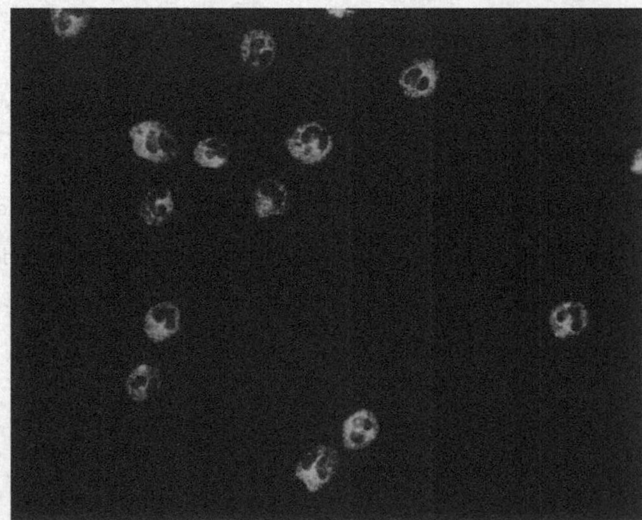

Figure 6.2
Cytoplasmic c-ANCA staining pattern on neutrophils fixed with ethanol.

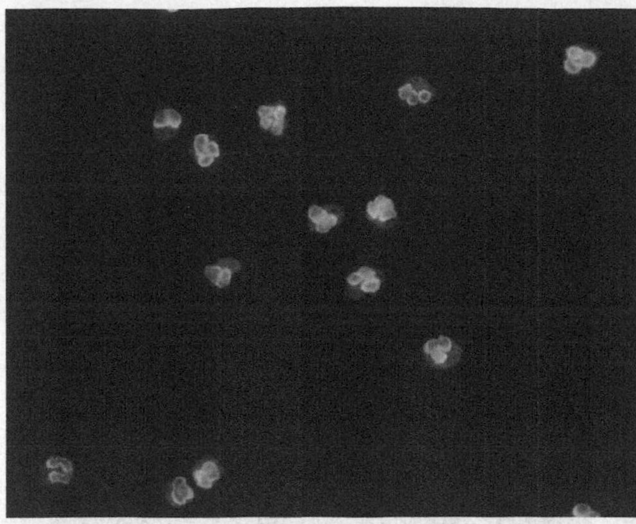

Figure 6.3
Perinuclear p-ANCA staining pattern on neutrophils fixed with ethanol.

although this relationship holds true in most patients, it is possible to find sera which give a p-ANCA on immunofluorescence that react with PR3 and c-ANCA sera which react with MPO. In addition, some patients show 'mixed' patterns and demonstrate positivity to both MPO and PR3. It is therefore unwise to assign specificity to the anti-neutrophil cytoplasmic antibodies based on their immunofluorescent staining pattern.

Additional antibodies have been described which react with a p-ANCA or 'p-ANCA like' pattern on IIF and which do not react with MPO. These patterns have been classified by some investigators as atypical ANCA (a-ANCA or x-ANCA). Look at Figure 6.4 to see an example of an atypical ANCA. It is often difficult in the routine laboratory to differentiate these from a classical p-ANCA on immunofluorescence. Antibodies which may give these 'p-ANCA like' patterns on IIF include those directed against BPI, cathepsin G, lactoferrin, and elastase. These other antibodies have been linked to inflammatory bowel disease and ulcerative colitis—however, these varieties of antigens are not correlated with any features of disease.

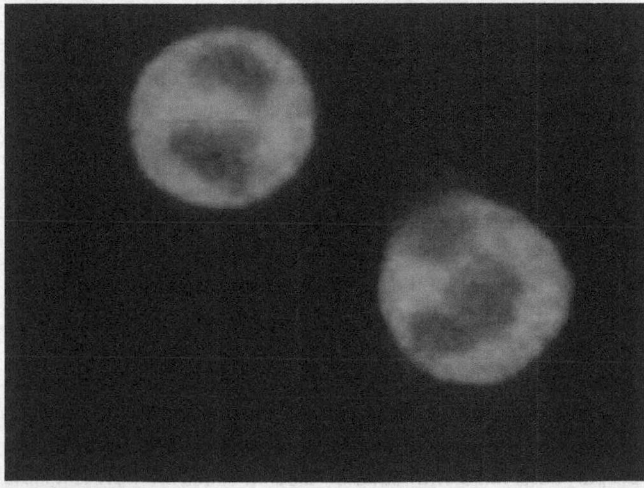

Figure 6.4
Atypical ANCA.

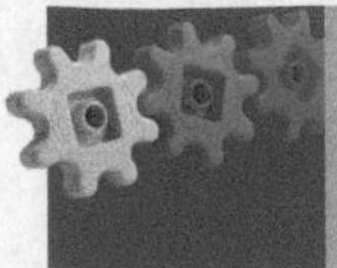

METHOD 6.1 *Fixation of neutrophils as a substrate for immunofluorescence*

The **fixative** used for human neutrophils as a substrate is important in the determination of the immunofluorescent pattern. There are two commonly used fixatives—ethanol and formalin.

When human neutrophils are fixed with ethanol, the ethanol causes the **cationic** neutrophil granule proteins, which include MPO and lactoferrin, to migrate to the negatively charged nuclear membrane. This produces the artefact of fixation, the p-ANCA pattern. The PR3 granules are not cationic and therefore do not migrate. This produces the granular pattern seen in c-ANCA as these granules remain in the cytoplasm of the neutrophils. Ethanol fixation is the most commonly used method in the clinical laboratory and is recommended by the international consensus on ANCA diagnosis. It enables the two patterns to be distinguished, allowing screening to determine the need for further confirmation using assays specific for the detection of MPO and PR3.

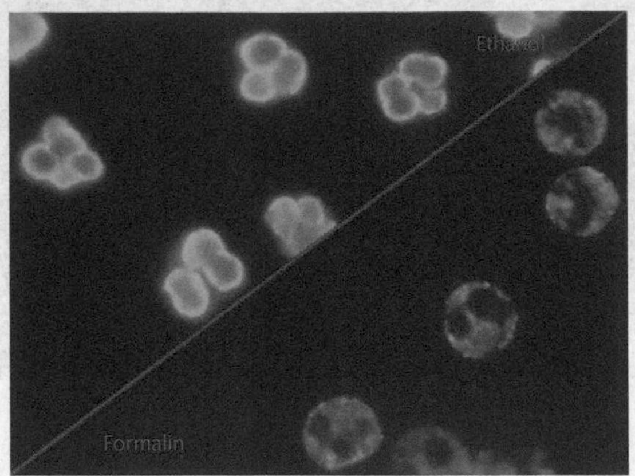

Figure 6.5
Perinuclear p-ANCA staining pattern on neutrophils fixed with both ethanol and formalin.

Historically, formalin fixation was used to enable the scientist to determine whether the p-ANCA pattern seen on ethanol slides was caused by the staining of MPO, or whether this was due to other interfering antibodies such as anti-nuclear antibodies (ANA). This was more commonly used before assays were available for specific testing with the level of sensitivity and specificity currently available. When formalin is used as the fixative, all granules are fixed into the cytoplasm of the neutrophil, therefore both p-ANCA and c-ANCA have the same granular appearance of immunofluorescence. Look at Figure 6.5 to see the difference between a p-ANCA pattern on the two fixatives.

Fixative
A compound (such as ethanol or formaldehyde) that preserves or stabilizes tissues and cells for microscopic study.

Cationic
Referring to a positively charged molecule.

As the neutrophil has a multi-lobed nucleus, it is to be expected that anti-nuclear antibodies will also be detected on immunofluorescence, as well as antibodies to other cellular structures. It can be difficult to distinguish the presence of anti-nuclear antibodies, especially in a homogenous pattern from a true p-ANCA. Look at Figure 6.6 to see what a homogenous pattern ANA looks like on a neutrophil. Experienced immunofluorescence readers can often determine the presence of an ANA, or, if it is clinically necessary, the ANA screening assay can be tested in conjunction with all ANCA testing to control for this.

Alternatively some people have suggested that instead of using a pure neutrophil suspension, a whole white cell suspension which contains lymphocytes should be used for IIF testing. The lymphocytes will act as a control since they will be stained by ANA but will not react with ANCA antigens since lymphocytes do not contain the specific enzymes. However whilst these approaches may help in the differentiation between a pure ANA and a pure p-ANCA, it is likely they will be of little use in the cases where both sets of antibodies coexist. Therefore many scientists have taken the pragmatic approach of testing all positive sera for specific antibodies thus reducing the risk that positive sera will be missed due to the misinterpretation of the immunofluorescent pattern. Commercial preparations for immunofluorescence are varied, but the majority are neutrophil preparations fixed with ethanol. Biochip slides are now available

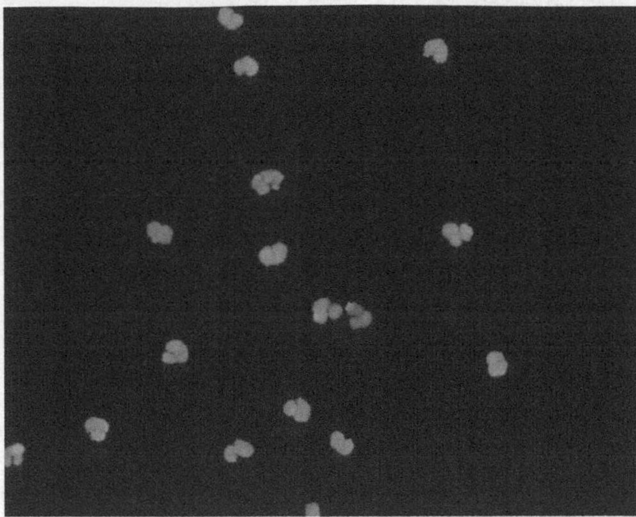

Figure 6.6
Homogenous ANA staining of human neutrophils.

which can contain a mixture of substrates on one slide such as neutrophils fixed by ethanol and formalin, purified preparations of myeloperoxidase and proteinase 3, and HEp-2 cells for the detection of anti-nuclear antibodies. These preparations, whilst more expensive, can provide more information at the screening stage, reducing the amount of confirmatory testing required.

Cross reference
You can read in more detail about anti-nuclear antibodies and the tests performed in Chapter 5.

Whilst indirect immunofluorescence was the original technique for the detection of ANCA, the advent of assay systems for the detection of specific antibodies has reduced their importance in arriving at the final characterization of the antibody. The primary usage in the clinical laboratory of IIF tests is for screening purposes, to exclude negative samples from further testing.

It has been reported that some antibodies to PR3 may give a negative result on IIF. These are usually seen in patients with GPA (Wegener's) who are undergoing treatment. However, this should be borne in mind and in cases where there is a high suspicion of disease it may be justified to measure both MPO and PR3 even if the immunofluorescence is negative.

6.9.2 Anti-proteinase 3 (PR3)

Proteinase 3 (PR3) is a multifunctional protein found in the primary granules of neutrophils, as well as in other phagocytic cells. It is a serine protease enzyme. Antibodies to PR3 are most commonly found in >95% of GPA (Wegener's granulomatosis) cases. It has been reported, however, that this frequency may depend on the extent of the disease. In patients where the granulomatosis disease is restricted to the nasal cavity or another single organ (e.g. the eye), the frequency of positivity may be as low as 10%, whereas in patients with systemic and renal involvement the frequency will exceed 90%. Antibodies to PR3 may also be found in other forms of systemic vasculitis and in systemic infections, although the frequencies in these diseases are low.

Levels of anti-PR3 correlate in many patients with disease activity and thus can be used as a surrogate marker on which to monitor therapeutic needs. However this relationship is not clear. It has been reported that patients with persistently positive anti-PR3 levels are more likely to suffer clinical relapse, and that the change from negative to positive anti-PR3 also has a high risk of predicting relapse, but that changes in level can be seen in many patients without any change in clinical activity.

Antibodies to PR3 produce a cytoplasmic staining pattern (c-ANCA) when tested by indirect immunofluorescence on ethanol-fixed or formalin-fixed granulocytes. It should however be noted that this pattern-specificity association occurs in only 90–95% of sera and that some p-ANCAs can be due to anti-PR3. Look at Figure 6.2 to see the c-ANCA pattern on neutrophils.

6.9.3 Anti-myeloperoxidase (MPO)

Myeloperoxidase (MPO) is an enzyme found in the primary cytoplasmic granules of neutrophils, and is involved in peroxidation reactions within the cytoplasmic vacuoles associated with the killing of ingested micro-organisms.

Antibodies directed against MPO are found most commonly in microscopic polyangiitis (about 70–80% of patients). They are also associated with destruction of the glomeruli within the kidney in a condition termed rapidly progressive glomerulonephritis (RPGN). This may occur as part of a systemic vasculitis or in a form where the vasculitis is limited to the kidney.

Antibodies to MPO may also be found in GPA (approximately 5% of cases) and rarely in other forms of systemic vasculitis and autoimmune rheumatic diseases such as rheumatoid arthritis and SLE. In addition they have also been found in up to 20% of patients with Goodpasture's disease in conjunction with anti-GBM antibodies.

Antibodies to MPO produce a perinuclear-staining pattern (p-ANCA) when tested by indirect immunofluorescence on ethanol-fixed granulocytes. This is an artefact caused by the fixation process and if other fixatives are used, e.g. formaldehyde or formalin, then antibodies to MPO give the same staining pattern as those to PR3. This differential staining pattern may be of limited use in classifying the reactive antibody on indirect immunofluorescent testing. It should however be noted that this pattern-specificity association occurs in only 90–95% of sera and that some p-ANCAs can be due to anti-PR3, whilst some c-ANCAs can be due to anti-MPO. Look at Figure 6.3 to see the p-ANCA pattern on neutrophils.

Cross reference

The international guidelines for ANCA testing can be found in Savige et al. (1999, 2003).

Key Point

The international guidelines on ANCA testing recommend that antibodies to PR3, MPO, and GBM be tested on all patients in whom a diagnosis of MPA, GPA, EGPA, or anti-GBM disease is suspected.

Anti-PR3 and anti-MPO can be measured specifically using a number of different systems including ELISA, chemiluminescence, and addressable bead laser immunoassay (ALBIA). Each of these techniques relies on the coating of the purified antigen to a solid phase, the subsequent binding of circulating antibodies, and the detection of these bound antibodies using a labelled **conjugate**. All of these systems are capable of producing assay systems which will give clinically valid results. The most critical aspect of these assays is probably the integrity of the antigen and it has been noted that PR3 in particular is prone to degradation, which affects its antigenicity. The effect of this on assay systems can be seen by studies which have shown considerable variation in the frequency of these antibodies in a group of patients with clinically defined GPA. This is an important aspect of the selection of an assay for clinical use, as a poorly reactive antigen will lead to false negative results.

Conjugate

The term generally used to describe an immunoglobulin that has a marker attached, such as an immunofluorescent label or an enzyme. These immunoglobulins are used to label human antibodies in techniques such as IIF or ELISA.

In addition to this aspect, anti-PR3 ELISA assays have been formulated in two different ways. Most commonly these assays use a direct binding format where the antigen is bound directly to the surface of the plate. Some assays, however, use a sandwich format where monoclonal antibodies are bound to the plate and antigen subsequently bound to these via the antigen binding sites. It has been argued that these assays present the antigen in a different plane and thus different epitopes are visible to the circulating antibodies. Studies comparing these two formats of assays have indicated that capture ELISAs may be more sensitive in relation to diagnosis and more informative in relation to the monitoring of disease activity.

SELF-CHECK 6.3

What specificities of ANCA are associated with systemic vasculitic syndromes?

SELF-CHECK 6.4

Why is it important to test for ANCA and anti-GBM urgently in patients presenting with acute kidney failure?

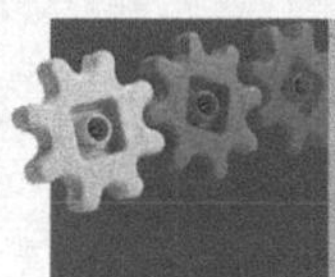

METHOD 6.2 Methods used in detecting autoantibodies in autoimmune kidney diseases

ANCA screen

- Indirect immunofluorescence using ethanol-fixed human granulocytes.
- Indirect immunofluorescence using formalin-fixed human granulocytes.

Anti-PR3

- ELISA using biochemically pure proteinase 3 or recombinant protein using either direct or capture ELISA methodology.
- Chemiluminescence using biochemically pure proteinase 3.
- Dot or line blotting using purified or recombinant antigens.
- Western blotting using cell homogenates.
- Addressable bead immunoassay using purified or recombinant antigens.

Anti-MPO

- ELISA using biochemically pure MPO.
- FPIA using biochemically pure MPO.
- Dot or line blotting using purified MPO.
- Western blotting using cell homogenates.
- Addressable bead immunoassay using purified MPO.

Anti-GBM

- ELISA using biochemically pure antigen.
- Chemiluminescence using biochemically pure antigen.
- Dot or line blotting using purified antigen.
- Addressable bead immunoassay using purified antigen.

Anti-PLA2R

- ELISA using recombinant phospholipase A2 receptors.
- Indirect immunofluorescence using human cell line HEK293 expressing phospholipase A2 receptors.

There are many different commercial preparations available for the detection and identification of these antibodies. The variations in technology and in the antigen sources can lead to discrepancies in the results obtained between different technologies. It is often common practice to use more than one technique in the clinical laboratory to confirm the presence of these antibodies, due to the clinical importance of the result.

6.9.4 Anti-glomerular basement membrane (GBM) antibodies

Autoantigen
A self-antigen that is the target of an immune response, such as in autoimmune disease.

Anti-GBM antibodies can be detected by indirect immunofluorescence using primate kidney sections as a substrate. The major problem with this technique is that it is well recognized that a number of potential **autoantigens** exist within the glomerular basement membrane and using IIF it is not possible to differentiate between them. Given that only one of these antigens is associated with Goodpasture's syndrome, this leads to the possibility that positive reactions may be assigned to non-Goodpasture's antigen reactivity. It is therefore sensible that IIF testing only be regarded, at best, as a preliminary screen to eliminate negative sera prior to more extensive testing on more specific systems. This is no longer a practice that is common in the routine clinical laboratory. There are a number of systems available for the detection of antibodies specific to the alpha-5 chain of type IV collagen—these include ELISA, chemiluminescence, and immunoblot techniques. It is standard practice to use more than one technique in the laboratory to confirm the presence of anti-GBM antibodies, due to the clinical importance of these results.

Anti-glomerular basement membrane (GBM) antibodies are strongly associated with a form of severe rapidly progressive kidney vasculitis known as Goodpasture's disease. There is some evidence that the antibodies are more closely associated with the kidney disease, as they are rarely seen in patients with lung haemorrhage alone.

Anti-GBM antibodies can be found in association with anti-myeloperoxidase (MPO) antibodies (approximately 20% of cases), and occasionally with anti-proteinase 3 (PR3) antibodies. The antigenic target of anti-GBM is the alpha-3 chain of collagen type IV. Anti-GBM antibodies in the absence of Goodpasture's disease are reactive with other epitopes found on the alpha-3 chain of type IV collagen, the other alpha chains, entactin, and laminin.

False positive antibodies are most commonly found in sera from patients with other autoimmune diseases and in chronic inflammatory diseases. It is estimated that approximately 1% of normal sera may contain antibodies to these non-Goodpasture's antigens. Because of this it is important that when assessing an assay for anti-GBM antibodies, close attention is paid to the nature of the antigen and that appropriate control groups are used to determine the specificity of the assay.

Since prognosis is closely associated with prompt diagnosis and treatment, requests for anti-GBM antibodies are usually urgent and positive results should be notified to the requesting clinician as soon as possible.

6.9.5 Phospholipase A2 receptor (PLA2R) antibodies

Phospholipase A2 receptor (PLA2R) antibodies are a novel antibody in the Clinical Immunology laboratory. As noted earlier in Section 6.6, these antibodies are important in determining whether a membranous nephropathy is due to either a primary or secondary cause. This information is critical to the clinician as treatment options differ depending on the cause.

Antibodies to PLA2R are directed against a type 1 transmembrane receptor expressed on the surface of podocytes. The function of these receptors on podocytes is unknown.

There are two commercial assays currently available for the clinical laboratory—a standard ELISA preparation and an immunofluorescent technique. A recombinant cell-based indirect immunofluorescent assay is available using HEK293 human cells which express PLA 2 receptors. Both assays can be used to determine both the presence of antibodies and their concentration using titration. The ELISA assay gives a more accurate result for the concentration of antibodies present, with sensitivity and specificity greater than 95%, and tends to be more financially viable. The immunofluorescent technique requires a high level of expertise in the reader.

Titration of the antibodies is of clinical importance, as levels of circulating antibody correlate well with disease activity and clinical outcome.

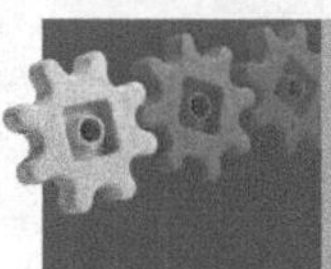

METHOD 6.3 Quality control of assays for the detection of antibodies in autoimmune kidney disease

For ANCA screening on neutrophils and the detection of antibodies to MPO, PR3, and GBM there is an established NEQAS scheme.

There is no current NEQAS scheme for PLA2R antibodies. To overcome the need for an external quality control scheme under the ISO15189 criteria, many Clinical Immunology laboratories participate in a sample exchange scheme with other laboratories offering this test.

Quality control protocols should be determined in light of the recommendations within the 2003 Addendum to the International Consensus Statement. Internal quality control samples should be regularly tested for all patterns including atypical and staff should be regularly monitored for their ability to recognize all patterns including those rarer ones. Regular competency testing of slide readers is important to ensure competence and consistency of manual interpretation of both antibody pattern and concentration.

It is important that quality control material assesses the assay at the point of determination, the cut-off point of the assay, and not just using material of strong positivity. This should be taken into consideration when determining the uncertainty of measurement of the assay.

The screening dilution for ANCA testing is not standardized in the UK and is determined by the commercial preparations. More commonly, companies now provide kits for immunofluorescence containing substrates and conjugates that have been optimized for use. If a laboratory is using substrates and conjugates from separate sources, a chequerboard must be performed for each lot number of reagents received to ensure that the sample and conjugate dilutions are optimized.

There have been documented issues with the quality of fixation of commercial neutrophil preparations resulting in the misidentification of ANCA patterns on immunofluorescence. Laboratories should account for this during batch testing procedures by using a known library of antibody patterns.

Laboratories should have a standardized gating protocol for which patterns are reflexed for further testing. This should include both typical and atypical patterns.

Ultimately when performing immunofluorescent assays, it is important to take into account the volume of samples passing through your laboratory services and whether you have the staff skill mix and expertise to maintain the competency to perform these assays. There are a number of automated technologies to perform the specific autoantibody assays such as MPO, PR3, and GBM, as described in Method 6.2.

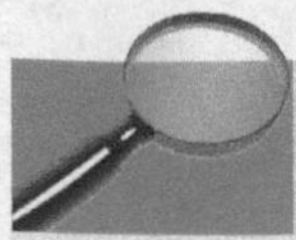

CASE STUDY 6.1 Pulmonary renal syndrome

Patient history

A 47-year-old female was seen in clinic, presenting with a three-week history of lethargy, dyspnoea (shortness of breath), cough, **haemoptysis** (coughing up blood), and dark urine. She did not have any chest pain or other cardio-respiratory symptoms. She had no recent history of infection or fever. She had no classical risk factors for venous thromboembolism. Patient was a smoker.

Results (1)

- Hypertensive: 161/92
- Peripheral oedema
- Crepitations throughout both lung fields
- No lymphadenopathy, rash, scleritis, arthritis, synovitis, or ENT findings
- Haemoglobin LOW 8.4
- WBC normal range
- Urea HIGH 40 (NR 2.5–7.8 mmol/L)
- Creatinine HIGH 580 (NR 55–110 μmol/L)
- Raised CRP
- Urinalysis
    - Blood + + +
    - Protein + + + +

Significance of results (1)

The patient appears to have a vasculitis which is affecting both lungs and kidneys. The urea and creatinine levels are consistent with renal failure, supported by high levels of blood and protein in the urine.

Results (2)

- ANA negative
- C3 1.59 (NR 0.7–1.7 g/L), C4 0.27 (NR 0.16–0.54 g/L)
- Rheumatoid factor negative
- Cryoglobulin negative
- ANCA IIF and ELISA negative
- Anti-GBM positive: titre 201 iu/ml (NR <25)

Significance of results (2)

The GBM antibodies were confirmed to target the a5 chain of type IV collagen using a commercial immunoblot.

Presence of anti-GBM antibodies suggests diagnosis of anti-GBM disease.

The patient had a renal biopsy to confirm this diagnosis.

Treatment (1)

- Commenced haemodialysis
- Daily plasma exchange for 14 days
- Pulsed i.v. cyclophosphamide
- High dose oral corticosteroids

Treatment reduced the titration of anti-GBM antibodies.

- Then converted to azathioprine (borderline positivity)

Weaned from all immunosuppression after 9 months (sustained negativity).

Patient eventually went on to receive a live donor transplanted kidney following smoking cessation.

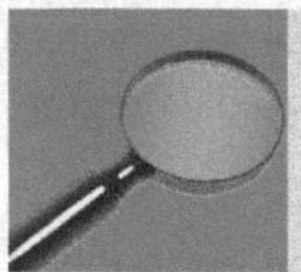

CASE STUDY 6.2 ANCA: Anti-neutrophil cytoplasmic antibodies

Patient history

A 57-year-old man presented to A&E with a three-week history of fever, fatigue, muscle pain, night sweats, and a weight loss of 6kg. On admission it was noted that his urine contained blood and a chest X-ray showed evidence of lung granuloma formation.

Results (1)

- Creatinine borderline raised 115 (NR 55–110 μmol/L)
- Urea raised 12 (NR 2.5–7.8 mmol/L)
- ANCA immunofluorescence showed a positive (+ + +) c-ANCA pattern
- Anti-MPO 3 (NR <25U/ml)
- Anti-PR3 167 (NR <25U/ml)
- Anti-GBM 2 (NR <25U/ml)

Significance of results (1)

The raised urea and creatinine are suggestive of renal failure, supported by the blood in his urine.

The c-ANCA seen on immunofluorescence is confirmed as anti-PR3. Antibodies to PR3 are associated with granulomatosis with polyangiitis (MPA) formerly known as Wegener's granulomatosis. This is consistent with the lung granuloma formation seen on X-ray and **haematuria**.

Haematuria
Blood in urine.

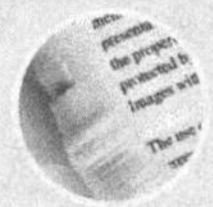

Chapter summary

- ANCA-associated vasculitic syndromes, anti-GBM disease, and membranous nephropathy often present with similar symptoms. The laboratory findings are essential to direct diagnosis and treatment.
- Granulomatosis with polyangiitis (GPA; Wegener's granulomatosis) is a systemic vasculitic disease which predominantly affects the upper airways, lungs, and kidneys.
- Anti-proteinase 3 antibodies are usually associated with a c-ANCA pattern on indirect immunofluorescence and are found most commonly in GPA.
- Microscopic polyangiitis (MPA) is a systemic vasculitic disease of small arteries and capillaries.

- Anti-myeloperoxidase antibodies are usually associated with a p-ANCA on indirect immunofluorescence pattern and are found most commonly in MPA and rapidly progressive glomerulonephritis (RPGN).
- Eosinophilic granulomatosis with polyangiitis (EGPA; Churg–Strauss) is an eosinophilic rich and necrotizing systemic vasculitic disease of the small and medium arteries and capillaries.
- EGPA is usually associated with anti-MPO antibodies and p-ANCA.
- In anti-GBM disease, kidney survival is directly related to the time between disease onset and the commencement of treatment.
- Anti-GBM antibodies are found in patients with anti-GBM disease.
- PLA2R antibodies are important in determining whether the cause of membranous nephropathy is primary or secondary, which enables the clinician to target treatment effectively.

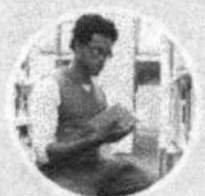

Further reading

- **Jennette JC *et al.* (2013) *Revised International Chapel Hill Consensus Conference Nomenclature of Vasculitides*. *Arthritis Rheum*, 65 (1), 1–11.**
- **Savige J *et al.* (1999) *International consensus statement on testing and reporting of antineutrophil cytoplasmic antibodies (ANCA)*. *Am J Clin Pathol*, 111, 507–13.**
- **Savige J *et al.* (2003) *Addendum to the international consensus statement on testing and reporting of antineutrophil antibodies*. *Am J Clin Pathol*, 130, 312–8.**

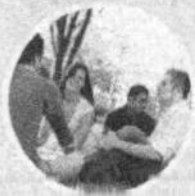

Discussion questions

6.1 Describe the methods for detection of antibodies in autoimmune kidney disease and comment on their relative advantages and disadvantages.

6.2 Describe the symptoms and laboratory findings associated with ANCA and anti-GBM related diseases.

6.3 Describe the evidence that suggests that MPO and PR3 antibodies may play a role in the pathogenesis of ANCA-associated vasculitis.

6.4 How are PLA2R antibodies tested and how do they assist the clinical diagnosis?

6.5 Describe the treatments and prognosis for the ANCA-associated vasculitides.

Answers to self-check questions are provided in the book's Online Resource Centre.

Visit www.oxfordtextbooks.co.uk/orc/hall2e

7

Organ-specific autoimmunity

Learning Objectives

After studying this chapter you should be able to:

- outline the common features of organ-specific autoimmune diseases
- explain the clinical features of the organ-specific autoimmune diseases
- outline the assays and techniques used to test for organ-specific autoimmune diseases
- discuss the limitations of these techniques
- outline the treatment of organ-specific autoimmune diseases.

Introduction

During development the body learns what is 'self' and either eliminates any immune cells recognizing 'self' or turns them off, a process called tolerance.

Cross reference

You can read in more detail about the mechanisms of tolerance in a core immunology textbook, such as Murphy (2011), Male et al. (2012), or Owen et al. (2013).

You should note that not all self-reactive mechanisms are eliminated but in normal circumstances are strictly controlled. There are a number of situations where self-reactivity is useful. These include tumour surveillance and clearing infection. A good example of the latter function is the presence of 'natural' IgM antibodies (coded by germline genes) which recognize apoptotic cell-associated molecular patterns on cell surfaces resulting in deposition of complement and the phagocytosis of the apoptotic cell.

For convenience, autoimmune diseases can be broken down into those that are organ specific and organ non-specific, the latter also being referred to as systemic autoimmune diseases. This division is more apparent than real as many patients have diseases from both categories. This chapter focuses on some of the more common diseases which are related to specific organs within the body.

Cross reference

You can find more examples of organ-specific autoimmune diseases in Chapter 8.

In order to develop autoimmune disease three criteria need to be fulfilled. Firstly, the patient needs to be genetically susceptible to the disease. Often there are associations between a

Human leukocyte antigen (HLA)
A genetically determined series of markers (antigens) present on human white blood cells (leukocytes) and on tissues that are important in histocompatibility.

Cross reference
You can read in more detail about the structure and function of the major histocompatability complex and HLA in Chapter 13 of this book and in the *Transfusion and Transplantation Science* textbook of the OUP series.

Epitope
The region on an antigen that is recognizable by the immune system.

Cytokine
Proteins produced by cells of the immune system that act as regulatory proteins and intercellular mediators facilitating the immune response.

Cross reference
For an example of pathogenic auto-antibody see anti-TSH receptor, and for a marker auto-antibody see anti-thyroglobulin antibody in Section 7.1.

particular disease and specific **human leukocyte antigen (HLA)** genes. This is because in order to develop autoimmune T cell or T-dependent B cell responses, the antigen has to be 'seen'. Certain HLA haplotypes are required to allow presentation of the appropriate peptide, thus increasing the likelihood of that individual developing an autoreactive clone. Also within this sphere are endogenous factors such as hormone balance. Women are more often affected by autoimmune disorders than men. The exact mechanism is not yet understood but oestrogen appears to effect gene expression that alters the activation and survival of B cells, which in turn predisposes to the breaking of tolerance. Thus the higher oestrogen levels found in women may explain why women are more often affected by autoimmune disorders than men. Another factor that appears to play a part, at least in some autoimmune disorders, is 'X-inactivation'. Females, with two X-chromosomes (one maternal and one paternal), would expect to activate these at random and hence express them on a 50:50 basis. This is not always the case and in some disorders (e.g. autoimmune thyroid disease) there is evidence that one chromosome is utilized much more than the other. This skewing of expression might mean that X-linked antigens from the less activated chromosome are insufficiently expressed to induce tolerance.

Secondly, the patient requires some form of trigger to break tolerance. Often this trigger is unknown but infections are commonly thought to be involved. Evidence for this has been hard to acquire in humans. However, there are animal models that show an antibody response developing to a part of a protein in the virus (an **epitope**) can also react with a similar epitope on a native protein (sometimes called 'molecular mimicry'). A good example of molecular mimicry can be seen in rabbits immunized with a peptide derived from hepatitis B virus polymerase, which then develop a response to rabbit myelin basic protein and subsequent inflammation of the central nervous system. Finally, the patient requires an element of bad luck, as even identical twins brought up in the same environment do not always both get the disease. This is probably explained by splice variants (alternative splicing of genes resulting in multiple proteins, such that the same genetic code can still produce different protein phenotypes).

Autoimmune diseases are mediated in most cases by T cells. T cell responses are difficult to evaluate in the laboratory because there are no routine assays for T cell responses that equate directly to looking at the product of B cells (i.e. antibody). To assess specific T cell responses the isolated T cells must be incubated with stimulating antigen. Evidence of T cell stimulation is provided either by measurement of **cytokine** production (e.g. interferon) or, after several days, cell proliferation. Although there are assays that can determine the presence of T cells reactive to some infections, there are as yet no routinely available assays for autoimmune T cells. Therefore, we often have to rely on indirect evidence of autoimmunity. The presence of self-reactive antibodies (auto-antibodies) is a useful way of demonstrating autoimmunity. Sometimes the antibodies are directly pathogenic, that is, they cause the disease. Sometimes the antibody is just a 'marker': the presence of the antibody indicates autoimmunity without itself actually causing harm.

You should also be clear on the difference between autoimmune *phenomena* and autoimmune *disease*. Auto-antibodies may be detected in some members of the normal, healthy population. It is important, therefore, to interpret any laboratory findings carefully, taking note of the clinical context in which they are found. Also note that the transient appearance of auto-antibodies, particularly during and after a viral infection, is a common occurrence. Most patients do not go on to develop autoimmune disease, although some do. After the infection and associated cell destruction has been cleared, tolerance is re-established and the auto-antibodies again become undetectable. Where this balance is not restored the patient may go on to develop autoimmune disease. Those with persistent antibody on retesting are more likely to develop the associated autoimmune disease in the future.

In the rest of this chapter we will look in more detail at autoimmune diseases that involve a number of different organs: the thyroid gland, small intestine, stomach, pancreas, and adrenal glands. In each case we will consider the clinical features, the immunobiology of the disease and the laboratory tests which may be of help in the diagnosis or monitoring of the disease.

Key Points

- **Detection of auto-antibodies is not a guarantee of an autoimmune disease.**
- **Auto-antibodies are frequently an effect of autoimmune disease, not the cause.**

SELF-CHECK 7.1

What are the three requirements which need to be fulfilled to acquire an autoimmune disease?

7.1 Autoimmune thyroid disease

7.1.1 Thyroid function

To understand the different autoimmune thyroid diseases you must first understand the thyroid's central role in controlling metabolism. The thyroid gland produces hormones that are released into the bloodstream and affect most, if not all, organs and tissues in the body. These effects include the control of the rate at which the body utilizes energy, the growth and structure of bones, and sexual development.

Cross reference

For more information on the symptoms of thyroid disease see Clinical correlation 7.1.

In disease the thyroid may become overactive (**hyperthyroidism**) leading to a 'fast metabolism' or underactive (**hypothyroidism**) leading to a 'slow metabolism'.

Hyperthyroidism

Excessive production of thyroid hormones caused by overactivity of the thyroid gland.

Hypothyroidism

A reduction in the production of thyroid hormones caused by underactivity of the thyroid gland.

The production of thyroid hormones thyroxine (T_4) and triiodothyronine (T_3) are critical to thyroid function. Thyroxine is formed on tyrosine residues of a thyroid protein, thyroglobulin. Iodine is bound to tyrosine by the action of an enzyme (thyroid peroxidase, TPO). Two iodinated tyrosine residues are combined to make T_3 or T_4. Look at Figure 7.1 to see how the structures of tyrosine, T_3, and T_4 are related. Production of thyroid hormones is regulated by another

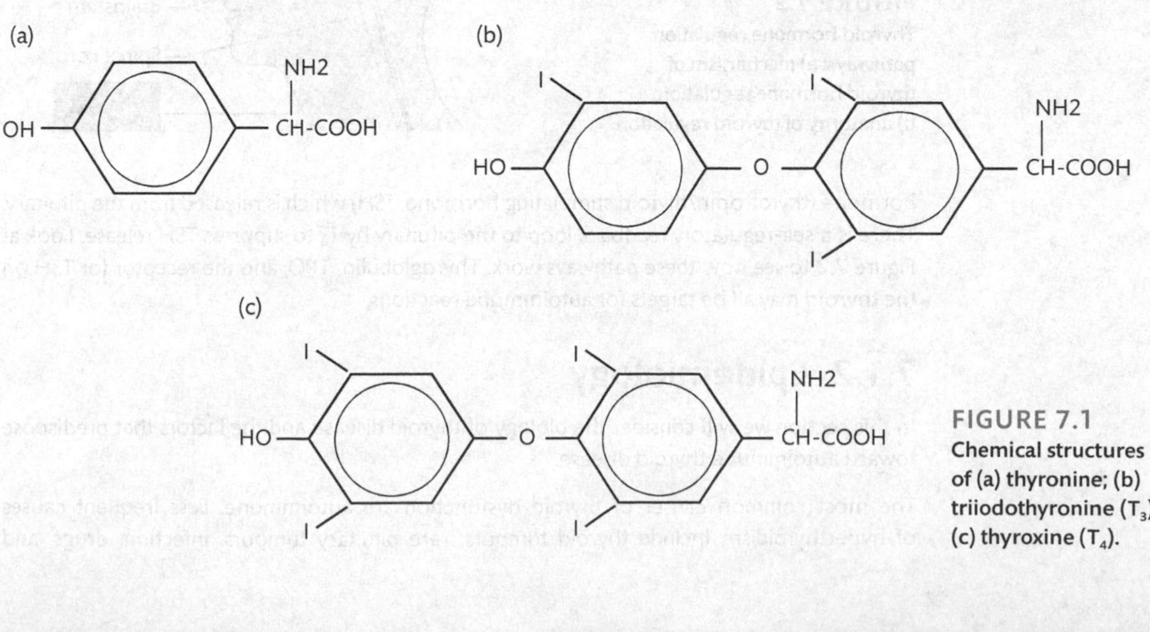

FIGURE 7.1 Chemical structures of (a) thyronine; (b) triiodothyronine (T_3); and (c) thyroxine (T_4).

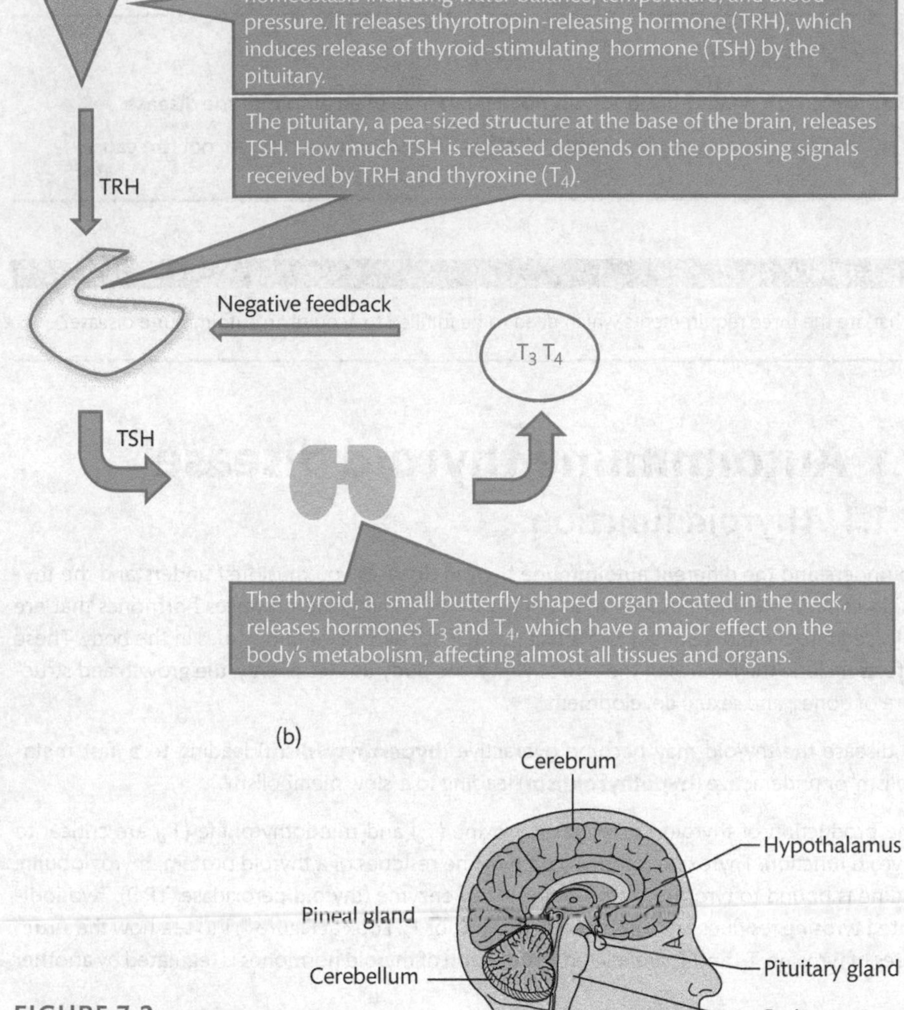

(a)
The hypothalamus, a small cone-shaped part of the brain, controls homeostasis including water balance, temperature, and blood pressure. It releases thyrotropin-releasing hormone (TRH), which induces release of thyroid-stimulating hormone (TSH) by the pituitary.
The pituitary, a pea-sized structure at the base of the brain, releases TSH. How much TSH is released depends on the opposing signals received by TRH and thyroxine (T_4).
TRH
Negative feedback
T_3 T_4
TSH
The thyroid, a small butterfly-shaped organ located in the neck, releases hormones T_3 and T_4, which have a major effect on the body's metabolism, affecting almost all tissues and organs.
(b)
Cerebrum
Hypothalamus
Pineal gland
Cerebellum
Pituitary gland
Brainstem
Spinal cord
Thyroid

FIGURE 7.2
Thyroid hormone regulation pathways: a) mechanism of thyroid hormone regulation; b) anatomy of thyroid regulation.

hormone (thyrotropin/thyroid stimulating hormone, TSH) which is released from the pituitary. There is a self-regulatory feedback loop to the pituitary by T_4 to suppress TSH release. Look at Figure 7.2 to see how these pathways work. Thyroglobulin, TPO, and the receptor for TSH on the thyroid may all be targets for autoimmune reactions.

7.1.2 Epidemiology

In this section we will consider the biology of thyroid disease and the factors that predispose toward autoimmune thyroid disease.

The most common causes of thyroid dysfunction are autoimmune. Less frequent causes of hyperthyroidism include thyroid tumours, rare pituitary tumours, infection, drugs, and hyperactive nodular disease (which may be a genetic defect in TSH receptor). Less frequent causes of hypothyroidism include birth defects, infection (DeQuervain's thyroiditis), secondary hypothyroidism (for example due to pituitary disease), and tertiary hypothyroidism (due to a problem with the hypothalamus).

SELF-CHECK 7.2

Why would diseases of the pituitary or hypothalamus cause thyroid disease?

Autoimmune thyroid disease may result in an underactive thyroid (hypothyroidism) or an overactive thyroid (hyperthyroidism). Approximately 2% of the population in Europe and North America are affected with an autoimmune thyroid disease. Autoimmune thyroid diseases are five to ten times more common in women than men. The most common are autoimmune hyperthyroidism (Graves' disease) and autoimmune hypothyroidism (Hashimoto's and atrophic thyroiditis). Look at Clinical correlation 7.1 for more detail.

In autoimmune thyroiditis, the thyroid is infiltrated with T cells. These appear to damage the thyroid through several mechanisms: direct cytotoxicity, cytokine production, and induction of **apoptosis** via interleukin-1–induced Fas ligand expression on thyroid cells. Whether auto-antibodies also have a role in the disease process (**pathogenesis**) in autoimmune thyroiditis remains uncertain. However, in Graves' disease the main function of $CD4^+$ T cells infiltrating the thyroid appears, after antigen recognition, to be to help B cells produce pathogenic auto-antibodies.

Most cases are **idiopathic** (that is, we do not know the cause of the disease) but some cases are induced by drugs. A good example of this is an iodine-containing drug, amiodarone, used for the treatment of heart disease. Up to 20% of patients on amiodarone get drug-induced **thyrotoxicosis** (hyperthyroidism). Other drugs that may induce thyroid disease include lithium (for psychiatric disorders) and alpha interferon. Patients with pre-existing anti-TPO antibodies are particularly susceptible to developing thyroid disease.

Apoptosis
Programmed cell death.

Pathogenesis
The origination and development of a disease.

Idiopathic
Of an unknown cause.

Thyrotoxicosis
The condition resulting from an excess of thyroid hormones.

Several other environmental factors are known to affect autoimmune thyroid disease. High iodine intake is known to increase the risk of both Graves' disease and hypothyroidism. Tobacco smoking is a minor risk factor for Graves' disease. Surprisingly, smoking confers a protective effect against Hashimoto's thyroiditis. Moderate alcohol intake also decreases the risk for developing overt Graves' disease or Hashimoto's thyroiditis. There is some evidence that low selenium and low vitamin D levels may increase the risk of developing autoimmune thyroid disease, but the data are inconclusive. Infection has been implicated in the development of autoimmune thyroid disease. The role of *Yersinia enterocolitica* remains unproven. There is stronger evidence that hepatitis C infection is associated with an increased risk for autoimmune thyroid disease.

The genetic predisposition in thyroid disease is becoming clear. The major association in Graves' disease in Caucasians is with the class II HLA protein, HLA-DR3. Expression of HLA-DR3 is also a risk factor for other autoimmune diseases. Studies in twins indicate other genes must also play a role. The *CTLA-4* gene (coding for a protein (CTLA-4, also called CD152) which inhibits co-stimulation of T cells) is the second major susceptibility gene. In addition, there is evidence that many other genes also confer susceptibility including *PTPN22*, *CD40*, *FCRL3*, *IL2RA*, and *FOXP3*.*CTLA-4* polymorphisms are also associated with hypothyroidism and other related disorders, including type 1 diabetes and Addison's disease. We know, therefore, that several autoimmune diseases share the same genetic predispositions and, as a consequence, several autoimmune diseases may be found together in the same patient. The best example of this is autoimmune polyglandular syndrome. You can see examples of other autoimmune diseases associated with autoimmune thyroid disease in Clinical correlation 7.2.

Cross reference
You can find out more about diabetes in Section 7.4.1, Addison's disease in Section 7.4.2, and autoimmune polyglandular syndromes in Section 7.4.3.

Key Point

Women are more likely to develop autoimmune diseases than men.

CLINICAL CORRELATION 7.1

Autoimmune thyroid diseases

Hyperthyroidism

Hyperthyroidism leads to a 'fast metabolism'. Symptoms include nervousness, insomnia, palpitations, warm moist skin, and intolerance to heat.

Graves' disease
Autoimmune hyperthyroidism.

Graves' Disease.

Graves' disease is characterized by a diffuse goitre (swelling of the thyroid gland) with hyperthyroidism or ophthalmopathy (eye involvement, often resulting in bulging eyeballs (exophthalmus)) or both. Smoking increases the risk of developing the ophthalmopathy.

Hypothyroidism

Hypothyroidism leads to a 'slow metabolism'. Symptoms of hypothyroidism include fatigue, weight gain, coarse dry hair, dry skin, hair loss, and intolerance to cold. There are several subtypes of autoimmune hypothyroidism.

Hashimoto's thyroiditis and atrophic thyroiditis

These two forms of chronic autoimmune thyroiditis differ only in the presence or absence of goitre; Hashimoto's thyroiditis (with goitre) and atrophic thyroiditis (without goitre). Together these are the most common form of hypothyroidism.

Post-partum thyroiditis

Parity (having borne children) is a small risk factor for developing autoimmune thyroid disease. One hypothesis is that this results from exposure to small amounts of foetal material that crosses the placenta (microchimerism).

Silent thyroiditis is a transient disorder which presents with hyperthyroidism or hypothyroidism. This may present as post-partum thyroiditis in approximately 5% of women during the first year after parturition. However, around 20% of these women develop permanent hypothyroidism over the next decade.

Sub-clinical hypothyroidism

Sub-clinical hypothyroidism is a laboratory-based diagnosis. Sub-clinical hypothyroidism is characterized by high TSH (usually 5–10 mU/L (normally < 5mU/L)) with normal serum free T_4. It is primarily a disease of elderly women. In patients who also have anti-thyroid peroxidase antibodies there is a high risk of progression to overt hypothyroidism.

Focal thyroiditis

Focal thyroiditis (infiltration by lymphocytes) is seen in 30% of thyroid glands at autopsy. Focal thyroiditis is often asymptomatic but may develop into hypothyroidism in some individuals.

Juvenile lymphocytic thyroiditis

Juvenile lymphocytic thyroiditis presents as a chronic disorder, often with non-toxic goitre, but with sub-clinical hypothyroidism and growth retardation in some. Spontaneous recovery occurs in some children.

CLINICAL CORRELATION 7.2

Diseases associated with autoimmune thyroid disease

Autoimmune thyroid disease is often found together with other autoimmune diseases. Some are chance findings. Many are found more often than expected by chance alone and these are listed here. Figures (where they are given) are estimates of the frequency of the associated disease. The presence of the related antibodies is often much higher. For example parietal cell antibodies (seen in pernicious anaemia) are found in 20–40% of patients with autoimmune thyroid disease and anti-nuclear antibodies (seen in connective tissue diseases) in 20–30%.

- **Pernicious anaemia (5–20%)**
- **Addison's disease (1–2%)**
- **Systemic lupus erythematosus**
- **Rheumatoid arthritis**
- **Primary biliary cirrhosis**
- **Coeliac disease (3–5%)**
- **Myasthenia gravis (an autoimmune disease in which auto-antibody-mediated destruction of acetylcholine receptors at the neuromuscular junction leads to profound weakness and fatigability)**
- **Lymphocytic hypophysitis (lymphocytes infiltrating the pituitary gland resulting in an underactive pituitary)**
- **Autoimmune polyglandular syndromes (about 4% of type 1 and 75% of type 2 have autoimmune thyroid disease).**

Cross reference

You should refer to Chapter 5 for further information on anti-nuclear antibodies.

SELF-CHECK 7.3

What are hyperthyroidism and hypothyroidism? What is the effect of each on the body's metabolism?

7.1.3 Testing for autoimmune thyroid disease in the clinical laboratory

We have seen how the various types and subtypes of autoimmune thyroid disease present both clinically and that some of these have characteristic auto-antibodies. In this section we will explore how the laboratory is able to help in making the diagnosis and the limitations of the assays available.

Initial screening in many cases is by serum analysis for serum TSH to indirectly assess thyroid function. TSH is raised in hypothyroid disorders and suppressed in hyperthyroidism. If TSH is abnormal a further test of thyroid hormones, usually free T_4, is performed. Most T_4 is bound to proteins; free T_4, the metabolically active fraction, is not. However, there are other causes of disrupted thyroid function tests, including pituitary dysfunction and severe disease such as sepsis. The autoimmune nature of the disease will only be confirmed by the presence of circulating auto-antibodies or by biopsy of the thyroid gland. Look at Method 7.1 for a breakdown of the auto-antibodies seen in thyroid disease. Biopsy of the thyroid gland shows infiltration by lymphocytes.

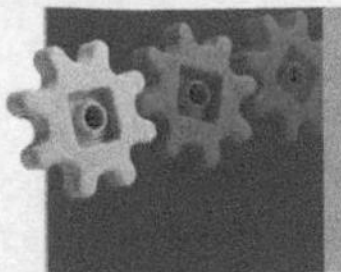

METHOD 7.1 Auto-antibody testing for autoimmune thyroid disease

Three main anti-thyroid antibodies have been described: anti-TSH receptor antibody (TSHRAB), anti-thyroglobulin, and anti-thyroid peroxidase (anti-TPO). Many techniques have been used to detect anti-thyroid antibodies including immunofluorescence (now rarely used for anti-thyroid antibodies), particle agglutination, radioassay, and ELISA. Of these, ELISA has become the most widely used for anti-TPO and anti-thyroglobulin assays. ELISA has distinct advantages over the agglutination and immunofluorescence assays in that it is less subjective, easier to automate, and gives fully quantified results.

TSHRAB may be inhibitory or stimulatory when they mimic the effect of TSH on the thyroid, thus causing hyperthyroidism. This is one of the occasions when the antibody is pathogenic, that is it causes disease. The most widely used assay for TSHRAB measures the inhibition of binding of iodine-125 to soluble TSH receptors by the antibodies. These thyroid binding inhibition assays have a sensitivity of 70–90% and a specificity of 90–95% for untreated Graves' disease. Most TSHRAB assays on the market cannot distinguish between thyroid-stimulating and thyroid-inhibiting antibodies. Results need to be interpreted with care in a clinical setting.

Anti-TPO antibodies are found in 60–80% of patients with Graves' disease and 90–95% of patients with Hashimoto's or atrophic thyroiditis. You should note that this antibody may be found in both hyper- and hypothyroid disease and again the result requires interpretation in the clinical setting.

Anti-thyroglobulin antibodies are rarely seen in the absence of anti-TPO antibodies. For this reason they are generally not used in the diagnosis of autoimmune thyroid disease. Anti-thyroglobulin antibodies may interfere in assays for thyroglobulin in serum. Serum thyroglobulin measurement is used to monitor patients with differentiated thyroid cancer. In this group of patients it is therefore important to know whether they have anti-thyroglobulin antibodies. Anti-thyroglobulin antibodies are found in about 20% of patients with thyroid carcinoma.

Other antibodies may be seen in autoimmune thyroid disease; 40% of patients will have anti-nuclear antibody.

Anti-thyroid antibodies may also be seen in other organ-specific autoimmune disease, such as type 1A diabetes and pernicious anaemia.

SELF-CHECK 7.4

What are the three protein targets for auto-antibodies in autoimmune thyroid disease?

7.1.4 Treatment for autoimmune thyroid disease

We have seen how the laboratory can help in determining the type and cause of the thyroid disease. We have also noted that this is limited by the sensitivity and specificity and that knowing the clinical context is crucial to interpretation of the results. Treatment is then tailored to correct the disrupted metabolism.

In Graves' disease the purpose of therapy is to reduce the activity of the thyroid; there are a number of therapeutic options. Radioactive iodine has been used effectively. However, radioactive iodine can have the side effect of destroying too much of the thyroid, resulting in hypothyroidism. Indeed, a few patients, mostly elderly, actually get worse after treatment with radioactive iodine.

Anti-thyroid drugs (propylthiouracil and carbimazole) interfere with thyroid hormone production by preventing the binding of iodine to tyrosine. Anti-thyroid drugs also have an immunomodulatory action which reduces the release of pro-inflammatory molecules from thyroid cells.

The treatment of the ophthalmopathy associated with thyroid disease has proved difficult. Smoking cessation and strict euthyroid hormone status are the most important factors; many individuals require no therapy, but irradiation of the orbit, steroids, or decompression surgery may be required for some patients. In the future, it is possible that biological anti-inflammatory drugs that have proved effective in other autoimmune diseases might have a role here also.

Anti-thyroid receptor antibodies can be used to monitor response to anti-thyroid drugs. Declining concentration of TSHRAB in patients on long-term anti-thyroid drugs suggests remission. Patients with very low or undetectable TSHRAB at the end of treatment are likely to have long-term remission. However, those patients with positive TSHRAB at the end of therapy are only three times more likely to relapse than those patients in whom the antibody is undetectable. As a result, using the criterion of positive TSHRAB to predict relapse is likely to misclassify 25% of patients as regards to their subsequent outcome.

In future, there may be scope for use of more directed therapy, particularly in the ophthalmopathy of Graves' disease, which has a significant inflammatory component.

For most patients with hypothyroidism, treatment is relatively simple: the deficient hormone is replaced. For most levothyroxine, a synthetic form of T_4, taken orally is effective. Fluctuating requirements for levothyroxine may be a result of problems with absorption and could indicate the presence of coeliac disease. In addition, it has been suggested that vitamin D supplementation might be beneficial in some cases.

The development of other autoimmune diseases is common in patients with autoimmune thyroid disease. The patient should be watched carefully for these and annual testing for relevant antibodies might be appropriate. This is particularly true for pernicious anaemia, where anti-gastric parietal cell antibodies provide a sensitive screen.

Cross reference

You can see more information on pernicious anaemia in Section 7.3.

7.1.5 Summary

Autoimmune thyroid disease is common. It may result in over activity (e.g. Graves' disease) or under activity (e.g. Hashimoto's thyroiditis). Thyroid dysfunction is assessed first by TSH and thyroxine measurements. Auto-antibody analysis may help to confirm the diagnosis, although

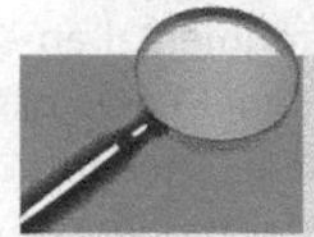

CASE STUDY 7.1 A troubled infant

Patient history

- **24-year-old female.**
- **History of Graves' disease.**
- **Gave birth to healthy male infant at 38 weeks gestation.**
- **A week post-partum the baby, who was low weight, became increasingly irritable.**

Results

- **Infant T4>50 TSH–undetectable**
- **Mother euthryoid**
- **TPO antibody positive–mother**
- **TSHRAB antibody positive–mother.**

Significance of results

- **The baby has the biochemistry of neonatal Graves' disease.**
- **The mother has both TPO and TSH receptor antibodies.**

The baby was treated for neonatal Graves' disease with carbimazole and propylthiouracil and made a good recovery.

How do you think the baby has acquired Graves' disease?

If the doctors adopted a 'watch and wait' policy, how long do you think it will be before the baby shows significant improvement?

sensitivity is only 70–95%. Treatment for hyperthyroidism is by anti-thyroid dugs. Treatment for hypothyroidism is by hormone replacement.

7.2 Coeliac disease

Enteropathy
A disease of the intestinal tract.

Hypersensitivity
The reaction that causes reproducible signs or symptoms, following exposure to a defined stimulus, in a susceptible individual.

Coeliac disease is a gluten sensitive **enteropathy** (disease of the intestine). Coeliac disease is an immunologically mediated **hypersensitivity** response (Type IV) to gluten, a complex of gliadin and glutelin proteins, found in wheat. The disease manifests as an atrophy of the small intestinal villi, giving a classic 'flat mucosa'. The patient has an inability to absorb nutrients leading to malabsorption. Classic symptoms are weight loss, fatigue, diarrhoea, and anaemia.

7.2.1 Epidemiology

Cross reference
You can read more about the four types of hypersensitivity in Chapter 3.

Coeliac disease is a common disease in Europe and USA affecting all age groups. The incidence varies geographically from 1:4000 in southern Europe to 1:100 in North Europeans and is twice as common in females as in males. It is seen in 5–15% of family members. This rises to 70% in identical twins. The disease can manifest at any age, with a peak onset in early childhood.

Coeliac disease is HLA associated, with over 95% patients expressing the HLA-DQ2 protein. However, the association of DQ2 with coeliac disease is complex as there are several isoforms of DQ2, of which DQ2.2 and DQ2.5 are strongly associated with coeliac disease. The DQ2.5 isoform is able to bind and present deamidated gliadin. The DQ2.2 isoform does not have both the required subunits, but in combination with DQ7.5 can express a protein on the cell surface almost identical to that expressed by DQ2.5. Almost all the remaining 5% of patients with coeliac disease express HLA-DQ8.

Cross reference
Further detail on the genetics of coeliac disease (including allelic data) may be found in Sollid et al. (2000).

You should note that this genetic background provides a susceptibility to coeliac disease but does not predict who will eventually develop the disease. For example about 25–30% of North American and European Caucasian populations carry the HLA-DQ2.5 isoform and about 10% carry HLA-DQ8, but only 1% of the population develop coeliac disease.

Coeliac disease and the closely related disorder dermatitis herpetiformis are unusual when compared to many other autoimmune diseases because we know the environmental antigen that triggers the disease. In keeping with some other disorders (e.g. some cases of drug-induced lupus) removal of the trigger leads to resolution of the disease. Therefore coeliac disease, although usually included in the autoimmune diseases, is better thought of as a hypersensitive immune reaction triggered by an exogenous antigen. The trigger is the alpha-gliadin fraction of gluten found in cereals, in particular in wheat. Other proteins from cereals (e.g. hordein from barley, avenin from oats) may cause similar problems but much less frequently.

Tissue transglutaminase is an enzyme thought to be involved in tissue repair. Tissue transglutaminase cross-links glutamine residues to lysine or, at low pH or when there is no recipient amino acid, removes $-NH_2$ groups (deamidation) from glutamine residues. The reaction is shown in Figure 7.3. Alpha-gliadin is rich in the amino acid glutamine. There are some peptides of gliadin that are resistant to breakdown and are also rich in glutamine. You can see the structure of these peptides in Figure 7.4. Once deamidated by tissue transglutaminase, the peptides bind strongly to the HLA-DQ2 or HLA-DQ8 molecules on antigen presenting cells. $CD4^+$ T cells recognize these gliadin peptides and subsequently produce pro-inflammatory cytokines, including gamma-interferon. The ensuing inflammatory response releases other tissue-damaging molecules and ultimately induces the changes in the crypts and villi (which you will find illustrated later in the chapter in Figure 7.7).

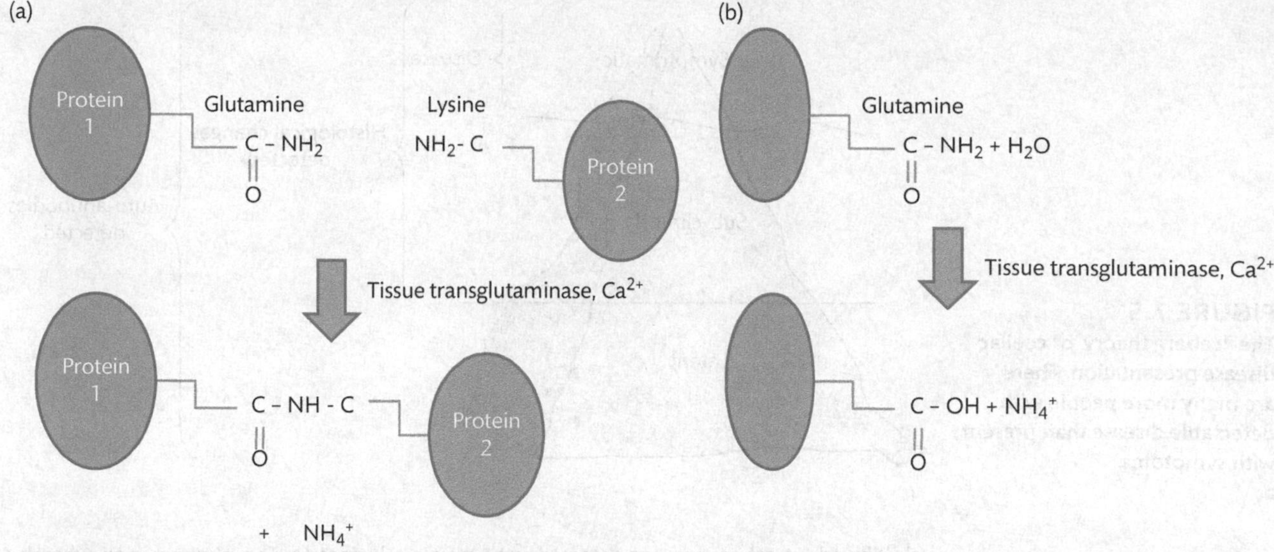

FIGURE 7.3

Deamidation of glutamine residues by tissue transglutaminase: (a) crosslinking of two proteins; (b) deamidation of proteins when no lysine acceptor is available.

Clinically, there are three types of disease onset:

- Classical (typical) form:
  - childhood onset of symptoms
  - failure to thrive
  - bloating
  - diarrhoea.
- atypical forms:
  - adult onset
  - anaemia (especially women of childbearing age).
- Asymptomatic (silent) form.

It is not unusual for a disease to express itself in different ways in different patients. It appears from various studies that auto-antibodies and other autoimmune phenomena may be present in people for many years before the onset of symptoms. The patients give the impression of being 'primed', and only when a second stress on the immune system occurs (e.g. infection) does tolerance get broken. Hence some patients present with the classical symptoms in

31 L-G-Q-Q-Q-P-F-P-P-Q-Q-P-Y 43
31 L-G-Q-Q-Q-P-F-P-P-Q-Q-P-Y-P-Q-P-Q-P-F 49
44 -P-Q-P-Q-P-F-P-S-Q-Q-P-Y 55

FIGURE 7.4

Immunogenic peptides derived from breakdown of α-gliadin. Gliadin is rich in glutamine and proline (as seen in the peptides shown) and very resistant to degradation by gut enzymes. Peptides pass intact across the epithelial barrier where they are deamidated by tissue transglutaminase. The deamidated peptides are processed by macrophages and presented to the immune system. L, leucine; G, glycine; Q, glutamine; P, proline; F, phenylalanine; Y, tyrosine.

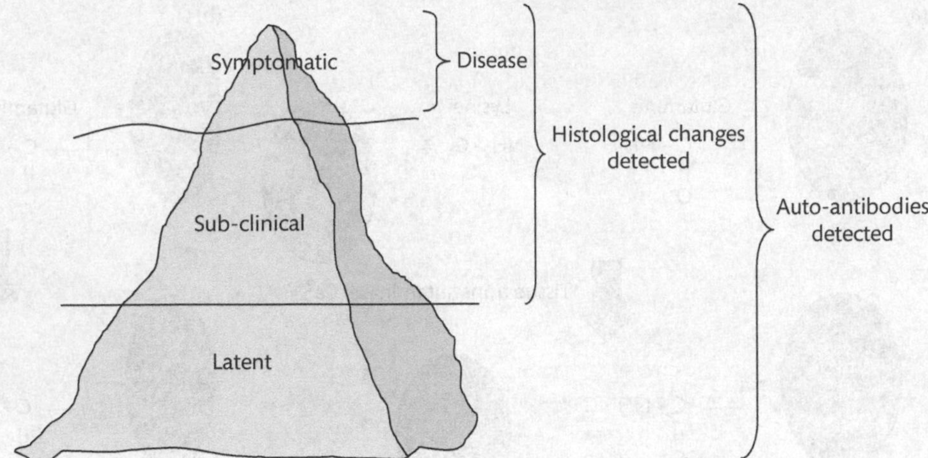

FIGURE 7.5
The 'iceberg theory' of coeliac disease presentation. There are many more people with detectable disease than present with symptoms.

childhood yet others are not detected until their ninth decade. The phenomenon whereby many people have undetected disease and a few have severe symptoms is sometimes referred to as 'the coeliac iceberg'. Look at Figure 7.5 to see how this works. A similar model could equally well be applied to other diseases where there is a long time between onset of the disease and onset of symptoms. It is worth reiterating here the point made in the introduction that some patients with auto-antibodies never go on to develop clinical disease.

Cross reference

We look at autoimmune diabetes type 1A in more detail in Section 7.4.1.

Like autoimmune thyroid disease, coeliac disease is frequently found in association with other diseases, many of which are also autoimmune in nature. Look at Clinical correlation 7.3 for a detailed list of other diseases associated with coeliac disease.

CLINICAL CORRELATION 7.3

Diseases associated with coeliac disease

Coeliac disease is often found together with other autoimmune and non-autoimmune diseases. These include:

- **dermatitis herpetiformis**
- **insulin-dependent diabetes mellitus (type 1A diabetes)**
- **autoimmune thyroid disease**
- **systemic lupus erythematosus**
- **IgA nephropathy**
- **IgA deficiency**
- **primary biliary cirrhosis**
- **common variable immune deficiency**
- **Down syndrome.**

Key Point

It is a common feature of autoimmunity to have diseases which overlap.

7.2.2 Testing for coeliac disease in the clinical laboratory

We have seen that coeliac disease results from an interaction between gliadin and the immune system. In this section we will look at the antibodies and auto-antibodies generated as a part of that response and the use of these antibodies in the diagnosis of coeliac disease. We will also explore the use of biopsy to visualize the morphological changes that take place in coeliac disease.

There are a number of serological techniques available for the testing of coeliac disease. Three are still in general use. Some laboratories still offer all three antibodies but as sensitivity and specificity improves for the newest markers, the older ones (such as anti-reticulin antibody) are being replaced.

We are now going to look at the three key techniques. These are:

1. Endomysium antibodies.
2. Gliadin antibodies.
3. Tissue transglutaminase antibodies.

You will notice that there are two categories of antibody detected; those to an external antigen (anti-gliadin) and those to internal antigens (auto-antibodies: anti-endomysium, anti-tissue transglutaminase). In addition to the mechanisms we saw earlier CD4⁺ T cells also control B cell responses. The major immune response in coeliac disease takes place in the gut, a site where mucosal immunity is most important. For this reason IgA responses predominate and are the more important in diagnosis. Anti-gliadin antibodies are a result of the normal immune response to a foreign antigen. Why the auto-antibodies arise is less well understood. One proposed mechanism is that the deamidated gliadin peptides may become covalently bound to tissue transglutaminase, thus creating a new antigen (**neoantigen**) which is then seen as foreign by the immune system. It has been shown that the major antigen contributing to anti-endomysium (and indeed, anti-reticulin and anti-jejunum antibodies, which are not used routinely but are described, particularly in the older literature) is in fact tissue transglutaminase. Thus, tissue transglutaminase is the major auto-antigen of coeliac disease.

Neoantigen
A newly acquired and expressed antigen; often present after a cell is infected by an oncogenic virus.

Details of the three most widely used methods are given in Method 7.2.

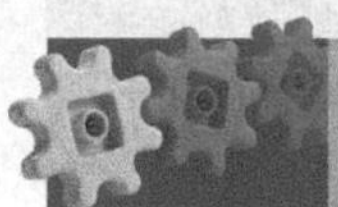

METHOD 7.2 Serological testing of coeliac disease

There are three main serological markers for coeliac disease. We will look at each in turn. IgA class antibodies have a much higher specificity for coeliac disease than the corresponding IgG class antibodies. There are two main guidelines for the investigation of coeliac disease in children and guidelines from the National Institute for Clinical Excellence referring to both children and adults; these are outlined in Clinical correlation 7.4.

In recent years, anti-tissue transglutaminase has become the preferred screening test for a number of reasons. As an ELISA it has the benefit of being fully automated. This has become important as demand for coeliac disease testing has increased. It can be made fully quantifiable, although there is no agreed international standard as yet. Some commercial ELISAs are over-sensitive and so positive results may be confirmed by anti-endomysium. The specificity of anti-tTG is greatly superior to the older anti-gliadin ELISA.

Endomysium antibodies

The most reliable marker is endomysium antibodies. Endomysium antibodies were first described by Chorzelski et al. (1983). Endomysium is connective tissue found between microfibrils. The test has high sensitivity and specificity.

IgA antibodies to endomysium are detected by indirect immunofluorescence. As such it is a labour intensive, subjective assay requiring specially trained staff to interpret the results. It is also susceptible to false negative results when in high titre or when found with anti-smooth muscle antibodies. Look at Figure 7.6 for examples on different tissue substrates.

	Sensitivity	Specificity
IgA endomysium antibody	84–100%	94–100%

Gliadin antibodies

Gliadin antibodies, which can be detected using ELISA, are less sensitive and specific. For this reason they are no longer recommended for screening for coeliac disease (see Clinical correlation 7.4). You should note, however, that there are newer assays to deamidated gliadin which have promise for the future.

	Sensitivity	Specificity
IgA anti-gliadin	84–100%	70–90%
IgG anti-gliadin	50–70%	60–75%

Tissue transglutaminase antibodies

Tissue transglutaminase (tTG) is the major auto-antigen in coeliac disease and is the target for endomysium antibodies. It is a protein cross-linking enzyme, which upon wounding is released from cells to aid in tissue repair. Antibodies to tissue transglutaminase were first described by Dieterich et al. (1997). IgA antibodies to tTG are measured by ELISA.

Antibodies to tissue transglutaminase have higher sensitivity (> 95%) and specificity (> 90%) than do gliadin antibodies. Quantified levels of anti-tTG correlate well with coeliac disease activity. Transglutaminase antibodies are therefore useful to monitor response to therapy.

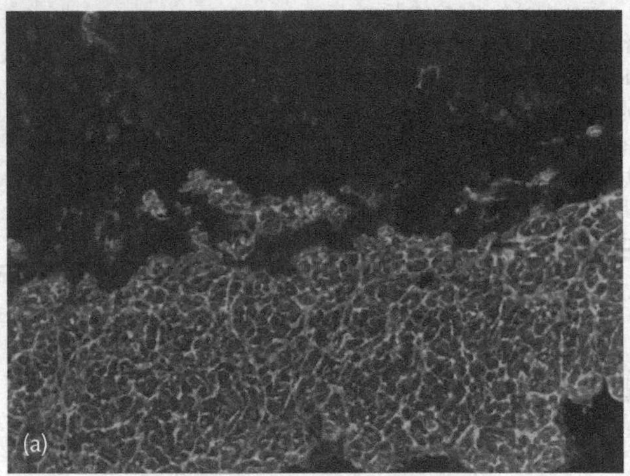

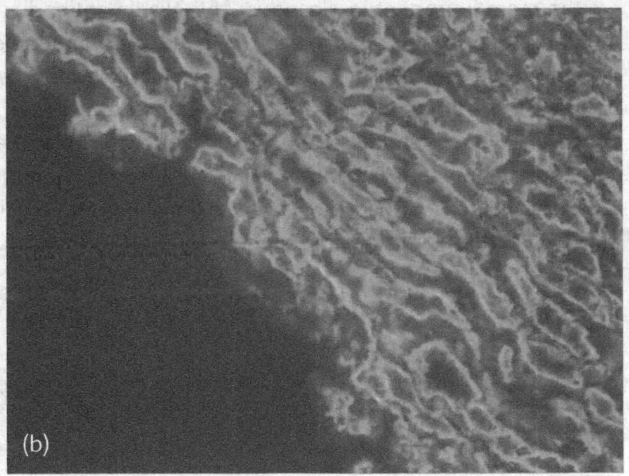

FIGURE 7.6
Indirect immunofluorescence staining of anti-endomysium antibodies on (a) monkey oesophagus; and (b) human umbilicus. Magnification ×400.

Online Resource Centre
To see an online video demonstrating ELISA, log on to www.oxfordtextbooks.co.uk/orc/fbs

Cross reference
You can look up sensitivity and specificity in the *Biomedical Science Practice* textbook of this series.

CLINICAL CORRELATION 7.4

Guidelines for coeliac disease

In 2005 guidelines were published by the North American Society for Pediatric Gastroenterology and Nutrition for the diagnosis and treatment of coeliac disease in children. The guidelines recommend that coeliac disease 'be an early consideration in children with FTT (failure to thrive) and persistent diarrhoea'. The recommended testing strategy was to screen with IgA class tissue transglutaminase antibody and confirm with biopsy. This has led to a move away from gliadin antibody testing, previously used in the diagnosis of coeliac disease in children.

More recently, the European Society for Pediatric Gastroenterology, Hepatology, and Nutrition guidelines modified this advice. Anti-tTG is recommended as the initial screening test. If the anti-tTG is high (> 10 times the upper limit of the reference range) and this is verified by a positive anti-endomysium antibody then it may be possible to make the diagnosis of coeliac disease without biopsy and to start a gluten-free diet. The guidelines advise checking the patient's HLA type is HLA-DQ2/DQ8 as a further confirmation of the likely diagnosis.

In 2009 NICE recommendations were issued for services in the UK. These were updated in 2015. The key recommendations for Immunology laboratories were that initial screening should be by IgA anti-tissue transglutaminase, anti-endomysium antibodies should be used to confirm equivocal anti-tTG, and anti-gliadin should no longer be used.

Cross reference

See Hill et al. (2005), Husby et al. (2012), and NICE (2015) for detailed guidelines.

The current final tool for diagnosis is still an intestinal biopsy, as described in Method 7.3. This is still considered to be the 'gold standard' test. There are advantages and disadvantages to this technique. The main advantage of biopsy is that you can look directly at the affected tissue rather than relying on indirect indications of disease. The disadvantage is that the patient needs to be sedated and the technique is invasive. Whilst small, there are always risks of adverse reactions to drugs. It is an invasive procedure which can be uncomfortable for the patient.

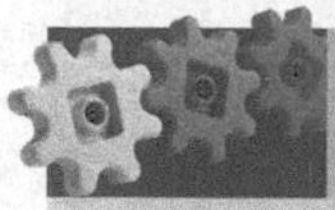

METHOD 7.3 The intestinal biopsy

The intestinal biopsy is still considered the gold standard technique to confirm a diagnosis of coeliac disease.

- A tube is passed down the patient's throat and through the stomach to the small bowel (usually the duodenum).
- A device is then fed through this tube that can snip off a small piece of bowel and be withdrawn.
- The biopsy is snap frozen in liquid nitrogen.
- The biopsy is cut into thin sections (4–6 μm).
- Sections are stained and examined under a microscope to look for changes that are seen in coeliac disease.

In normal small bowel there are villi—finger-like projections which increase the surface area available for the absorption of nutrients. In severe coeliac disease these are absent over much of the small bowel mucosa (also called coeliac sprue). There are intermediary states. One popular system for grading the damage to the small bowel is the Marsh classification. There are also variants of this system. You should look at Figure 7.7 for more detail of the original classification. The disease can be focal or patchy and so multiple biopsies should be obtained.

Although this is considered the gold standard technique you should remember that other disorders can also lead to a 'flat gut'. These include infection, for example by *Giardia lamblia* (a protozoan) and some immunodeficiency syndromes. In order to be certain that the patient has coeliac disease, the patient must be put on a strict gluten-free diet. After about 3 months the gut should have largely recovered. Until recently, guidelines recommended that a second biopsy was required to prove this. However, it is now not thought necessary, provided that the auto-antibodies (endomysium antibodies, tissue transglutaminase antibodies) are no longer detectable in the serum.

7.2.3 IgA deficiency in coeliac disease

We have seen how the most useful serologic tests look for IgA class antibodies. We also saw (in Clinical correlation 7.3) that coeliac disease is associated with IgA deficiency. Clearly IgA deficient patients will not develop IgA class immune responses to gliadin or tissue transglutaminase. In this section we explore the extent of the problem and the implications of this association for the diagnosis of coeliac disease.

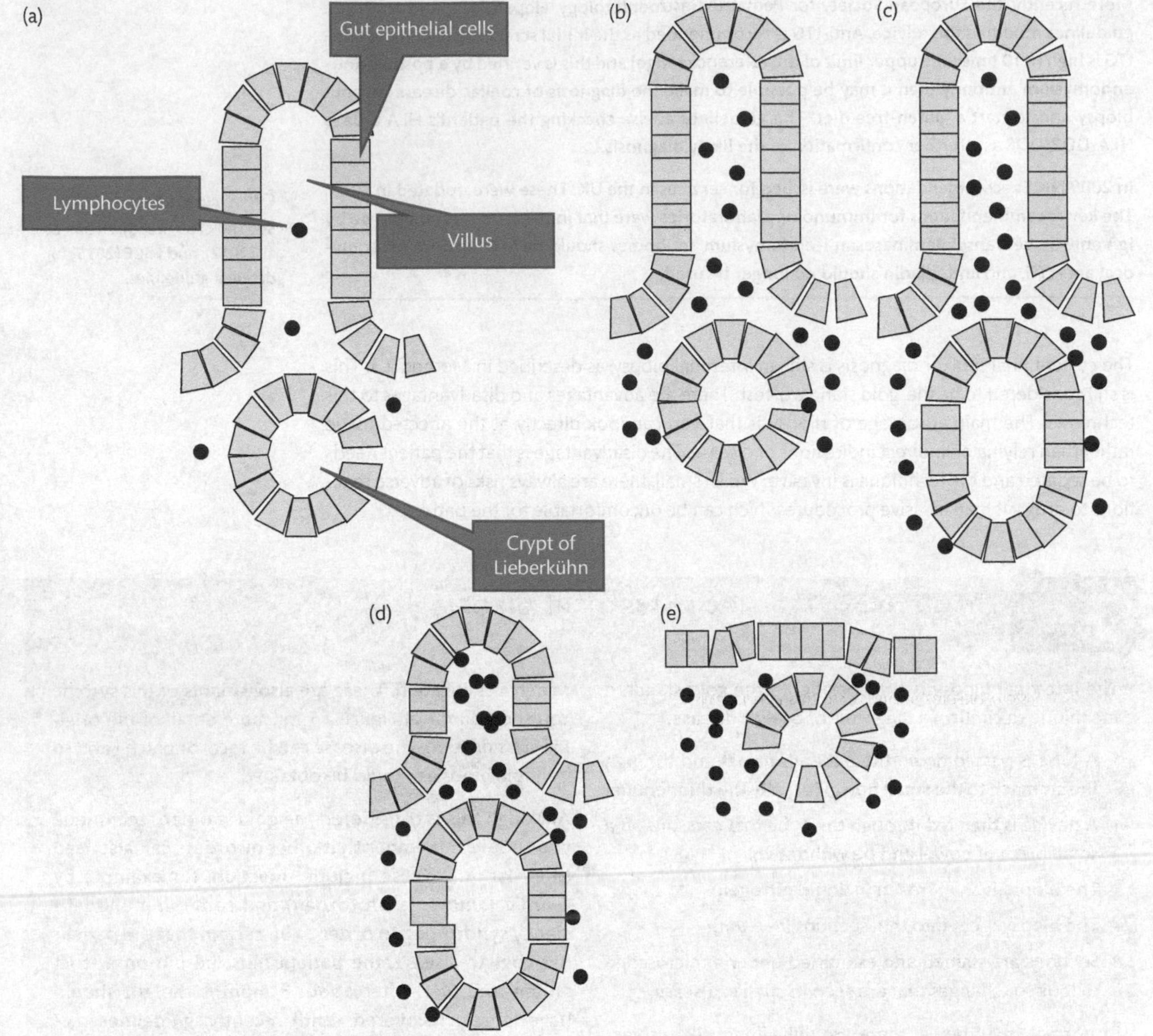

FIGURE 7.7

Histological changes seen in the small bowel of patients with coeliac disease. The diagrams show increasing severity from normal to total villous atrophy (the Marsh classification). (a) Marsh grade 0 (pre-infiltrative). The mucosa is normal; note the tall villus and the shallow crypt of Lieberkühn. Very few lymphocytes are present (< 25 per 100 enterocytes). (b) Marsh grade 1 (infiltrative). The overall architecture is essentially unchanged, but infiltrating intraepithelial lymphocytes are present. There are more than 25 lymphocytes per 100 enterocytes. (c) Marsh grade 2 (infiltrative hyperplastic). Lymphocytic infiltration and proliferation of crypts can be seen. Note that the crypts are now deeper as cell proliferation increases (crypt hyperplasia). (d) Marsh grade 3 (flat destructive). The villus is now shorter or even absent in places (subtotal or total villus atrophy). Crypts are still plentiful and deep but damage to enterocytes is evident. This appearance is commonly seen in untreated coeliac disease. (e) Marsh grade 4 (atrophic hypoplastic). Destruction of the normal mucosa is almost complete. This is the classic 'flat gut' of coeliac disease. Notice that crypts are small and reduced in number or even absent. Lymphocytes are numerous.

IgA deficiency is a common finding in the UK. About 1 in 500–700 blood donors are IgA deficient. In most people this does not cause any obvious problems. However, people with IgA deficiency are more prone to develop autoimmune disease. Genetic studies have shown that the HLA-A1,Cw7,B8,DR3,DQ2 haplotype confers a susceptibility to develop selective IgA deficiency, although the reasons for this are unclear. As we have seen most coeliac disease patients also express HLA-DQ2. Thus individuals with the HLA-DQ2 phenotype are more susceptible to both disorders than those without HLA-DQ2. IgA deficiency is about ten times more common in patients with coeliac disease than in the general population.

IgA deficient coeliac patients will not have IgA class antibodies to gliadin, endomysium, or tissue transglutaminase. However, most IgA deficient coeliac patients will have IgG class antibodies. Despite the lower specificity, it is helpful in IgA deficient patients to check for IgG class antibodies, and this has been recommended by NICE.

7.2.4 Treatment of coeliac disease

We have seen how the diagnosis of coeliac disease is confirmed by the laboratory. In theory, treatment is relatively simple.

The treatment for coeliac disease is to remove the gluten from the patient's diet. By removing the stimulus the whole inflammatory process in the gut can be reversed and normal gut mucosa restored. Furthermore, the autoimmune phenomena all die away. Look at Case Study 7.2. This is an example of how by removing the gluten stimulus from the patient's diet, the serological markers can be affected. In practice, as wheat is used in many manufactured food products, complete avoidance is sometimes difficult to achieve.

Patients with coeliac disease are twice as likely to get cancer as the general population. In particular, enteropathy associated T cell lymphoma is a rare but important complication of coeliac

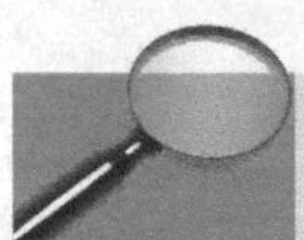

CASE STUDY 7.2 Gluten-free diets

Patient history

- **31-year-old female.**
- **Complains of bloating, abdominal pain, and fatigue.**
- **Starts a low carbohydrate diet and reports feeling much improved.**

Results

- **FBC, B_{12}, and folate—within normal limits**
- **Iron status—within normal limits**
- **U&E, LFT, and bone—within normal limits**
- **tTG antibody >15 u/ml [Reference range <12 u/ml]**
- **Endomysial antibody weak positive.**

The GP advised that the results were consistent with coeliac disease on a gluten-free diet and advised the patient to continue.

If the coeliac screen results were inconclusive, what advice could you give to the GP if they were still concerned about coeliac disease?

disease. This immune system cancer is most likely to arise in the jejunum but may be found elsewhere. The risk of getting this cancer is much lower if the patient keeps to a gluten-free diet. One way of checking if the patient is keeping to their diet is to monitor the auto-antibodies. Auto-antibodies return after the immune system is rechallenged with gluten. If the patient is suspected of non-compliance, or if new symptoms develop, the auto-antibody test should be repeated.

7.2.5 Summary

Classically, coeliac disease presents as a gluten sensitive enteropathy in young children with failure to thrive, often with diarrhoea. More often now it presents more subtly in adults, often with anaemia a feature. Characteristic antibodies are present to gliadin, endomysium, and tissue transglutaminase. Of these, IgA anti-endomysium has the best diagnostic reliability. However, anti-tissue transglutaminase antibodies are technically easier and provide a quantified answer which may be useful in monitoring treatment. Therefore, anti-tissue transglutaminase is has taken over as the standard first-line investigation. Treatment is by removal of gluten from the diet.

7.3 Pernicious anaemia

Vitamin B_{12} is an essential requirement for the production of red blood cells. In pernicious anaemia absorption of vitamin B_{12} is impaired. Normally, a cofactor, intrinsic factor, is released from parietal cells in the stomach. This binds to vitamin B_{12}. Further down the gut the vitamin B_{12}–intrinsic factor complex binds to receptors in the terminal ileum, leading to active transport of vitamin B_{12} across the gut epithelium (look at Figure 7.8 for more detail). In individuals

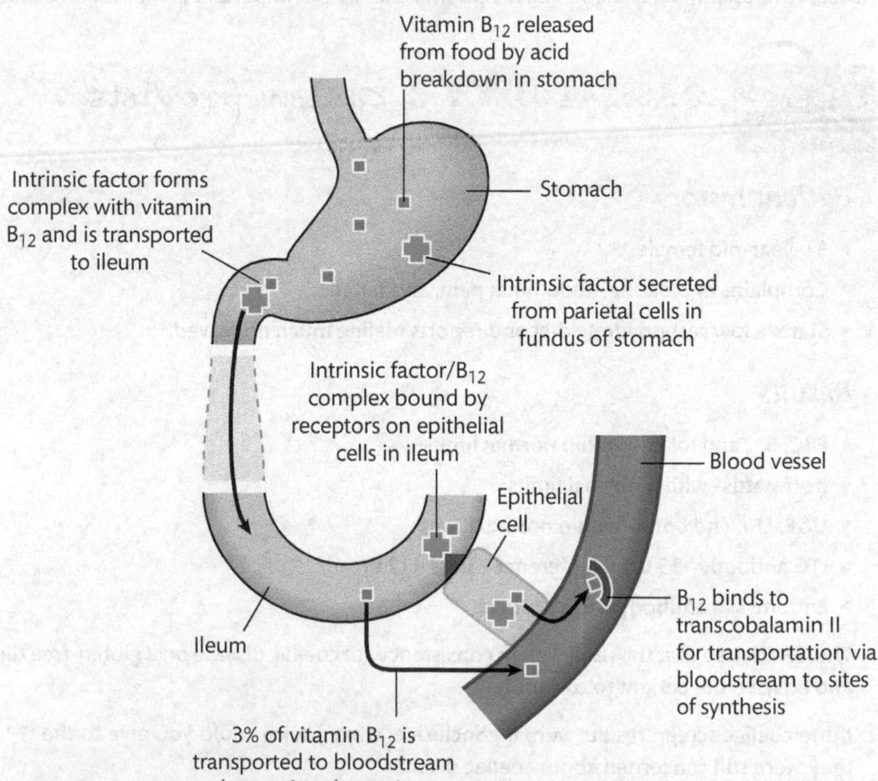
Vitamin B12 released from food by acid breakdown in stomach
Intrinsic factor forms complex with vitamin B12 and is transported to ileum
Stomach
Intrinsic factor secreted from parietal cells in fundus of stomach
Intrinsic factor/B12 complex bound by receptors on epithelial cells in ileum
Blood vessel
Epithelial cell
B12 binds to transcobalamin II for transportation via bloodstream to sites of synthesis
Ileum
3% of vitamin B12 is transported to bloodstream by passive absorption

FIGURE 7.8
The importance of intrinsic factor in the absorption of vitamin B_{12}.

with pernicious anaemia, parietal cells are destroyed. Consequently, intrinsic factor is deficient and so vitamin B_{12} is not absorbed. The patient develops a form of anaemia with large red cells (macrocytes) low in haemoglobin (megaloblastic anaemia). The most common presenting symptom is fatigue. A further complication seen in some patients is numbness or tingling in the hands and feet (peripheral neuropathy). This occurs because a lack of vitamin B_{12} leads to nerve damage.

7.3.1 Epidemiology

In this section we will look at the biology of disease of pernicious anaemia and atrophic gastritis.

Pernicious anaemia is the end stage of autoimmune **gastritis** (also called type A chronic atrophic gastritis). Autoimmune gastritis affects the corpus of the stomach, which contains the parietal cells. Autoimmune gastritis is characterized by an inflammatory infiltration by lymphocytes of the main body of the stomach. Parietal cell antibody is a marker for autoimmune gastritis. It is most commonly seen in persons over 60 years of age. In North America and Europe pernicious anaemia is said to be the most common cause of vitamin B_{12} deficiency. Pernicious anaemia is found in 2% of persons over 60 years of age. It affects women twice as often as men. It may take 20–30 years for atrophic gastritis to develop into pernicious anaemia.

Gastritis
Inflammation of the stomach lining.

The anaemia is caused by a deficiency of vitamin B_{12}. This results from two mechanisms. Primarily, the destruction of parietal cells in the stomach leads to a lack of intrinsic factor, which, as we can see in Figure 7.8, is necessary for efficient vitamin B_{12} absorption. As a secondary mechanism, intrinsic factor auto-antibodies can further impair the absorption of vitamin B_{12}, either by preventing B_{12} binding to intrinsic factor or by interfering with the binding of intrinsic factor to receptors in the ileum.

There is a second form of atrophic gastritis (type B) caused by *Helicobacter pylori*. It is interesting to note that antibodies to parietal cells are found in 20–30% of patients with *H. pylori* infection. This has led to the hypothesis that *H. pylori* might be the environmental trigger for the development of pernicious anaemia.

7.3.2 Testing for pernicious anaemia in the clinical laboratory

We will now consider the tests available to confirm the diagnosis of pernicious anaemia.

Given that the key feature of the disease is anaemia we must first establish that we are looking at the right sort of anaemia. Many patients suffer from iron deficiency anaemia and this usually results in small red cells being made in the bone marrow (**microcytic anaemia**). In both B_{12} deficiency and folate deficiency large red cells are made (**macrocytic anaemia**). This is as a result of delayed DNA synthesis, as both B_{12} and folate are required for thymidylate synthesis. However, RNA synthesis is unaffected and cytoplasmic development continues; a larger than normal cell results. Most modern blood count analysers allow the distinction to be made very easily.

Microcytic anaemia
An anaemia in which the red blood cells are smaller in volume than normal (reduced mean corpuscular volume [MCV]).

Macrocytic anaemia
An anaemia in which the red blood cells are larger in volume than normal (raised mean corpuscular volume [MCV]).

If the patient has macrocytic anaemia, tests for folate and vitamin B_{12} are performed. Deficiencies, particularly folate, may be due to poor diet. However, vitamin B_{12} deficiency may also be due to autoimmune disease—the pernicious anaemia we are considering here. Characteristic autoantibodies are found in pernicious anaemia; anti-parietal cell antibody and anti-intrinsic factor antibody. Look at Method 7.4 for details of the serological tests used in the diagnosis of pernicious anaemia. You will see that, although they may provide supporting evidence, serological tests are not sufficiently sensitive or specific for us to be sure of the diagnosis.

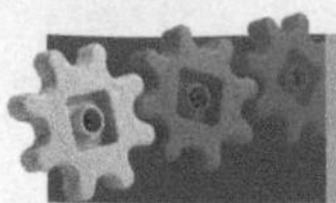

METHOD 7.4 Serological testing for pernicious anaemia

Two tests are commonly used to support a diagnosis of pernicious anaemia: anti-parietal cell antibody and anti-intrinsic factor antibody.

Anti-parietal cell antibodies are most commonly detected by indirect immunofluorescence using rat or mouse stomach as substrate.

Look at Figure 7.9 to see what anti-parietal cell staining looks like. As the antigen is now defined (H^+-K^+-ATPase), it is also possible to use ELISA. However ELISA is more expensive than immunofluorescence and is not yet widely used in the UK.

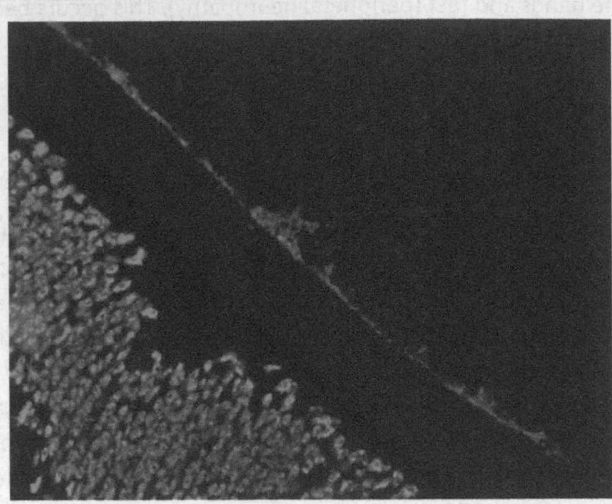

FIGURE 7.9
Indirect immunofluorescence staining of anti-parietal cell antibody in mouse stomach.

Parietal cell antibodies are found in > 90% of persons with pernicious anaemia. However this percentage decreases with disease progression, possibly due to reduced antigen drive as the parietal cells are destroyed. Parietal cell antibodies are found in about 50% of patients with only atrophic gastritis. Parietal cell antibodies are also found in 30% of non-anaemic first degree relatives of patients with pernicious anaemia.

There are two types of intrinsic factor antibody. Type 1 (blocking) antibodies recognize the vitamin B_{12} binding site, whereas type 2 (binding) antibodies recognize a remote site. Type 1 antibodies affect transport of vitamin B_{12} whereas type 2 antibodies do not. ELISA is most commonly used to detect intrinsic factor antibody. ELISA detects both type 1 and type 2 antibodies.

Intrinsic factor antibodies have higher specificity for pernicious anaemia, but lower sensitivity, being found in 40-70%, depending on the study. Type 1 antibodies are found in around 70% of patients with pernicious anaemia and type 2 in about one third. They are rare in patients with only atrophic gastritis.

The presence of both antibodies is strong support for a diagnosis of pernicious anaemia. You should note, however, that the two antibodies are not always found together. Some patients with pernicious anaemia will have only one of the two antibodies. Furthermore, most commercial kits do not recognize the difference, so this distinction is somewhat academic in routine practice.

It was previously possible to look directly at vitamin B_{12} absorption using an assay called the Schilling test. This assay compares the absorption of radioactive B_{12} (labelled with radioactive cobalt), with and without intrinsic factor, by looking for B_{12} excretion in the urine. The ability to absorb more of the B_{12}-intrinsic factor complex, compared to free B_{12}, indicates pernicious anaemia. Poor absorption of both would indicate malabsorption for another reason (e.g. coeliac disease). It is no longer routinely available because of the radioactivity exposure to large numbers of people, poor renal function may affect the result, and the results of the test rarely affect management of the disease.

7.3.3 Treatment of pernicious anaemia

We have seen how the laboratory can help in confirming the diagnosis of pernicious anaemia. The treatment is simple and cheap.

The key to treatment of B_{12} deficiency is to replace the missing vitamin B_{12}. This may be either by oral replacement (pills) or by injection. Before replacement therapy was discovered this disease was invariably fatal. High dose oral vitamin B_{12} works in patients with dietary insufficiency, but is less effective in pernicious anaemia; however, a small amount of vitamin B_{12} is passively absorbed across the gut wall (as we can see in Figure 7.8) and this is sometimes used in developing world countries. Most patients in the developed world receive intramuscular injections. Provided that treatment is started early enough and continued lifelong the patient should have a normal lifespan. However, some patients may have permanent nerve damage before treatment is started.

7.3.4 Summary

Pernicious anaemia is caused by the destruction of parietal cells by T cell infiltration and subsequent cytokine excretion (as described in Section 7.3.1 above). The destruction of parietal cells in the stomach leads to lack of intrinsic factor and hence to vitamin B_{12} deficiency. Pernicious anaemia is the end result of atrophic gastritis. It may take many years for pernicious anaemia to develop. Antibodies to parietal cells are seen in both atrophic gastritis and pernicious anaemia. Antibodies to intrinsic factor are more specific but less sensitive for pernicious anaemia. Treatment is by vitamin B_{12} replacement.

7.4 Autoimmune endocrinopathies

Any organ in the body may be a target for autoimmunity. In this part of the chapter we will look at some examples where hormone secreting organs are involved.

7.4.1 Diabetes

Diabetes mellitus is a disorder of carbohydrate metabolism. It is characterized by high blood glucose (hyperglycaemia). Normally, glucose is controlled by insulin, a hormone released from the pancreas. Look at Figure 7.10 for detail on the structure and function of the pancreas. As we will see, diabetes may be autoimmune in nature but many cases are not autoimmune. In this

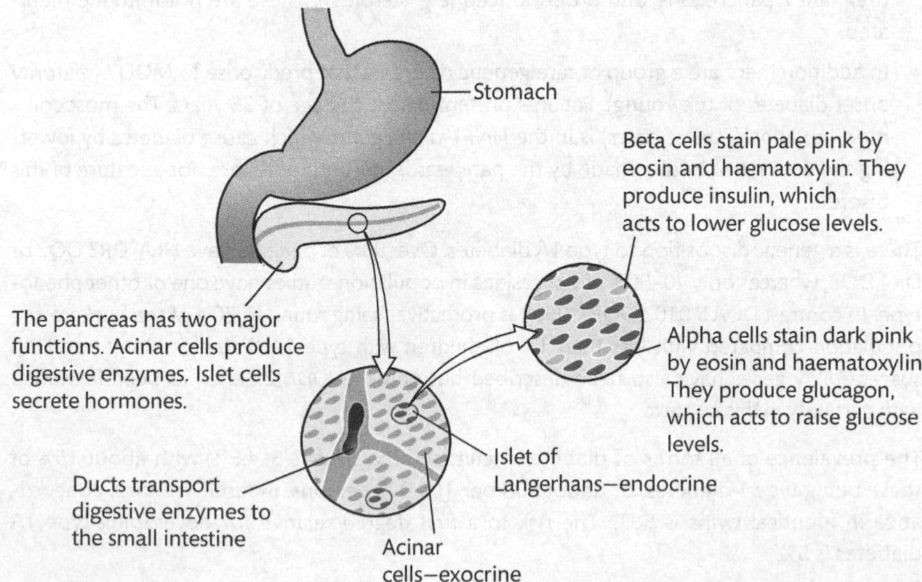
Stomach
Beta cells stain pale pink by eosin and haematoxylin. They produce insulin, which acts to lower glucose levels.
The pancreas has two major functions. Acinar cells produce digestive enzymes. Islet cells secrete hormones.
Alpha cells stain dark pink by eosin and haematoxylin. They produce glucagon, which acts to raise glucose levels.
Islet of Langerhans–endocrine
Ducts transport digestive enzymes to the small intestine
Acinar cells–exocrine

FIGURE 7.10
Structure of the pancreas, showing the exocrine and endocrine areas and the location and function of α and β cells in the islets of Langerhans.

section we will be concentrating on the major autoimmune variant of diabetes, looking at the biology of the disease, the serological tests that help to confirm the autoimmune nature of the disease, and therapy.

Epidemiology

Diabetes is broken down into subtypes according to the aetiology of the disease. Look at Clinical correlation 7.5 for details on the clinical findings seen in diabetes.

- Type 1A (the subject of this part of the chapter) is immune-mediated diabetes (formerly 'juvenile onset' or 'insulin-dependent diabetes mellitus'). This is the major autoimmune subtype of diabetes. It tends to present in younger people (under the age of 40 years) and accounts for about 10–15% of all diabetes. In type 1A the beta cells in the islets of the pancreas are destroyed. The exact mechanism in humans is still not completely understood. By the time patients present, the disease has been established for months or years with some 80% of beta cells being destroyed. Extensive mononuclear cell infiltrates can be seen. These infiltrating cells include CD8$^+$ cytotoxic T cells with specificity for beta cell antigens which are thought to be an important mechanism of beta cell destruction.
- Type 1B is non-immune-mediated diabetes with severe insulin deficiency.
- Type 2 is late onset (formerly non-insulin-dependent) diabetes. It is much more common in western populations than type 1 diabetes, accounting for 85–90% of all cases. Most cases of type 2 diabetes are not mediated by immune mechanisms. Onset of type 2 diabetes is usually in older people (over 40 years old), often in association with obesity. In this form of diabetes the mechanisms are metabolic rather than autoimmune. The pancreas does not produce sufficient insulin for the body's needs. In addition insulin is not used efficiently (so-called 'insulin resistance').
- There is a subgroup (about 10%) of type 2 diabetes in which antibodies to islet cells are found (i.e. autoimmunity is a feature of this subgroup). This subgroup is sometimes called 'latent autoimmune diabetes of adults' (LADA). LADA is similar in many ways to type 1A diabetes. Patients with LADA often become insulin dependent over time.
- There are also forms of diabetes associated with other conditions (examples include pregnancy, pancreatitis, and drug-induced (e.g. steroids)). These are not immune mediated.
- In addition there are a group of rare genetic disorders that predispose to MODY (maturity onset diabetes of the young). Patients present before the age of 25 years. The most common mutation (70% of cases) is in the *HNF1-alpha* gene, which cause diabetes by lowering the amount of insulin made by the pancreas. Auto-antibodies are not a feature of this disorder.

There is a genetic disposition to type 1A diabetes. Over 90% of patients have HLA-DR3,DQ2 or DR4,DQ8, whereas only 40–50% of Caucasians in population studies have one or other phenotype. In contrast DQA1*0102,DQB1*0602 is protective, being found in 20% of the background population compared with less than 1% of children with type 1A diabetes. Many non-HLA susceptibility genes have also been described but only the *IDDM2* gene has been identified with certainty in this context.

The prevalence of all forms of diabetes mellitus in the UK is 3.5–4.5%, with about 15% of these being type 1 diabetes, or about 600 per 100 000 persons. In family studies, concordance in identical twins is 50%. The risk to a first degree relative for developing type 1A diabetes is 5%.

In terms of environmental factors, only congenital rubella infection has been proven to be associated with type 1A diabetes. Other potential triggers, such as bovine milk ingestion or enteroviral infection, remain unproven.

CLINICAL CORRELATION 7.5

Clinical findings in type 1A diabetes

The main problems seen in diabetes stem from damage to blood vessels. Glucose binds to proteins, increasing rigidity. Endothelial progenitor cells, essential for blood vessel repair, become too rigid to move to sites of damage. Damage to small blood vessels (microvascular damage) may lead to renal disease and blindness. Damage to large blood vessels (macrovascular disease) may lead to atherosclerosis (hardening and narrowing of the arteries). Atherosclerosis in turn may cause strokes or coronary heart disease.

Early symptoms are related to high blood sugar and low insulin. Patients pass large amounts of urine and have increased thirst. The low insulin levels affect metabolism and patients do not store fat or protein properly. So, despite an increased appetite patients lose weight. Patients become fatigued and are prone to infections of the bladder and skin.

Infection can increase the requirement for insulin.

The most severe presentation is diabetic coma. This can happen when the blood sugar falls too low. This form of coma results from low blood sugar when the patient is over-treated with insulin. It is treated with infusion of glucose or glucagon.

Coma can also happen when the blood sugar gets too high and the patient becomes dehydrated. In these circumstances the patient's metabolism becomes deranged. Ketones are generated and the blood pH falls (ketoacidosis). It is a life-threatening condition. The patient requires prompt treatment: fluids to rehydrate the patient and insulin to reverse the ketoacidiosis.

Testing for type 1A diabetes in the clinical laboratory

In this section we will consider some of the assays that confirm the presence of diabetes in general and then the autoimmune tests that can confirm the presence of autoimmune diabetes specifically.

Diabetes is a disorder of glucose metabolism and therefore the most useful first-line test is a measurement of blood glucose. It is also possible to challenge the patient with a solution of glucose and monitor blood glucose over a period of hours (the 'glucose tolerance test'). In a normal person blood glucose becomes elevated but rapidly returns to normal. In a diabetic patient the glucose rises higher than normal and takes longer to return to normal.

Measurement of blood glucose is key to monitoring response to therapy. There are home monitors available for patients to check their control of glucose levels. A second useful monitoring tool is the glycosylated haemoglobin (HbA1c). The more circulating glucose, the more will be bound to haemoglobin. HbA1c levels fluctuate less than glucose and give a better measure of overall glucose load. Good control is indicated when the HbA1c is less than 7.5%, that is less than 7.5% of total haemoglobin has glucose bound to it. The range for a normal non-diabetic person is about 3.5–5.5%.

Cross reference

You can look up the use of positive and negative predictive values in the *Biomedical Science Practice* textbook of this series.

Many auto-antibodies have been linked to type 1A diabetes. Only a few have so far proved to be useful in clinical practice. Although auto-antibodies are frequently found in type 1A diabetes there is no evidence to suggest they are causative of the disease. For details on testing for these, look at Method 7.5.

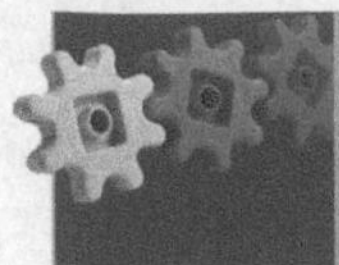

METHOD 7.5 Auto-antibody testing for type 1A diabetes

Islet cell auto-antibodies (ICA)

ICA were first described in 1974 using human pancreas as substrate in an indirect immunofluorescence test. Now it is more usual to use monkey pancreas as this is commercially available. The Juvenile Diabetes Foundation (JDF) developed an international standard for this assay. Look at Figure 7.11 to see what anti-islet cell staining looks like.

At the onset of type 1A diabetes approximately 70–75% of Caucasians are ICA positive (sensitivity 70%) with a specificity of > 95%. With destruction of the beta cells, and thus the concomitant depletion of antigen, ICA levels fall and are rarely found after the first year of disease. The positive predictive value for type 1A diabetes is 85% for ICA above 40 units of the JDF standard.

Islet-cell antibodies can also be seen in patients with an overlapping neurological disorder called stiff person syndrome. In stiff person syndrome the auto-antibodies are directed against glutamic acid decarboxylase (GAD). GAD is one of a number of proteins contributing to ICA staining. All the major type 1 diabetes antigens (GAD, IA-2, and the more recently described zinc transporter ZnT8A) are related to the secretory apparatus of the pancreatic beta cells.

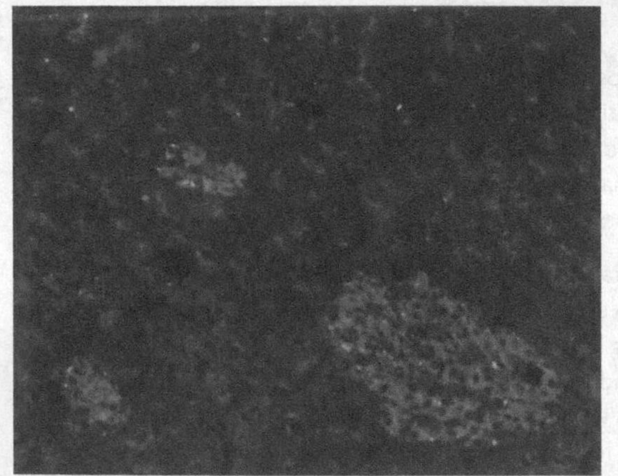

FIGURE 7.11
Indirect immunofluorescence staining of anti-islet cell antibody on monkey pancreas.

Glutamic acid decarboxylase (GAD) antibodies

GAD is an enzyme involved in the control of release of insulin. It is also found in tissues other than pancreas, including the cerebellum and sympathetic ganglia. Antibodies to GAD are common in type IA diabetes, with a sensitivity of about 80–85%. They are most often detected by ELISA or radioassay. Anti-GAD can also be detected by indirect immunofluorescence, and may be the dominant ICA reactivity. Commercial ELISA assays are now available for anti-GAD. This is less technically demanding than IFA and is now becoming the preferred assay for screening for type 1 diabetes. GAD antibodies are found mostly in adult patients. The antibodies to GAD found in type 1A diabetes and in stiff person syndrome are directed against different epitopes on the GAD molecule.

IA-2 (insulinoma-like antigen-2) antibodies

IA-2 is composed of two proteins, IA-2A (a tyrosine phosphatase-related protein, islet antigen 2, also known as ICA512) and IA-2β (phogrin). IA-2, like GAD, is found in nervous tissue and pancreas. Sensitivity for type 1A diabetes is about 75%. It is detected by radiobinding assay.

Insulin antibodies

Auto-antibodies to insulin may be present for many years prior to onset of type 1A diabetes. Insulin auto-antibodies are more often seen in children than adults and are often the first antibody seen in young children. They may be detected by either ELISA or radioassay. These assays do not measure the same population of antibodies. The radioassay results are better at predicting development of type 1A diabetes.

Insulin auto-antibodies are also found in many other autoimmune diseases including Graves' disease, Hashimoto's thyroiditis, Addison's disease, and pernicious anaemia.

All of these auto-antibodies may be present for years before the onset of disease. Studies of family members have shown the more auto-antibodies you have the more likely you are to develop type 1 IDDM.

Treatment of type 1A diabetes

In this section we will consider the treatment of autoimmune diabetes. Note that other therapies are used in diabetes, e.g. for the management of lipids, blood pressure, and other aspects of the disease generally, which will not be covered here.

The key to treatment of type 1A diabetes is insulin replacement. This has been by porcine insulin in the past. Some patients reacted to this non-self antigen by making antibodies specific to porcine insulin. These antibodies made the insulin ineffective. Notice that these anti-porcine insulin antibodies (to an extrinsic antigen) are different to the *auto*-antibodies directed against human insulin (an intrinsic antigen). Nowadays most therapeutic insulin is human recombinant insulin, largely avoiding this problem. It is administered by injection. For some patients with poor control an insulin pump is used to provide a more constant supply of insulin. Different formulations (fast, medium, or long acting) are used, for example, to balance the need for more insulin at mealtimes against the lesser requirement of sleep. One recent development is the use of inhaled insulin which may be used instead of injections before meals.

In future, transplantation may be a therapeutic option. Some patients have had successful pancreas transplants. Others have been transplanted with isolated islets. However, there are drawbacks to this approach. First, the patients need immunosuppression to prevent transplant rejection. Second, there is a lack of suitable donors. Some patients have a partial success in that they reduce their need for insulin, achieving better glycaemic control with less risk of hypoglycaemia.

As with other organ-specific autoimmune diseases there is an increased risk of developing further disorders, particularly autoimmune thyroid disease, pernicious anaemia, and coeliac disease. For these reason many clinics now monitor diabetes patients annually for the development of antibodies seen in these disorders.

Summary

Autoimmune type 1A diabetes is a disorder of glucose metabolism. It is caused by lack of insulin due to destruction of beta cells in the pancreas. Treatment is by replacement of insulin, usually by injection.

7.4.2 Autoimmune Addison's disease

Addison's disease is caused by a failure of the adrenal glands. The classic feature of Addison's disease is hyperpigmentation (darkening of the skin). This is most noticeable on the knuckles, knees, ankles, and creases in the palm of the hand. Salt craving is common.

Epidemiology

In this section we will consider the biology of Addison's disease and the factors that predispose toward autoimmune Addison's disease.

Addison's disease is characterized by deficient production of adrenocortical hormones, both mineralocorticoids and glucocorticoids. There is a concomitant increase in secretion of adrenocorticotrophic hormone (ACTH) from the pituitary. In the Western world, autoimmunity is the most common cause of adrenal failure, accounting for 70–80% of cases. The next most common cause is tuberculosis. Addison's disease affects approximately 1 in 10 000 persons. Other rare causes include adrenal cancer, fungal infections, and haemorrhage (for example after trauma). There are also cases of secondary adrenal insufficiency caused by disease of the pituitary (particularly pituitary cancer). The pituitary, as well as controlling thyroid function (see Figure 7.2), controls cortisol release by release of adrenocorticotrophic hormone (ACTH). ACTH triggers cortisol production in the adrenals. ACTH levels are reduced in pituitary disease, leading to low levels of corticosteroid release from the adrenals.

Addison's disease may be an isolated disease, but is often found with other autoimmune diseases in the autoimmune polyendocrine or polyglandular syndromes. Many patients with autoimmune Addison's disease (50–60%) develop other autoimmune diseases, such as type 1A diabetes or autoimmune thyroid disease. Other disease associations are shown in Clinical correlation 7.6. The disease mechanism is not fully understood, but, as with many other autoimmune diseases, it is thought to be T cell mediated. In autoimmune Addison's disease the auto-antibodies seen are not thought to contribute to the destruction of the adrenal gland.

The main clinical feature is hyperpigmentation. This results indirectly from the increase in levels of ACTH. ACTH derives from the same pro-hormone as melanocyte stimulating hormone, MSH. MSH stimulates production of melanin, the dark pigment in the skin.

Other symptoms include low blood pressure, anorexia, salt craving, weight loss, and fatigue. Why do we see salt craving as a symptom? Salt balance relies on another hormone released by the adrenal glands, aldosterone. When aldosterone falls too low the kidneys do not function properly to retain sodium and maintain blood pressure. It is the low aldosterone levels that lead to salt craving.

Key Point

Patients with Addison's disease frequently go on to develop other autoimmune endocrine disorders.

The main genetic association is with HLA-B8;DR3. Patients with HLA-DR3;DQ2 and HLA-DR4;DQ8 have a risk as high as 1 in 200–500. An atypical HLA molecule, MIC-A (to be exact the MICA-5.1 allele), is also strongly associated with Addison's disease.

CLINICAL CORRELATION 7.6

Diseases associated with Addison's disease

Addison's disease is very often found together with other autoimmune and non-autoimmune diseases. These include:

- **autoimmune thyroid disease (10–30%)**
- **type 1A diabetes (5–15%)**
- **pernicious anaemia**
- **autoimmune polyglandular syndromes**
- **hypoparathyroidism**
- **poor ovarian or testicular function.**

Hypoparathyroidism

Underactivity of the parathyroid, the gland that controls calcium levels in both blood and bone.

Testing for autoimmune Addison's disease in the clinical laboratory

We will now consider the tests available to confirm the diagnosis of Addison's disease. There are two approaches. Firstly, we need to confirm that the adrenal gland is not producing enough hormones. This is proven biochemically by artificially stimulating the adrenal gland and seeing how it reacts. Secondly, we need to show there is an autoimmune component. For details on testing for Addison's disease look at Method 7.6.

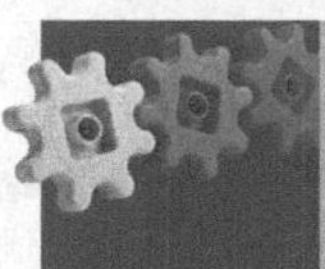

METHOD 7.6 Laboratory testing for autoimmune Addison's disease

Electrolytes

Low serum sodium is found in 90% of primary adrenal insufficiency cases.

Elevated serum potassium is found in 65%.

Low serum calcium is found in 50% of chronic cases

Short Synacthen test

We can look at adrenal function by challenging the patient with synthetic adrenocorticotrophic hormone (Synacthen or Tetracosactrin).

Serum samples are taken before injection of Synacthen and then at 30 minutes and 60 minutes after injection. Serum cortisol is measured. In a normal subject there will be a predictable increase in cortisol output. In patients with Addison's disease the output of cortisol is suppressed.

This can be a difficult test to interpret. If the patient has been taking glucocorticoids the response may be suppressed. In addition there are variations depending on the time of day the test is done (diurnal variation).

Adrenal cortex antibodies

Indirect immunofluorescence is still a popular method for looking for adrenal antibodies. It is positive in about 60% of patients with Addison's disease. Look at Figure 7.12 to see what anti-adrenal gland staining looks like.

The steroid 21-hydroxylase (P450c21) was shown to be an important auto-antigen in Addison's disease. Using radio-assay, antibodies to 21-hydroxylase are found in > 90% of patients with Addison's disease. False positive results are rarely seen.

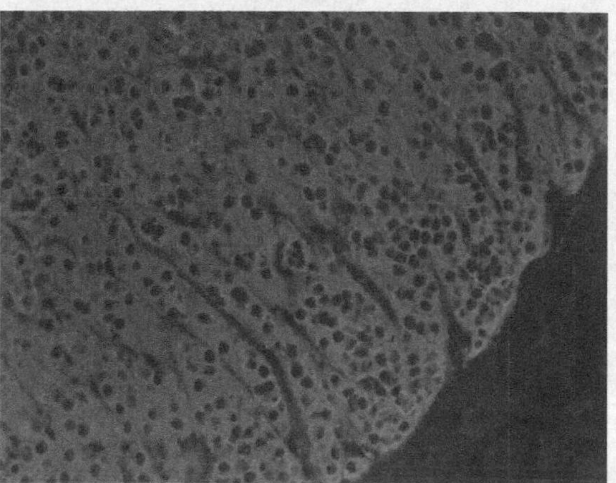

FIGURE 7.12
Indirect immunofluorescence staining of anti-adrenal gland antibody on monkey adrenal gland.

Treatment for autoimmune Addison's disease

The treatment for autoimmune Addison's disease focuses on hormone replacement. Both glucocorticoids and mineralocorticoids need to be replaced. Oral replacement is preferred where possible. In acute situations (e.g. patient collapse), intravenous hydrocortisone is used. Hydrocortisone is used to counter glucocorticoid deficiency. When the patient has an infection, has an accident, or is stressed, the dose of hydrocortisone needs to be increased to cope with this. Fludrocortisone is used to replace mineralocorticoid deficiency. The dose is adjusted according to the amount of salt craving and the blood pressure changes seen.

It is important to monitor patients regularly for other endocrine disorders which may develop during the course of the disease.

Summary

Autoimmune Addison's disease results in adrenal failure. Both glucocorticoid and mineralocorticoid hormones are reduced. Adrenal failure is confirmed by ACTH challenge and the effect this has on cortisol release. Auto-antibodies may be found to confirm the autoimmune nature of the disease. Treatment is by hormone replacement.

Cross reference

Look at Clinical correlations 7.2, 7.3, and 7.6 for examples of the multiple associations seen in autoimmune diseases.

7.4.3 Autoimmune polyglandular syndromes

As we have seen above, it is common for a patient to have more than one organ-specific autoimmune disease. In this part of the chapter we look at those syndromes where the disease associations are so strong that they are considered as a single entity.

Epidemiology

In this section we look at the clinical features found in APS-1 and APS-2, the genetic predispositions of each and the associations with other autoimmune disorders.

There are two main autoimmune polyglandular (or polyendocrine) syndromes (APS), called type 1 (APS-1) and type 2 (APS-2). APS-1 is a rare autosomal recessive disorder. It presents in childhood. APS-1 also has several other names, including APECED (autoimmune polyendocrinopathy-candidiasis-ectodermal dystrophy).Incidence varies according to the population studied; for example, prevalence is estimated at 1 in 500 000 inhabitants in North-western France. Look at Clinical correlation 7.7 for details of the clinical features of APS-1.

APS-1 is caused by mutation in the autoimmune regulator gene (*AIRE*). The *AIRE* gene is on chromosome 21q22.3. Over 50 different genetic variants have been described in APS-1 patients. *AIRE* expression is highest in the thymus. The AIRE protein is thought to have a role in transcription. Mouse models suggest AIRE is a critical regulator of self-antigen expression in the thymus. Alterations in this gene disrupt self-recognition. APS-1 was the first systemic autoimmune disorder to be found to be due to defects in a single gene. AIRE also regulates reactions against microbial agents, particularly against mycoses (fungal infections).

APS-2 is much more common than APS-1. It is found in about 1 in 20 000 persons. In contrast to APS-1 it usually presents in adulthood (age 20–60 years). Women are three times more frequently affected than males. The key features are Addison's disease, autoimmune thyroid disease, and type 1A diabetes. However, it is rare for APS-2 to present with several diseases simultaneously. More often the patient presents with one of the key disorders and the others develop with time. Look at Clinical correlation 7.8 for more details of the clinical features of APS-2.

Studies on susceptibility genes in APS-2 have produced variable results depending largely on the population studied. HLA-DRB1*03;DQB1*02 and HLA-DRB1*04;DQB1*03 appear to be associated with Addison's disease in APS-2 whilst HLA-DRB1*01;DQB1*05 confers protection from Addison's disease in APS-2. *AIRE* gene mutation is not found in this disorder.

CLINICAL CORRELATION 7.7

Clinical features of APS-1

The most frequent findings are mucocutaneous candidiasis (infection of the mucous membranes and skin with a fungus, *Candida*), hypoparathyroidism, and Addison's disease. At least two of these three should be present to make the diagnosis. Typically the disease presents in early childhood with mucocutaneous candidiasis as the first manifestation.

Mucocutaneous candidiasis is found in nearly all cases.

Hypoparathyroidism (under activity of the parathyroid glands) is found in 70–80% of patients with APS-1. This leads to disordered metabolism of calcium and phosphorus and therefore bone metabolism.

Addison's disease is found in 70–80% of patients with APS-1.

Other endocrine features include:

- **Premature ovarian failure in 60% of affected women.**
- **Testicular failure in men (though this is less common).**
- **Type 1A diabetes in 5–20% patients with APS-1.**
- **Autoimmune thyroid disease is uncommon, being seen in 10–15% of patients with APS-1.**

Non-endocrine features include:

- **Alopecia (hair loss).**
- **Vitiligo (loss of melanin).**
- **Autoimmune hepatitis.**
- **Pernicious anaemia.**
- **Corneal opacity.**
- **Enamel hypoplasia of teeth.**

Cross reference

For more detail, look at Sections 7.4.2 about Addison's disease, 7.3 about pernicious anaemia, 7.4.1 about type 1A diabetes, and 7.1 about autoimmune thyroid disease.

CLINICAL CORRELATION 7.8

Clinical features of APS-2

In order to be classified as having APS-2, the patient should have two of type 1A diabetes (55%), Addison's disease (45%), and autoimmune thyroid disease (75%)—either autoimmune hypothyroidism or Graves' disease.

Other autoimmune disorders seen in this complex include vitiligo (20%), pernicious anaemia (5%), hypogonadism, coeliac disease, and myasthenia gravis. Premature ovarian failure is seen in 60% of affected women.

Treatment for autoimmune polyglandular syndromes

The treatment of APS-1 includes replacement of deficient hormones and anti-fungal agents for the *Candida* infection. Hypoparathyroidism is treated with oral calcium and 1,25-dihydroxyvitamin D.

The treatment for APS-2 is based on the treatments for the individual components of the syndrome found in any given patient. The treatment can be complicated by the side effects of the drugs used. For example thyroxine has an effect on the liver, enhancing liver production of corticosteroids. This can mask problems with the adrenal glands. Conversely TSH secretion is inhibited by glucocorticoids from the adrenal gland. So treating one component of the disease may affect the therapy for another part.

In both APS-1 and APS-2 careful follow-up is required as patients may develop further autoimmune diseases with time.

Summary

There are two main types (APS-1 and APS-2). APS-1 is caused by mutations in the autoimmune regulator gene (AIRE). APS-2 is not.

APS-1 is characterized by candidiasis, hypoparathyroidism, and Addison's disease.

APS-2 is characterized by Addison's disease, autoimmune thyroid disease, and type 1A diabetes.

Treatment in both APS1 and APS-2 addresses the individual components of the disease.

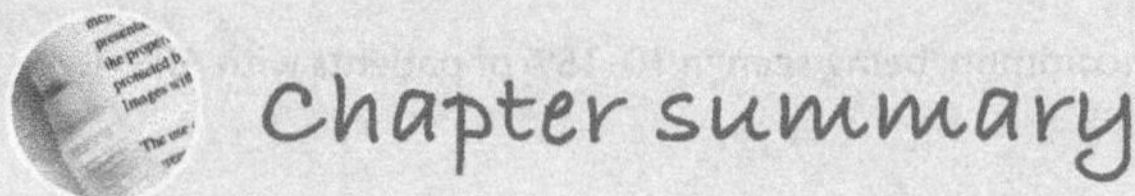

Chapter summary

- Organ-specific autoimmune diseases are common disorders.
- Organ-specific autoimmune diseases are more common in females than males.
- The presence of one autoimmune disease increases the risk of developing other autoimmune diseases.
- In part the overlap seen in organ-specific autoimmune disease is because certain genetic predispositions (HLA genes) are common to many.
- Characteristic antibodies ('disease markers') are often found.
- The characteristic antibodies may be pathogenic but more often are not.
- Indirect immunofluorescence and ELISA are the main laboratory tools for detecting auto-antibodies.
- Autoimmune disease requires an environmental trigger, but for most this is unknown.
- Coeliac disease is an exception, as gluten is known to be the trigger.
- Treatment is directed at replacing the lost factors (for example insulin in diabetes or vitamin B_{12} in pernicious anaemia) or modifying the immune response (for example removing the antigen (gluten) in coeliac disease)

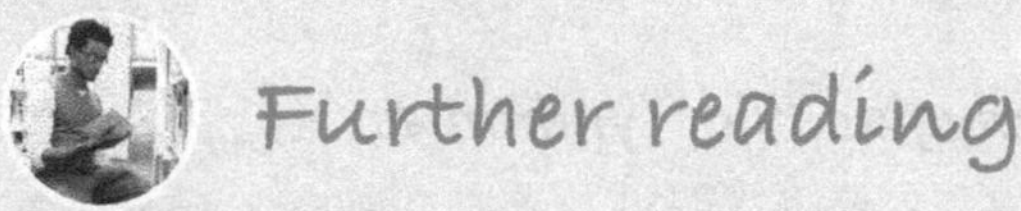

Further reading

- **Demers LM Spencer CA (eds) (2002) *Laboratory medicine practice guidelines. Laboratory support for the diagnosis and monitoring of thyroid disease*. National Academy of Clinical Biochemistry, http://www.nacb.org/. A comprehensive guide to testing for thyroid disease for both laboratory and medical personnel.**
- **Effraimidis G and Wiersinga WM (2014) *Mechanisms in endocrinology. Autoimmune thyroid disease: old and new players*. *Eur J Endocrinol*, 170 R241–52.**
- **Hill ID, Dirks MH, Liptak GS, *et al.* (2005) *Guideline for the diagnosis and treatment of celiac disease in children: recommendations of the North American Society for Pediatric Gastroenterology, Hepatology and Nutrition*. *J Paediatr Gastroenterol Nutr*, 40 1–19.**

- Hill PG, McMillan SA (2006) ***Anti-tissue transglutaminase antibodies and their role in the investigation of coeliac disease***. *Ann Clin Biochem*, **43** 105–17. A comprehensive review of the use of this recently introduced test.
- Husby S *et al.* (2012) ***European Society for Pediatric Gastroenterology, Hepatology, and Nutrition guidelines for the diagnosis of coeliac disease***. *J Paediatr Gastroenterol Nutr*, **54**, 136–60.
- Male D, Brostoff J, Roth D, Roitt I (2012). ***Immunology***. 8th Edition, Mosby, St Louis.
- Murphy K (2011) ***Janeway's Immunobiology***. 8th Edition, Garland Science, New York.
- NICE (2015) ***Coeliac disease: recognition, assessment and management***. NICE guideline 20, https://www.nice.org.uk/guidance/ng20
- Owen J, Punt J, Stranford S (2013) ***Kuby Immunology***. 7th Edition, W.H. Freeman, New York.
- Sollid LM, Spurkland A, Thorsby E (2000) HLA and gastrointestinal diseases. Chapter 17 in Lechler R, Warrens A (eds) ***HLA in Disease and Health***, pp. 249–62. Academic Press, London.

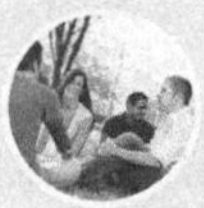

Discussion questions

7.1 What three criteria are needed to develop autoimmune disease?

7.2 What is the difference between autoimmune phenomena and autoimmune disease?

7.3 What are the autoimmune diseases associated with hypothyroidism and hyperthyroidism?

7.4 Why is it so important to know a patient's serum IgA level when performing tests for coeliac disease?

7.5 What are the two mechanisms that cause anaemia as a result of pernicious anaemia?

Answers to self-check questions are provided in the book's Online Resource Centre.

 Visit www.oxfordtextbooks.co.uk/orc/hall2e

8

Autoimmune skin disease

Learning Objectives

After studying this chapter you should be able to:

- explain the clinical features of autoimmune skin disease
- outline the assays and techniques used to test for autoimmune skin disease
- discuss the limitations of these techniques
- outline the treatment of autoimmune skin disease.

Cross reference

The skin is affected in a number of systemic autoimmune disorders described elsewhere in this book such as systemic lupus erythematosus, rheumatoid arthritis (see Chapter 5) and vasculitis (see Chapter 6). For an introduction to autoimmune disease you should read the introduction to Chapter 7.

Introduction

The skin is the largest organ in the body. It provides a protective barrier against the physical effects of trauma and hazardous chemicals, as well as providing a physical barrier to infection. In addition the skin has several other functions; it prevents loss of moisture, acts as a sensory organ, helps regulate temperature, protects against ultraviolet radiation and forms a part of the immune system.

In this chapter we will look at diseases where the skin is the main target organ. In particular we will examine the autoimmune bullous (blistering) skin diseases. You should note that not all of the blistering diseases are autoimmune in nature. There are disorders that are very similar in appearance but are caused by mutations in genes coding for the proteins that act as targets in autoimmune disease. In addition there are blistering skin conditions caused by infection. A good example of this is the **scalded skin syndrome**, which is caused by Staphylococcus and usually presents in infancy. In this condition a toxin from the Staphylococcus affects a structural protein in skin (called the **desmosome**), resulting in blistering. Herpes zoster is the virus which causes chicken pox and may reactivate as shingles. Shingles is another good example of infection-related blistering, as is Herpes simplex, the virus associated with the common cold sore. Blistering can also be a manifestation of T cell mediated drug hypersensitivity.

Scalded skin syndrome

Staphylococcal infection of the skin, leading to a generalized red blistering rash also known as bullous impetigo.

Desmosome

A specialized structure for cell-cell adhesion.

Cross references

You can read more about bacterial infections in the *Medical Microbiology* textbook of this series.

You can read more about drug hypersensitivity in Chapter 3.

8.1 Skin structure

Before we look at the diseases you will need an understanding of the structure of the skin. There are three main layers. The deepest is the **sub-cutis** (literally 'below the skin'), containing fibrous tissue, fat, blood vessels, and lymphatics. Above the sub-cutis is the **dermis**. The dermis contains many structures such as hair follicles and sebaceous (sweat) glands. The most superficial layer is the **epidermis**, which contains many of the target structures for autoimmune skin diseases. Look at Figure 8.1 to see the overall structure of the epidermis.

Sub-cutis
The deepest/innermost layer of the skin.

Dermis
The layer of skin between the epidermis and the sub-cutis.

Epidermis
The outermost layer of the skin.

Hemidesmosome
Stud-like structures on the inner layer of keratinocytes in the epidermis that allow cell adhesion to the extracellular matrix.

The basement membrane forms the link between the dermis and epidermis. The cells of the basal layer of the epidermis are joined to the basement membrane by a structure called the **hemidesmosome**. There are several protein components to this of which the most important as targets for autoimmune disease are BP180 (collagen XVII), BP230 (dystonin), laminin 332 (formerly called laminin-5), and collagen VII.

The cells higher in the epidermis (prickle cells and granular cells) are joined by a structure called the desmosome. The most important proteins are calcium-dependent cell adhesion molecules called cadherins, including desmogleins (named from the Greek *glein* meaning glue) and desmocollins. These are bound to intracellular anchoring structures such as desmoplakins and plakoglobins.

The type of blistering seen in the autoimmune dermatoses relates to the depth of the structure targeted by the autoimmune attack. Look at Figure 8.2 to see how different disorders blister at different levels of the skin. The blisters are formed by a complex interaction involving autoantibodies binding to the skin and the activation of complement. This in turn leads to activation of effector cells such as neutrophils, eosinophils, and mast cells.

Cross reference
See Chapter 4 for more information on complement activation.

SELF-CHECK 8.1

What are the three layers of the skin? In which layer are the blisters seen in the autoimmune skin diseases?

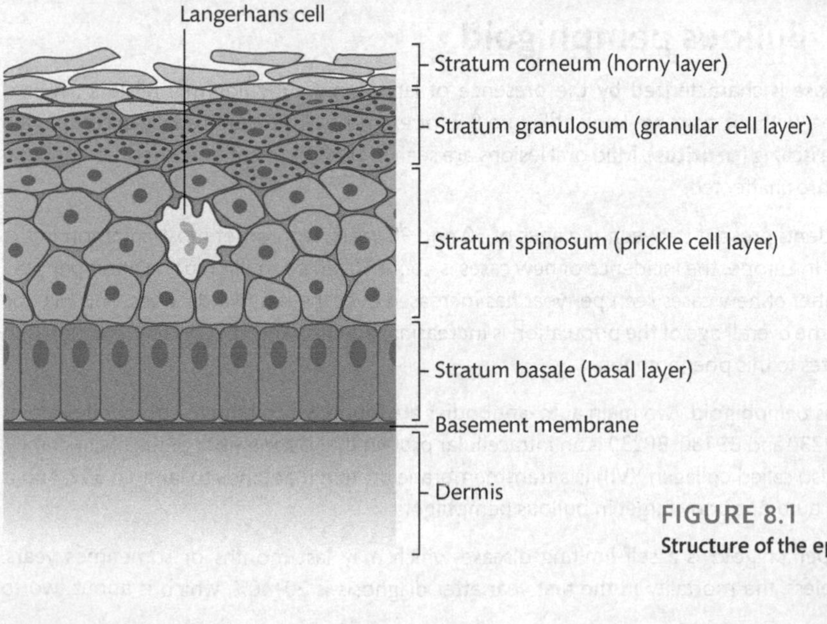

FIGURE 8.1
Structure of the epidermis.

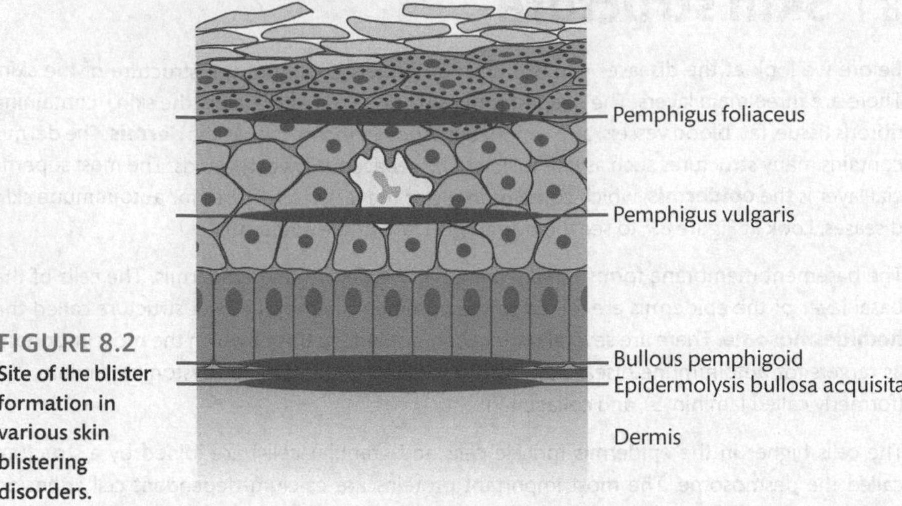

FIGURE 8.2
Site of the blister formation in various skin blistering disorders.

SELF-CHECK 8.2

Name a systemic autoimmune disease which can affect the skin.

SELF-CHECK 8.3

Name a blistering skin disease caused by an infection.

8.2 Pemphigoid diseases

Pemphigoid diseases are autoimmune diseases mediated by auto-antibodies directed against proteins within the skin at the point where the dermis and the epidermis meet. This connection between the dermis and epidermis is termed the **dermal-epidermal junction** (also called the hemidesmosome, as in Section 8.1).

Dermal-epidermal junction
The junction between the dermis and the epidermis.

8.2.1 Bullous pemphigoid

This disease is characterized by the presence of large tense subepidermal blisters (**bullae**) which heal without scarring. Look at Figure 8.3 for examples. These are usually accompanied by severe itching (**pruritus**). Mild oral lesions are seen in 10–20% of patients but other mucosal surfaces are unaffected.

Bullae
Large blisters containing serous fluid.

Pruritis
Itch.

Most patients present between the ages of 50 and 90 years, with onset most common in the over 70s. In Europe, the incidence of new cases is about 10–20 per million population per year. The number of new cases seen per year has increased over the last two decades. This may be because the overall age of the population is increasing, but it is likely that better detection also contributes to this phenomenon.

In bullous pemphigoid, two main auto-antibodies are found which bind to structural proteins called BP230 and BP180. BP230 is an intracellular protein that is a member of the plakin family. BP180 (also called collagen XVII) is a transmembrane protein that binds to laminin 332, and is the main auto-antibody target in bullous pemphigoid.

Bullous pemphigoid is a self-limiting disease which may last months or sometimes years. Nevertheless, the mortality in the first year after diagnosis is 20–40%, which is about two to three times higher than in healthy age-matched control subjects. Risk factors include old age, widespread disease, and high doses of oral steroids.

About a third of patients have some neurological association. Parkinson's disease, stroke, epilepsy, and multiple sclerosis have all been seen at higher incidence than in matched controls. This seems to be related to the finding that the auto-antibody targets of BP180 and BP230 are expressed in the central nervous system.

As with many other autoimmune diseases, it is not known whether environmental factors can trigger bullous pemphigoid. Trauma, burns, ultraviolet radiation, and the influenza vaccine have all been implicated.

Treatment depends on the extent of the disease. Localized or limited disease can be treated with topical corticosteroid (i.e. applied as a cream or ointment to the skin). Tacrolimus, an immunosuppressive drug used extensively in transplantation, can also be useful as a topical agent to treat bullous pemphigoid. More widespread disease is usually treated with oral prednisolone, a synthetic corticosteroid. Azathioprine, which acts as a terminator of DNA synthesis with resultant impairment of lymphocyte function, may be used to spare the amount of steroid required. This is important in reducing the severe and multiple side-effects of long-term steroid use.

Other drugs have been used but the evidence for efficacy is limited. These include mycophenolate mofetil, cyclophosphamide, and methotrexate. These are usually tried when other therapies have failed. Dapsone, an antimicrobial agent that also has some anti-inflammatory properties, can be used as an adjunct to steroids or other immunosuppressive therapy.

Cross reference

For descriptions of direct and indirect immunofluorescence see Methods 8.1 and 8.3.

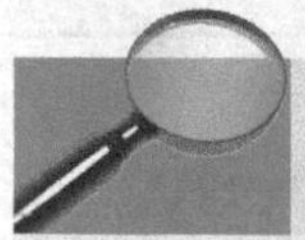

CASE STUDY 8.1 Bullous pemphigoid

Patient history

An 81-year-old female patient presented with a six-month history of a recurrent blistering rash mainly affecting the backs of the knees and upper calves (see Figure 8.3).

The rash was painful at the onset of lesions and would take 1–2 weeks to heal, and would not leave a scar. The roof of the lesions would always break off. The patient had been reviewed by Dermatology but unfortunately her rash was

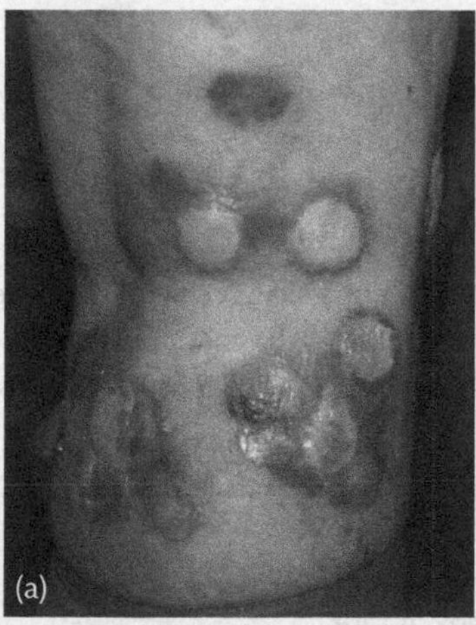

(a)

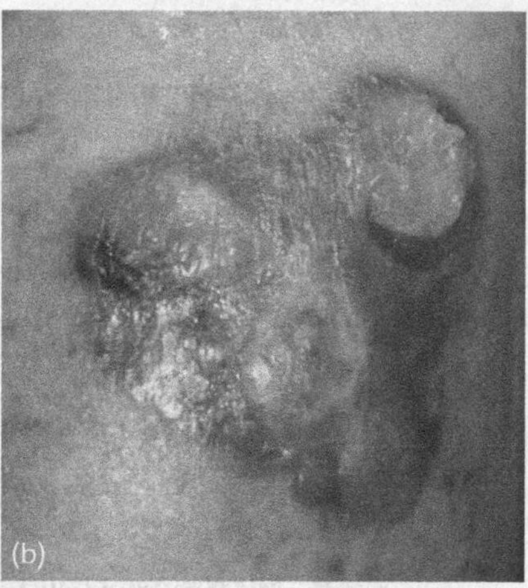

(b)

FIGURE 8.3
Bullous pemphigoid.

healing at the time, and the skin biopsy performed did not show evidence of basement membrane staining on direct immunofluorescence.

Results

Blood testing for bullous skin disease auto-antibodies was performed. This was positive for IgG anti-skin basement membrane antibodies. IgG and IgA intercellular antibodies were negative, as were IgA anti-skin basement membrane antibodies. IgG staining of split skin showed basement membrane immunofluorescence on the upper surface, consistent with bullous pemphigoid.

Significance of results

She was referred back to Dermatology with a confirmed diagnosis of bullous pemphigoid and was started on topical corticosteroid treatment in the first instance.

Key Points

- **Bullous pemphigoid is the most common of the autoimmune blistering diseases.**
- **The number of cases presenting per year has doubled in the last decade.**
- **Bullous pemphigoid is a disease of the elderly.**
- **Blisters are formed at the basement membrane.**
- **The major auto-antigen is the hemidesmosomal protein BP180 (collagen XVII).**

8.2.2 Mucous membrane pemphigoid (formerly cicatricial or scarring pemphigoid)

The mean age of onset for mucous membrane pemphigoid is 60–65 years of age. Incidence is approximately 1–2 cases per million people per year in Europe. There is an association with HLA-DQB1*0301. Most patients (85%) have lesions in the oral cavity. Fewer (65%) have involvement of the conjunctivae of the eye. The eye involvement can be very serious with decreased vision, photosensitivity, scarring, and eventual blindness. Other mucous membrane areas are less often affected.

Cross reference

You can read in more detail about HLA in Chapter 13.

In mucous membrane pemphigoid the target antigens vary. Patients may have auto-antibodies targeting BP180 (about 75% of cases), BP230 (about 25% of cases, usually with BP180 as well), laminin 332 (25% of cases), laminin 311, or $\alpha6\beta4$ integrin. In about 30% of cases with the anti-laminin 332 antibody a solid tumour is present.

Treatment is similar to that for bullous pemphigoid but clinical response is poor. The addition of intravenous immunoglobulin therapy has been favourable in some patients. The underlying pathogenesis of mucous membrane pemphigoid is not well understood.

Key Points

- **Mucous membrane pemphigoid is rare.**
- **The most commonly affected organs are the oral cavity and eye.**
- **The major auto-antigen is the hemidesmosomal protein BP180 (collagen XVII).**

8.2.3 Epidermolysis bullosa acquisita

Epidermolysis bullosa acquisita is a disease of adults. Incidence is 0.2–0.5 per million per year. There is an association with HLA-DRB1*1503 and African ancestry. The main auto-antibody detected is IgG directed against collagen VII. It is a chronic blistering skin disease which, unlike bullous pemphigoid, may cause scarring. About 50% of patients have oral lesions. It has been shown in mice that injecting antibodies from patients ('passive transfer studies') results in direct complement activation and subsequent neutrophil recruitment in the skin. This shows the antibodies to be **pathogenic**, that is they directly cause the disease. However, biopsies often show only mild or no histological inflammation. It has been suggested that the action of auto-antibody binding to collagen in this disorder might have a direct effect on the formation of the anchoring fibrils or might interfere with the binding to other structural proteins such as laminin 332.

Pathogenic
Causing disease.

Treatment is more difficult in epidermolysis bullosa acquisita, with the treatments used in bullous pemphigoid being less effective. In particular, systemic steroids are less effective than in other autoimmune blistering diseases. Colchicine, derived from the autumn crocus and used for the treatment of gout, is effective in high dose in some patients. Cyclosporin has also been effective in some patients who have not responded to other therapies. Plasmapheresis (see Method 8.2) and high dose intravenous immunoglobulin may be more effective.

Key Points

- **Epidermolysis bullosa acquisita is very rare.**
- **There is an association with African descent.**
- **About 50% of patients have oral lesions.**
- **The major auto-antigen is collagen VII.**

8.2.4 Pemphigoid gestationis

Pemphigoid gestationis (formerly called herpes gestationis) is a blistering skin disease associated with pregnancy. The incidence in Europe is 0.5–2.2 per million population per year. Pemphigoid gestationis usually occurs in the second half of pregnancy, although 10% of cases occur up to 4 weeks after birth. It usually lasts about 4–6 months and has a relatively benign course. However up to 5% go on to have bullous pemphigoid.

In pemphigoid gestationis the target antigen is the non-collagenous NC16A region of BP180. Antibodies against BP230 can also be found. The infant may also be affected by transplacental transfer of maternal antibody, which usually resolves spontaneously as maternal antibody levels decline.

Key Points

- **Pemphigoid gestationis is associated with pregnancy.**
- **Up to 5% of patients go on to have bullous pemphigoid.**

8.2.5 Linear IgA disease

Linear IgA disease is the most common bullous pemphigoid disease of children. It is also seen in adults over the age of 60 years. Oral ulcers are seen in 70% of cases. It can be drug induced, the most common trigger being the antibiotic vancomycin.

The major target antigen for the auto-antibody is BP180 but unlike the other pemphigoid diseases the antibody is of IgA class, not IgG. As many laboratories only screen for IgG class antibodies the diagnosis may be missed. Treatment for linear IgA disease is similar to bullous pemphigoid, with dapsone and corticosteriods being the mainstay. In drug induced cases, removing the offending drug is also required.

Key Point

Linear IgA disease may be drug induced.

SELF-CHECK 8.4

In what age group would you expect bullous pemphigoid to present?

SELF-CHECK 8.5

Can you name three different treatments used in the pemphigoid diseases?

SELF-CHECK 8.6

Can you name the auto-antibody antigenic targets in the different pemphigoid diseases?

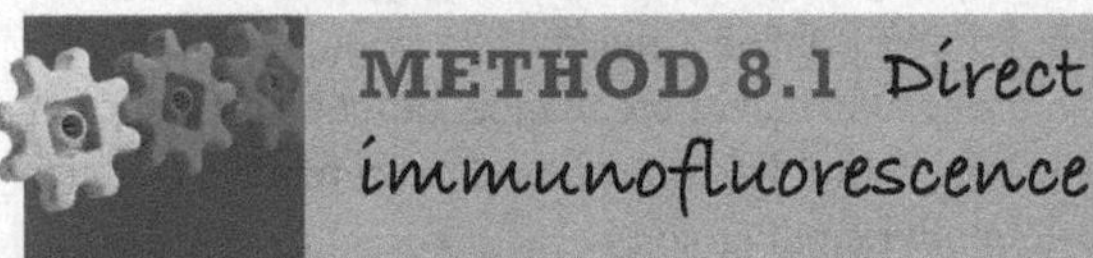

METHOD 8.1 Direct immunofluorescence

You can look directly at antibodies bound to the skin by taking a biopsy and directly looking for deposition of antibodies in the skin. This technique uses a conjugated antibody (either a fluorescent or enzyme labelled antibody) to IgG, IgA, or Complement C3 that is bound in the skin. This method is called direct immunofluorescence. You can see an example of this in Figure 8.4 from a patient with pemphigus foliaceus. The biopsy may not always be positive. For example about 20% of cases of mucous membrane pemphigoid are negative on biopsy.

Direct immunofluorescence is a little more sensitive than indirect immunofluorescence. For example, in pemphigus vulgaris oral biopsy is positive in about 90% of cases, compared with about 85% for indirect immunofluorescence.

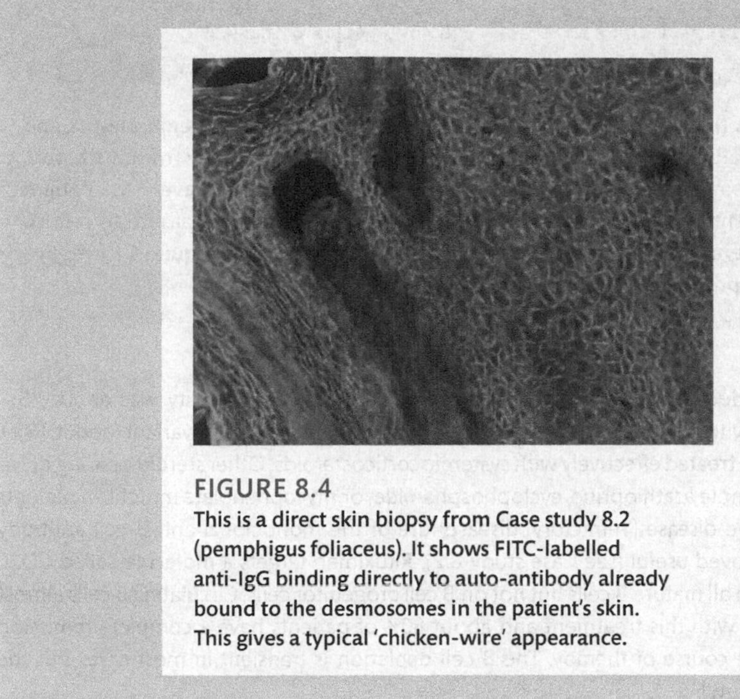

FIGURE 8.4
This is a direct skin biopsy from Case study 8.2 (pemphigus foliaceus). It shows FITC-labelled anti-IgG binding directly to auto-antibody already bound to the desmosomes in the patient's skin. This gives a typical 'chicken-wire' appearance.

Cross reference
See Case study 8.2 for details on the patient from whom the biopsy was taken.

8.3 Pemphigus diseases

Pemphigus diseases are autoimmune diseases mediated by auto-antibodies directed against protein structures linking cells (keratinocytes) together within the epithelium. These structures, which act as intercellular bridges, are called desmosomes.

8.3.1 Pemphigus vulgaris

This is the most severe form of pemphigus. It is most often seen in adults aged 30 to 50 years, and is less common than pemphigoid. It affects the skin and mucous membranes. It presents with flaccid intraepithelial blisters that are easily ruptured. Without treatment this is often a fatal disease. Owing to the breakdown of the skin, infection may breach the skin barrier resulting in sepsis which may prove fatal.

This is an antibody mediated disease. Some of the antibodies found are directed against cadherins. The main antigenic structure is made up of two proteins in the desmosome, called desmoglein 3 (130kDa cadherin) and plakoglobin. In 50–60% of cases antibodies may also be found to desmoglein 1, which is another cadherin protein in the desmosome. Desmoglein 3 is more highly expressed in the lower layers of the epidermis whereas desmoglein 1 is more highly expressed in the upper layers. In patients with only mucous membrane pemphigus vulgaris, anti-desmoglein 1 is not found. Other antibodies in addition to those mentioned can be found in pemphigus and the pathophysiology is complex. Nevertheless, antibodies to desmoglein 1 and desmoglein 3 are useful tools in the diagnosis of pemphigus.

Cross reference
Look at Method 8.1 and Method 8.3 where you can read more about the techniques used in the diagnosis of pemphigus.

Plasma exchange may be used to reduce the burden of antibody in the patient but needs to be used in combination with other therapies.

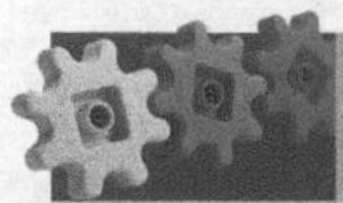

METHOD 8.2 Plasmapheresis

Plasmapheresis (plasma exchange) is a technique to remove the patient's plasma and replace it with albumin. This removes circulating pathogenic antibody from the blood, but does not remove antibody in the interstitium. Neither does it prevent the patient making more antibody. It is therefore only useful as a short-term measure to reduce antibody concentration while concurrent immunosuppression is required to reduce auto-antibody production, as described in Section 8.2.

Before the introduction of corticosteroid therapy in the 1950s mortality was about 75%. Mortality varies with subtype and is lower in the predominantly mucosal variant (about 15%). Most patients are treated effectively with systemic corticosteroids. Other steroid-sparing drugs are used, for example azathioprine, cyclophosphamide, or mycophenolate mofetil. In patients with unresponsive disease ('refractory' disease) use of the monoclonal anti-B-cell antibody rituximab has proved useful (see Case study 8.2). Rituximab targets a molecule called CD20 which is found on all mature B cells but not on B cell progenitor cells. Circulating B cells almost totally disappear with this treatment and about 80% of patients have a complete remission after just a single course of therapy. The B cell depletion is transient in most cases but the benefit is maintained.

Key Points

- **Pemphigus vulgaris is the most severe form of pemphigus.**
- **Mortality from pemphigus vulgaris is very high without treatment.**
- **Blisters are formed in the lower epidermis.**
- **The major auto-antigen is the desmosomal protein desmoglein 3.**

Cross reference

Look at Case study 8.2 to see an example of pemphigus foliaceus and the response to treatment.

8.3.2 Pemphigus foliaceus

Pemphigus foliaceus is the second most common form of pemphigus. The blisters are more superficial than pemphigus vulgaris and the mucous membranes are not involved. The antigen in pemphigus foliaceus is desmoglein 1.

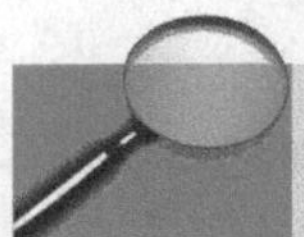

CASE STUDY 8.2 Pemphigus foliaceus

Patient history

A 63-year-old gentleman was referred by Dermatology for further management of severe, treatment unresponsive, serologically and biopsy confirmed pemphigus foliaceus, which had followed a relapsing and remitting course over the previous 8 years. He had a background of inflammatory bowel disease and ischaemic heart disease. He was on oral corticosteroids and had recently undergone a course of plasmapheresis for the skin disease. Over the

years he had tried and failed a number of treatments including dapsone, minocycline and nicotinamide, azathioprine, and intravenous and oral cyclophosphamide.

Treatment

A course of rituximab was planned. When the patient attended for the second of four weekly rituximab infusions he had very extensive cutaneous disease and was effectively erythrodermic (very extensive reddening of the skin). At this stage the extent of the skin disease was potentially life-threatening (see Figure 8.5). He required emergency admission for fluid, temperature, and blood glucose management, in addition to antibiotics. He subsequently completed the rituximab course and was discharged on mycophenolate mofetil and corticosteroids.

Response to treatment

He had a dramatic response following completion of the rituximab, such that all systemic immune suppression was weaned over the subsequent 2 years. The patient has had minimal cutaneous disease since, which has responded to topical corticosteroid therapy. Compare Figures 8.5 and 8.6 to see the response to rituximab.

At the time of treatment rituximab had been reported as effective therapy in a patient with paraneoplastic (cancer associated) pemphigus, the underlying malignancy being a B cell lymphoma, for which rituximab was licensed. There have since been further reports of the benefits of rituximab in the treatment of pemphigus, such that it is now an accepted treatment.

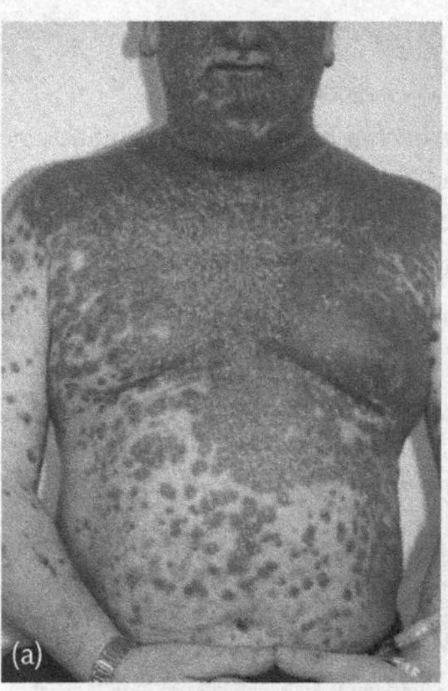

(a)

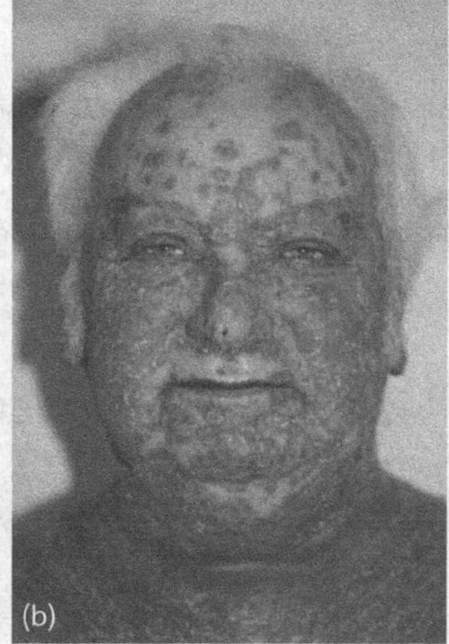

(b)

FIGURE 8.5
Pemphigus foliaceus pre-rituximab.

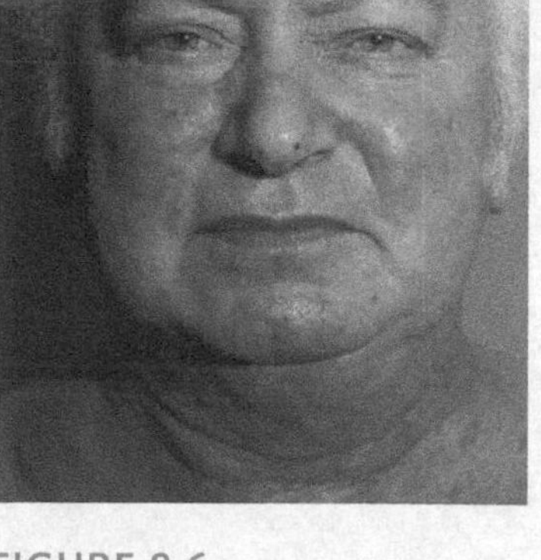

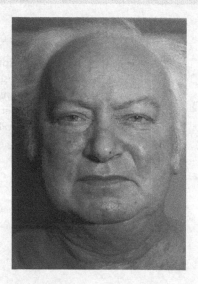

FIGURE 8.6
Pemphigus foliaceus post-rituximab.

The clinical picture is one of reddening of the skin (**erythema**), scaling, and crusting. The head, neck, and trunk are often involved with relative sparing of the limbs.

There are other forms of pemphigus foliaceus. In South America there is an endemic disease called 'fogo selvagem' (Portuguese for 'wild fire'). This is different to the non-endemic form. It may be initiated by bites of the black fly and seems to be made worse by ultraviolet radiation. There are also reports of drug induced forms of pemphigus foliaceus (for example by penicillamine or ACE inhibitors). Look at Case study 8.3. In all of these cases there is an autoimmune component, as antibodies to desmoglein 1 can be found in all forms of pemphigus foliaceus.

Cross reference

See Joly et al. (2007) for more on the use of rituximab in the treatment of pemphigus.

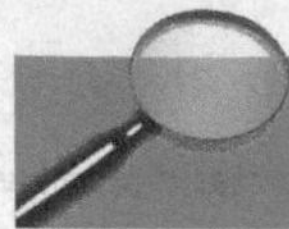

CASE STUDY 8.3 Pemphigus foliaceus

Patient history

A 68-year-old retired engineer, with a history of rheumatoid arthritis, presented to the Dermatology clinic with a widespread bullous and erosive facial rash after penicillamine had been prescribed for a flare of the joint disease (see Figure 8.7).

Results

The clinical differential diagnosis was of penicillamine induced pemphigus and cutaneous lupus. Biopsy was consistent with pemphigus, serology was also positive for anti-skin antibodies, lupus serology was negative, and complement levels normal. He had a poor response to azathioprine, ocular toxicity with hydroxychloroquine, itch with mepacrine, gastrointestinal side effects with mycophenolate, little benefit from topical tacrolimus, and poor response to cyclophosphamide.

Treatment

His disease was subsequently treated with plasma exchange, pulsed intravenous cyclophosphamide, high dose intravenous steroid, and rituximab. He had a very good response to the latter. He remains on low dose steroid for the rheumatoid arthritis but all other systemic immune suppression has been discontinued. He remains well at 4 years of follow-up.

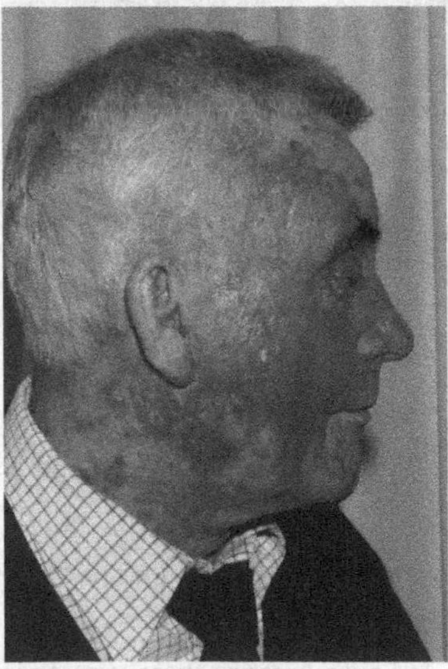

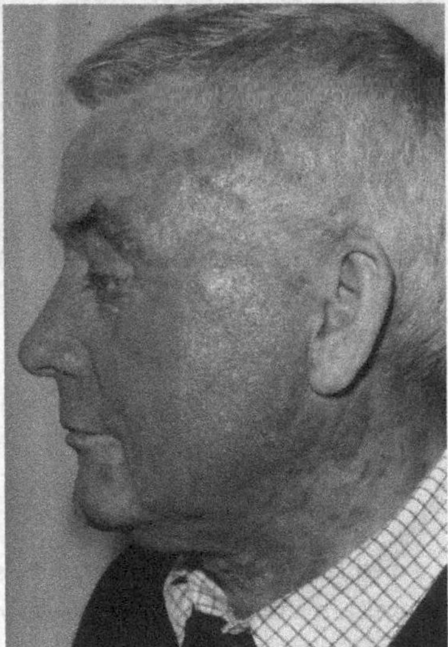

FIGURE 8.7
Drug-induced pemphigus.

Key Points

- **In pemphigus foliaceus blisters are formed in the high epidermis.**
- **The major auto-antigen is the desmosomal protein desmoglein 1.**

8.3.3 Paraneoplastic pemphigus

Paraneoplastic pemphigus typically presents with oral lesions in the presence of a primary neoplasm. It is usually a rapidly progressive disease and is usually fatal. The most common primary tumour is non-Hodgkin's lymphoma (NHL). Other tumours and conditions where paraneoplastic pemphigus is seen include chronic lymphocytic leukaemia, Castleman's disease, thymoma, sarcoma, and Waldenström's macroglobulinaemia.

The patients have antibodies to many different antigens including desmoglein 1, desmoglein 3, BP230, envoplakin, periplakin, desmoplakin 1, and desmoplakin 2. Characteristically the antibodies stain the intercellular spaces (desmosomal stain) and also the basal layer.

Cross references

You can read more about paraneoplastic diseases in Chapter 10.

You can read more about Waldenström's macroglobulinaemia in Chapter 2.

Look at Methods 8.1 and 8.3 for more detail on immunofluorescence.

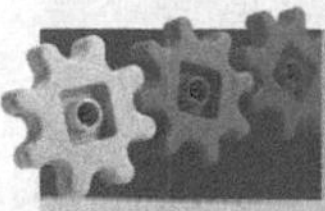

METHOD 8.3 Indirect immunofluorescence

You can look indirectly for circulating antibodies in the serum that will bind to primate tissue. This technique is known as indirect immunofluorescence. Patient serum is allowed to react with the appropriate tissue substrate. Unbound antibody is washed away and the bound antibody then labelled with a second, fluorescently labelled antibody, for subsequent microscopy.

Typically the substrate used for indirect immunofluorescence in the context of autoimmune skin disease is monkey oesophagus. Desmosomal stain has a 'chicken-wire' appearance whereas the basement membrane is a linear stain at the dermal-epidermal interface. Look at Figure 8.8 to see examples of skin desmosomal stain and basement membrane stain. You should note that the blood group A

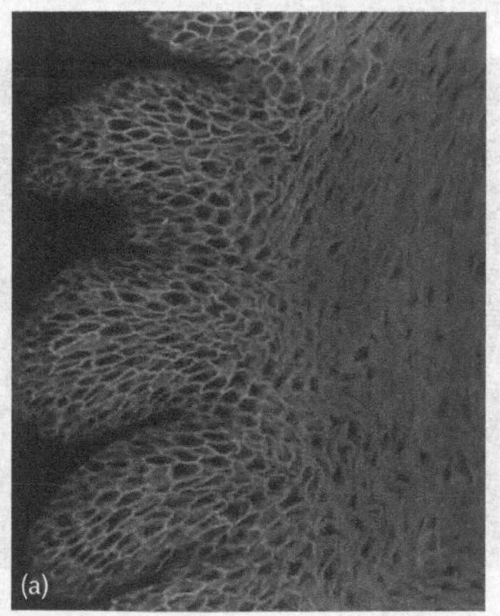

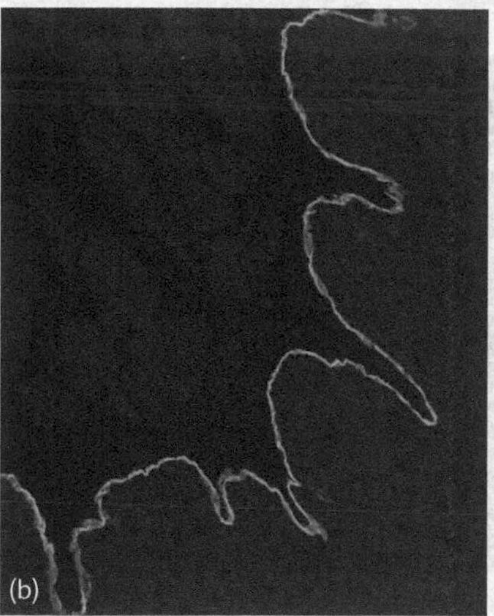

FIGURE 8.8

(a) Intracellular substance (desmosomes) in pemphigus vulgaris. (b) Basement membrane (hemi-desmosomes) in bullous pemphigoid.

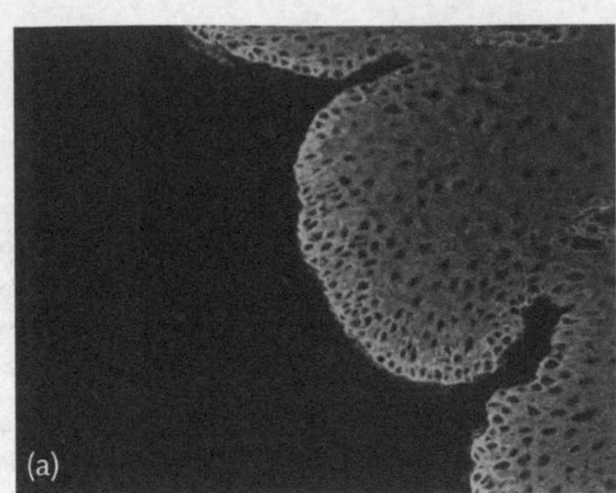

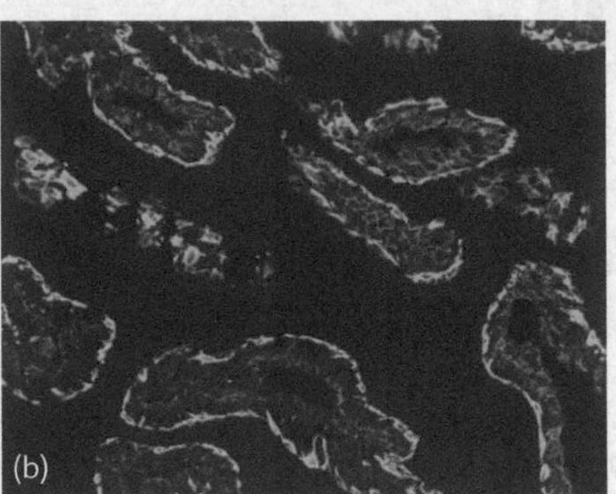

FIGURE 8.9
Paraneoplastic pemphigus. Indirect immunofluorescence on (a) monkey oesophagus and (b) rat bladder.

and B antigens may be expressed on the surface of primate epidermal cells. This can lead to a similar 'chicken-wire' staining pattern if the patient has anti-A or anti-B circulating in the serum. To avoid this it is best to absorb out the patient's anti-A and anti-B by using soluble AB substance in the dilution buffer before adding the serum to the tissue substrate. Distinguishing between desmoglein 1 and desmoglein 3 auto-antibodies is usually not possible using monkey oesophagus substrate. The antibodies associated with paraneoplastic pemphigus are more readily distinguished on rat bladder than monkey oesophagus. Look at Figure 8.9 to see this.

Alternative substrates may be used to better distinguish subsets of these patterns. Primate skin may be split along the basement membrane by treating it with 1 M saline before freezing and cutting the sections. The bullous pemphigoid antigens BP180 and BP230 are found on the upper (epidermal) surface of the 'split skin'. The collagen VII antigens are found on the lower (dermal) surface, and are associated with epidemolyis bullosa acquisita. Look at Figure 8.10

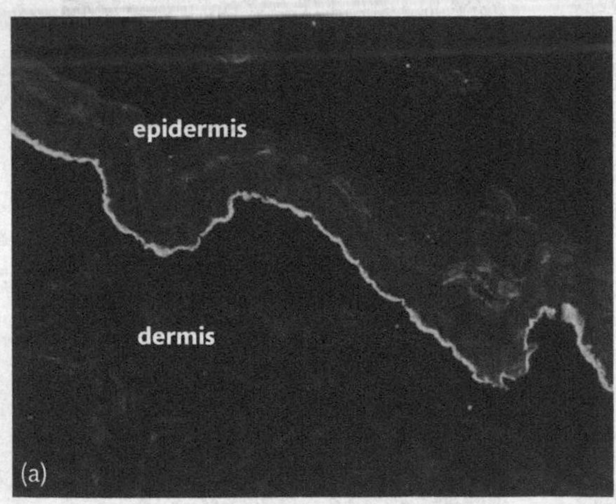

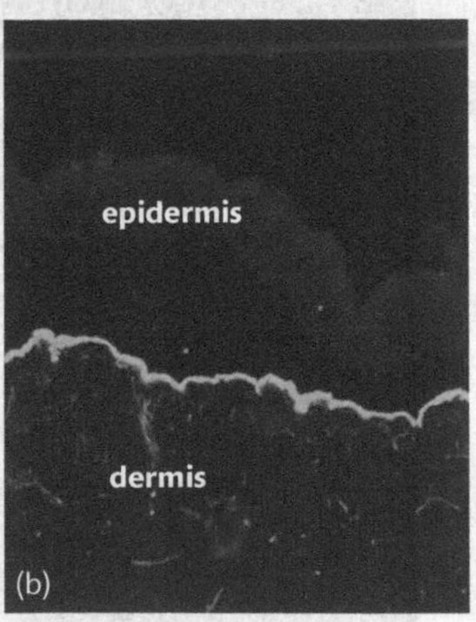

FIGURE 8.10
(a) Bullous pemphigoid. IIF on monkey split skin staining the upper surface of the basement membrane. (b) Epidermolysis bullosa acquisita. IIF on monkey split skin staining the lower surface of the basement membrane.

to see these patterns. About 45% of patients with mucous membrane pemphigoid stain both epidermal and dermal surfaces. This type of staining also occurs in about 5% of bullous pemphigoid cases and so is not entirely specific. Look at Figure 8.11 for an example of this pattern.

Not all patients will be positive by indirect immunofluorescence: 85% of patients with bullous pemphigoid have antibodies to BP180 and 60–70% have antibodies to BP230. In contrast, only 50–80% of patients with mucous membrane pemphigoid have detectable antibodies on split skin. Similarly, circulating collagen VII antibodies can only be demonstrated in about 50% of epidemolysis bullosa acquisita patients.

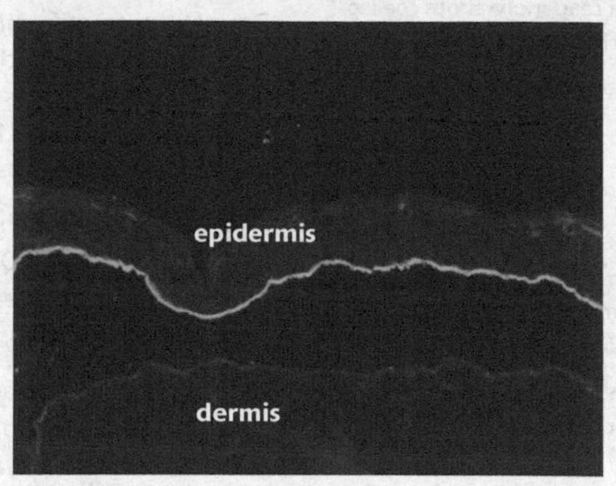

FIGURE 8.11
Mucous membrane pemphigoid. Indirect immunofluorescence on monkey split skin.

8.3.4 IgA pemphigus

IgA pemphigus is very rare. Two subtypes have been described. In sub-corneal pustular dermatosis the auto-antibodies are directed against desmocollin 1 and are seen deposited in the upper epidermis. In intra-epidermal IgA neutrophilic dermatosis the antigen remains unidentified in most cases. Auto-antibodies are seen either in the lower epidermis or throughout the whole epidermis. It is often associated with an underlying neoplasm (paraneoplastic).

SELF-CHECK 8.7

In what age group would you expect to find pemphigus vulgaris?

SELF-CHECK 8.8

What structure in the skin is targeted by auto-antibodies in pemphigus vulgaris?

SELF-CHECK 8.9

What is the auto-antibody antigenic target in pemphigus foliaceus?

8.4 Other autoimmune blistering skin disorders

We have seen how blistering skin diseases may be a direct result of antibodies to structures binding the skin cells together (desmosomes and hemidesmosomes). In this section we will consider two blistering conditions where mechanisms other than these are in place.

Cross reference

You can read more about coeliac disease in Chapter 7.

8.4.1 Dermatitis herpetiformis

Dermatitis herpetiformis is characterized by small blisters on the extensor surfaces (e.g. elbows or buttocks) which resemble the vesicles of herpes virus infections. These are very itchy (pruritic). The disease is one of the gluten-sensitive disorders and is related to coeliac disease. Indeed, on small bowel biopsy most patients with dermatitis herpetiformis have changes identical to those seen in coeliac disease.

Cross references

You can read more about other autoimmune diseases in Chapters 5, 6, and 7.

You can read more about HLA in Chapter 13.

Like coeliac disease there is a strong association between dermatitis herpetiformis and HLA-DQ2 and HLA-DQ8. Patients with dermatitis herpetiformis are also more likely to have other autoimmune diseases including autoimmune thyroid disease, systemic lupus erythematosus, dermatomyositis, Sjögren's syndrome, and rheumatoid arthritis.

In common with coeliac disease, antibodies are found to the extrinsic antigen gliadin (from wheat) and auto-antibodies are found to tissue transglutaminase (type 2) and endomysium. In addition, another auto-antibody is found directed against epidermal transglutaminase type 3. This enzyme is exclusively found in the skin.

Direct immunofluorescence techniques on skin biopsy can show the presence of IgA-containing complexes and collections of neutrophils in the apices just under the basement membrane in what are called dermal papillae. The complex is thought to be IgA auto-antibody bound to epidermal transglutaminase type 3 in the skin.

Cross reference

You can see an example of anti-endomysium antibody staining on immunofluorescence in Chapter 7, Figure 7.6.

Interestingly, in contrast to coeliac disease, selective IgA deficiency is rare in dermatitis herpetiformis. IgA anti-gliadin antibodies are found frequently in the circulation (about 70% of patients with dermatitis herpetiformis). In common with coeliac disease, IgA anti-endomysium antibodies are found in >90% of cases.

First line treatment is with dapsone, which is usually very effective. However, the most effective treatment, as with coeliac disease, is a gluten-free diet as no further medication is then required. As the gut symptoms are often mild in dermatitis herpetiformis many patients are reluctant to embrace a gluten-free diet.

8.4.2 Toxic epidermal necrolysis (Stevens–Johnson syndrome)

Cross reference

Look at Chapter 3 for more information on hypersensitivity reactions.

Unlike most other autoimmune blistering skin conditions toxic epidermal necrolysis is not mediated by auto-antibodies but is a delayed type 4 hypersensitivity reaction. Look at Case study 8.4.

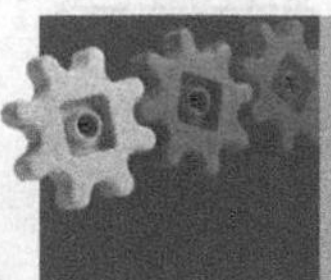

METHOD 8.4 Other methods for antibody detection

There are some antigens that have been purified for use in ELISA or line blotting techniques. See Table 8.1 for a breakdown of the antibodies found in autoimmune skin diseases that are available in diagnostic laboratories.

ELISA for BP180 NC16A subunit auto-antibodies has a sensitivity of 80–90% for bullous pemphigoid. ELISA for BP230 has a sensitivity of 60–70% for bullous pemphigoid. In addition antibodies to BP230 are found in about 4% of patients with itching skin disorders who do not have bullous pemphigoid.

TABLE 8.1 Commercially available assays for autoimmune blistering diseases and their clinical associations.

Immunofluorescence location	Antigen	Associated diseases
Intercellular substance (desmosome)	Desmoglein 1	Pemphigus vulgaris, pemphigus foliaceus, paraneoplastic pemphigus
	Desmoglein 3	Pemphigus vulgaris, paraneoplastic pemphigus
	Envoplakin	Paraneoplastic pemphigus
Basement membrane (hemidesmosome)	BP180 (specifically BP180 NC16A subunit)	Bullous pemphigoid, mucous membrane pemphigoid, pemphigoid gestationis
	BP230	Bullous pemphigoid, mucous membrane pemphigoid, pemphigoid gestationis, linear IgA disease (IgA class antibody)
	Collagen VII	Epidermolysis bullosa acquisita, mucous membrane pemphigoid
	Epidermal and tissue transglutaminase	Dermatitis herpetiformis

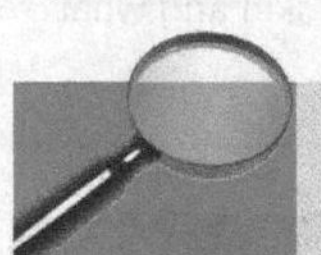

CASE STUDY 8.4 Toxic epidermal necrolysis (TEN)

Patient history

A 34-year-old HIV positive man presented with a painful, haemorrhagic, blistering rash, oral ulceration, fever, and difficulty swallowing to the extent that he was drooling saliva. This followed a change in his HIV therapy to include the non-nucleoside reverse transcriptase inhibitor nevirapine 12 days earlier, having developed side effects from previous treatment. The nevirapine dose was due to be increased at day 14. The blistering progressed to include at least 60% of the body surface area, consistent with a diagnosis of toxic epidermal necrolysis, a potentially fatal blistering condition.

Treatment

The offending drug, nevirapine was withdrawn and the patient received appropriate supportive care.

Response to treatment

Multidisciplinary supportive care is of utmost importance in the management of TEN. The patient made a full recovery but had pain on walking for 18 months after the episode in view of shedding of the skin from his soles. In such cases cytotoxic CD8 T cells with natural killer cell markers

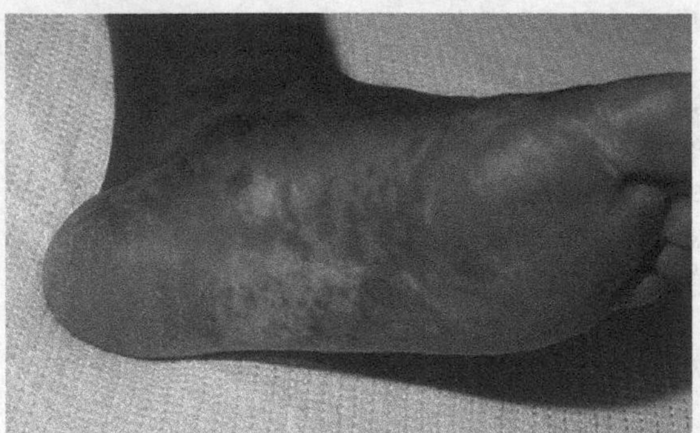

FIGURE 8.12
Toxic epidermal necrolysis blister.

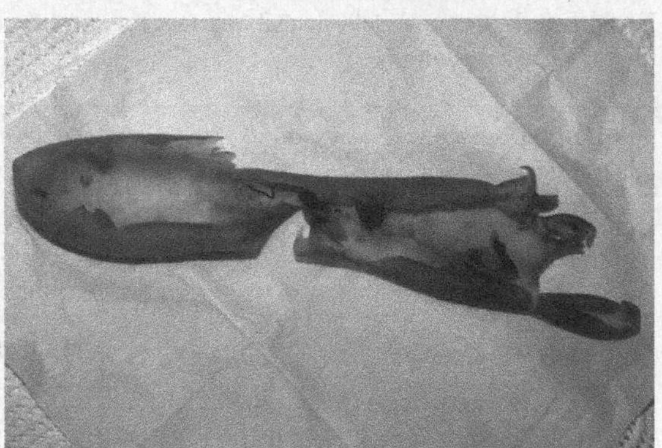

FIGURE 8.13
Toxic epidermal necrolysis shed skin.

are found in the blister fluid. Look at Figure 8.12 to see the haemorrhagic blistering lesions. Look at Figure 8.13 to see the extent of the cutaneous shedding, with skin loss from the soles and palms.

CLINICAL CORRELATION 8.1

Antibodies in pemphigus

It has been shown that the concentration of circulating antibodies in pemphigus is a good indicator of response to therapy. The concentration of antibodies varies in parallel with the disease activity in a patient. However, differing concentrations do not correlate well with disease severity in different patients. Curiously, despite the evidence that the antibodies are pathogenic (i.e. cause disease) concentration of antibody does not seem to be a good indicator of disease activity for the pemphigoid disorders.

SELF-CHECK 8.10

What are the three basement membrane patterns seen by indirect staining on split skin and what are the disease associations?

SELF-CHECK 8.11

Does antibody concentration correlate with disease severity in the bullous skin diseases?

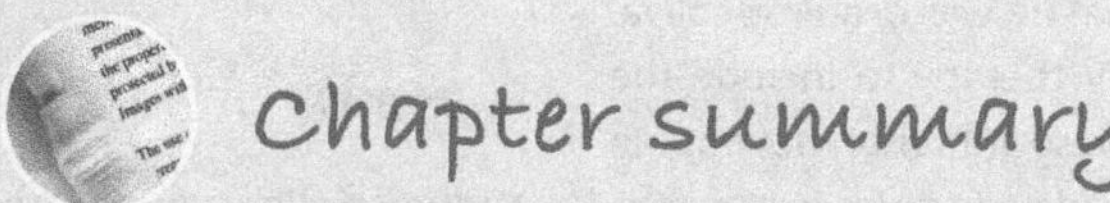

Chapter summary

- The major autoimmune blistering skin diseases are pemphigoid and pemphigus.
- In pemphigoid, auto-antibodies are directed against proteins at the dermal–epidermal junction.
- In pemphigus, auto-antibodies are directed against cell junctions in the epidermis.

- Specific auto-antibodies are associated with disruption of the skin structure leading to blistering.
- The presence of auto-antibodies may be demonstrated in biopsies (by direct immunofluorescence) or in serum (by indirect immunofluorescence or ELISA).
- Treatment can include steroids, either topical (directly to the skin) or systemic; steroid sparing systemic immune suppression; and for refractory disease, high dose intravenous immunoglobulin, plasmapheresis in conjunction with systemic immune suppression, or monoclonal antibody therapy targeting B lymphocytes.

Acknowledgements

The authors would like to thank all the patients who were kind enough to allow us to use their photographs in this chapter.

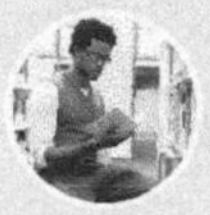

Further reading

- **Amagai M and Stanley JR (2012) *Desmoglein as a target in skin disease and beyond*. *J Invest Dermatol*, 132, 776–84.**
- **Grando SA (2012) *Pemphigus autoimmunity: Hypotheses and reality*. *Autoimmunity*, 45, 7–35.**
- **Joly P, Mouquet H, Roujeau J-C, *et al.* (2007) *A Single Cycle of Rituximab for the Treatment of Severe Pemphigus*. *N Engl J Med*, 357, 545–52.**
- **Mihályi L, Kiss M, Dobozy A, Kemény L, and Husz S (2012) *Clinical relevance of autoantibodies in patients with autoimmune Bullous dermatosis*. *Clin Dev Immunol*, 2012, 369–546.**
- **Nakajima K (2012) *Recent advances in dermatitis herpetiformis*. *Clin Dev Immunol*, 2012, 9141–62.**
- **Schmidt E, and Zillikens D (2013) *Pemphigoid diseases*. *Lancet*, 381, 320–32.**

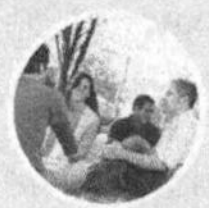

Discussion questions

8.1 How can the laboratory aid in the diagnosis of pemphigus and pemphigoid blistering skin disease?

8.2 What are the similarities and differences in treatment approach in pemphigus and pemphigoid blistering skin disease?

Answers to self-check questions are provided in the book's Online Resource Centre.

 Visit www.oxfordtextbooks.co.uk/orc/hall2e

9

Autoimmune liver diseases

Learning Objectives

After studying this chapter you should be able to:

- outline the common features of autoimmune liver diseases
- explain the clinical features of autoimmune hepatitis, autoimmune sclerosing cholangitis, and primary biliary cirrhosis
- outline the assays and techniques used to test for autoimmune liver diseases
- discuss the limitations of these techniques
- outline the treatment of autoimmune hepatitis, autoimmune sclerosing cholangitis, and primary biliary cirrhosis.

Introduction

The main autoimmune liver diseases are autoimmune hepatitis (AIH), autoimmune sclerosing cholangitis (ASC), and primary biliary cirrhosis (PBC). AIH and ASC are rare and may not be encountered in every laboratory.

Data on the incidence of the above diseases tend to be regional rather than national. The rarity of both AIH and ASC makes the gathering of incidence and prevalence data difficult. However, data are available; a report from a group in Oslo (Boberg et al. 1998) gives a mean annual incidence of AIH as 1.9/100 000 of the specific Norwegian population studied. It must be remembered that this is a regional figure and cannot be extrapolated on a European or global basis. The reason for this is that autoimmune disease is closely linked to genetic makeup and the huge variation seen in the human genome suggests an equally huge variation in incidence geographically. AIH is found in two serologically distinct forms known as type 1 and type 2. Possession of the human leukocyte antigen (HLA) DRB1*03 is associated with type1, and type 2 is associated with DRB1*07, in studies on Northern European populations.

Susceptibility to ASC in children is associated with the possession of HLA DRB1*1301in the UK population.

PBC is now included in the autoimmune group, although this was not always the case. This is a far more frequently encountered disease than either AIH or ASC and will be seen in most laboratories in the UK. The association of PBC and HLA DRB1*0801 was confirmed in a large-scale study of well-characterized PBC patients from the UK and Italy (Donaldson et al. 2006). This is not the case in China where the associated allele is HLA DRB1*0701 (Liu et al. 2006).

Cross reference

See Chapter 13 to read more on HLA disease association.

Key Point

The autoimmune liver diseases are autoimmune hepatitis (AIH) types 1 and 2, primary biliary cirrhosis (PBC), and autoimmune sclerosing cholangitis (ASC).

9.1 Autoimmune hepatitis (AIH)

AIH is an inflammatory liver disease characterized by a mononuclear cell infiltrate with interface **hepatitis**. This leads to the death of hepatocytes and their subsequent replacement by connective tissue, a process known as **cirrhosis**. The loss of hepatocytes leads in turn to the loss of hepatic function and ultimately hepatic failure. The 'autoimmune' adjective derives from the presence of auto-antibodies that accompany the disease process. The antigen specificity of these auto-antibodies is used in a classification of AIH into types 1 and 2. Interestingly, these auto-antibodies are not liver specific with the exception of anti-liver cytosol 1 (LC 1). The current view is that such auto-antibodies are **epiphenomena** and not directly responsible for hepatocyte damage. The treatment for AIH is **immunosuppression**, usually starting with corticosteroids and using more potent immunosuppressive agents as required. If this therapeutic approach fails then liver transplantation is the next option.

Hepatitis
Inflammation of the hepatocytes in the liver.

Cirrhosis
Irreversible change in liver tissue that results in the degeneration of functioning liver cells and their replacement with fibrous connective tissue.

Epiphenomenon
A secondary symptom that appears during the course of a disease, secondary to the existing disease symptoms.

Immunosuppression
A suppression of the immune system with a reduction in number, reactivity, expansion, or differentiation of T and/or B lymphocytes.

9.1.1 Incidence

AIH is a disease with a biphasic incidence; the first peak is seen in children and young adults and the second in the sixth and seventh decades of life. Type 1 AIH is found in both phases of the disease while type 2 is more commonly seen in children. As is seen in many autoimmune diseases, there is a female preponderance with as many as four out of five cases being female across both types. As a disease of childhood the incidence is some 7:1, female to male.

9.1.2 Histopathology

The histopathology of both type 1 and type 2 autoimmune hepatitis is identical and shows a mononuclear cell infiltrate of the hepatic portal tracts with interface hepatitis (inflammation of the hepatocytes) with hepatocyte **necrosis** (hepatocyte death). Look at Figure 9.1. As the necrosis intensifies the dead hepatocytes are replaced with fibrous tissue ultimately leading to cirrhosis. As a result of the loss of hepatocytes the liver enters a functional decline terminating in liver failure.

Necrosis
Unprogrammed cell death.

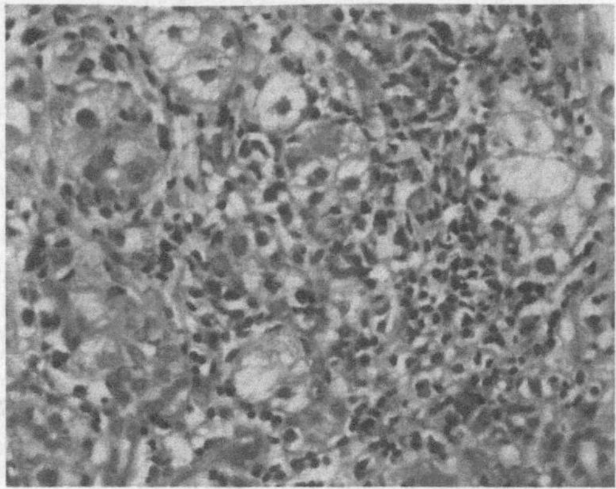

FIGURE 9.1
Margin of portal tract in autoimmune hepatitis. Reproduced by kind permission of Professor Bernard Portmann.

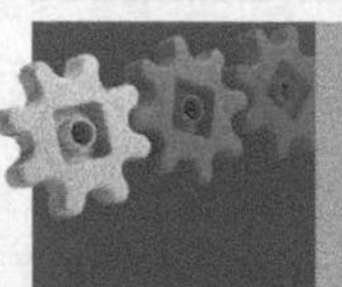

METHOD 9.1 Measuring auto-antibodies for autoimmune liver disease

Most commonly the screening for auto-antibodies in autoimmune liver disease is performed by indirect immunofluorescence (IIF), using an LKS substrate. This triple block consists of liver, kidney, and stomach sections from either mouse or rat. There are arguments for and against which tissue is the better to identify the different patterns seen using this technique. The conjugate used is an anti-human polyclonal IgG isotype.

The screening dilution varies from laboratory to laboratory, but is usually at 1/40 for adults. It is recommended to screen at 1/10 for paediatrics, as low titre antibodies can be clinically significant in this population.

Commercial ELISAs are available for some of the liver auto-antibodies such as M2 mitochondrial auto-antibodies and F-actin auto-antibodies. However, many laboratories are now moving towards confirming liver auto-antibodies using immunoblot techniques. The immunoblot strips often contain a group of the clinically significant antibodies, such as M2, LKM, LC 1, and F-actin.

SELF-CHECK 9.1

Why is it vital to differentiate between viral hepatitis and autoimmune hepatitis?

9.1.3 Serology—the auto-antibodies

The two serologically distinct forms of AIH present differently in the laboratory.

Type 1 is characterized by the presence of anti-smooth muscle antibody (SMA) and/or anti-nuclear antibody (ANA). Of historical interest, AIH was once known as 'lupoid hepatitis', mainly due to the presence of ANA.

The presence of anti-liver kidney microsomal antibody-1 (LKM 1) classifies type 2 AIH. In addition to the anti-LKM 1, the classical indicator auto-antibody of type 2 AIH, there is another auto-antibody of relevance, anti-liver cytosol-1 (LC 1). Anti-LC 1 is present in some 40% of anti-LKM-1 positive cases but is never detected in indirect immunofluorescence (IIF) due to its masking by the brighter fluorescence of the anti-LKM 1. It cannot be stressed too frequently that anti-LC 1 can and does occur without any other auto-antibody. Failure to detect this lone auto-antibody represents a crucially missed diagnostic opportunity.

Not all auto-antibodies are detected by the use of IIF. One such case pertinent to liver disease is that of anti-soluble liver antigen (SLA). It has been suggested by some authorities that the presence of anti-SLA establishes yet another type of AIH, AIH type 3. As anti-SLA is found in both types of AIH and in PBC/AIH overlaps, this classification is rarely used. Other assays are needed for the demonstration of anti-SLA.

Cross reference

See Section 9.4 to read more on AIH and PBC overlap syndromes.

Key Point

AIH type 1 and 2 are differentiated by their auto-antibody profiles.

Anti-smooth muscle antibody (SMA)

There is a group of IIF patterns associated with the auto-antibody known as SMA. This alone indicates that there is probably more than one target auto-antigen. The original classifcation of SMA by Bottazzo et al. (1976) describes three predominant patterns seen in rat kidney alone.

1. Vessel wall staining alone (SMA-V).
2. Glomeruli with some vascular staining (SMA-G).
3. Both vessels and glomeruli with intracellular fibres of renal tubules (SMA-T).

The group found that sera from patients with 'lupoid hepatitis' and 'chronic active hepatitis ANA negative' (both now described as AIH type 1) were positive for anti-SMA-G and anti-SMA-T antibodies. This positivity was lost in most cases after absorption with actin, indicating actin as a target auto-antigen. We now know that auto-antigenic target to be F-actin and antibodies to F-actin to be typical of AIH type 1. That is not to state that anti-F-actin is the only SMA found in AIH type 1 or that it is unique to AIH type 1.

The routine use of rodent liver, kidney, and stomach sections in IIF allows one to go beyond the Bottazzo classification (which is kidney based) and to look at smooth muscle auto-antibodies in the other tissues. The stomach is particularly useful in this respect. The staining of the transverse and longitudinal muscle bands of the stomach along with the staining of intragastric fibres is another manifestation of SMA seen in AIH type 1. This staining pattern is associated with anti-F-actin but not uniquely so. In some cases there is staining only of the longitudinal and transverse muscle bands which is not anti-F-actin but nevertheless is associated with AIH type 1. Also in AIH type 1 there is staining of the vessels of the kidney only with nothing seen in the stomach. Such a pattern is also seen in viral hepatitis and other viral infections and is usually of low titre. Anti-F-actin is the major SMA seen in AIH type 1 but only accounts for some 80% of the SMA positivity. The patterns are predominantly VGT which is taken to be anti-F-actin and VG, non-anti-F-actin. Hence, there is by implication more than one antigen responsible for the SMA pattern.

The non-anti-F-actin antibody patterns have been associated with desmin, vimentin, and myosin antibodies. Desmin, myosin, and vimentin are described as intermediate filaments.

The use of antigen-specific assays such as ELISA and immunoblot for anti-F-actin does not give 100% positivity in histologically proven AIH where SMA has been detected by IIF. This may be seen as further evidence that not all anti-smooth muscle antibody associated with AIH type 1 is anti-F-actin. Another substrate frequently used in IIF is the HEp-2 cell line and this shows anti-F-actin particularly well. When a strong positive anti-F-actin antibody is detected in HEp-2 cells it becomes self-evident as to why F-actin is described as a microfilamentous form of SMA.

Cross reference

You can read in more detail about the HEp-2 cell line in Chapter 5. The HEp-2 cell line is commonly used in the detection of anti-nuclear antibodies.

Look at Figure 9.2 to see what smooth muscle antibodies look like on kidney and stomach substrate and HEp-2 cells using indirect immunofluorescence.

Key Point

Anti-smooth muscle antibody has several molecular targets hence the different patterns seen in IIF.

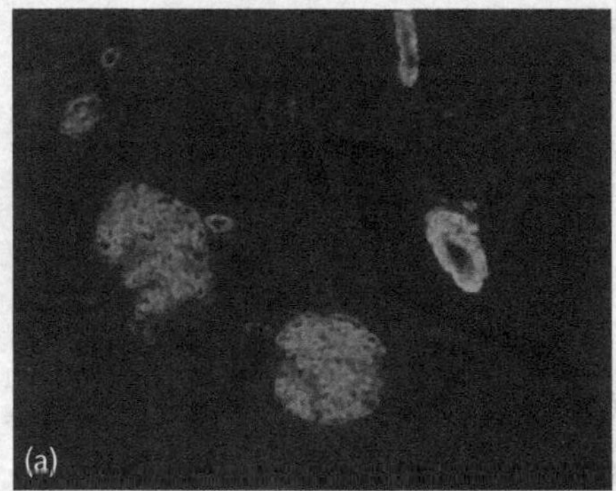

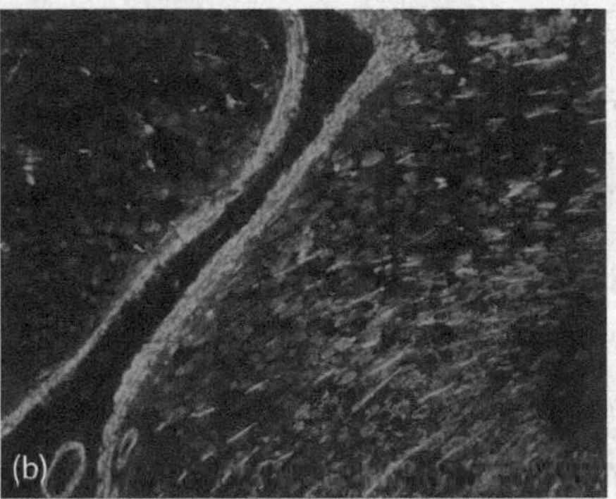

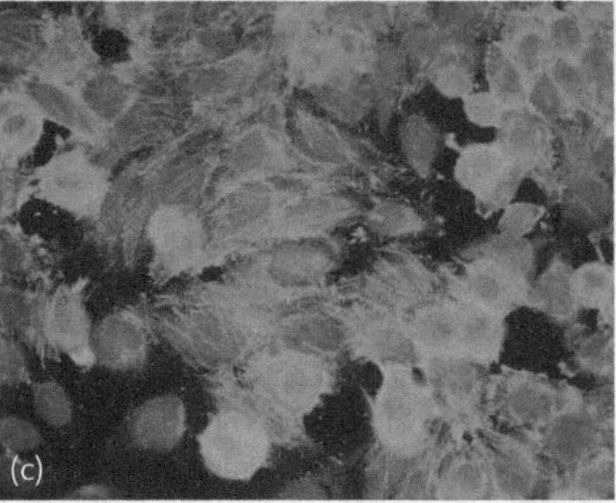

FIGURE 9.2

(a) Anti-smooth muscle antibody from the serum of an 8-year-old girl with AIH type 1. The section of rat kidney shows positive staining in both the glomeruli and blood vessels. This is anti-F-actin. (b) Anti-smooth muscle (serum from the same patient as Figure 9.2a). The section of rat stomach shows positive staining of one of the three major muscle bands of the stomach (bottom left to top centre) and two small vessels in the connective tissue between the bands. Note also the staining of the fine smooth muscle fibres within the mucosal area (right). (c) Smooth muscle antibody seen as a microfilamentous pattern on HEp2.

Anti-nuclear antibodies (ANA)

Anti-nuclear antibodies are the most commonly seen auto-antibody in clinical immunology. The usual substrate for the detection of ANA is the HEp-2 cell line or one of its derivatives. However, when searching for liver disease related auto-antibodies the substrate of choice is the rodent liver, kidney, and stomach (LKS) composite section. At the time of the serological classification of AIH it was the LKS substrate that was used and not the HEp-2 cell line to define ANA positivity. However, the International Autoimmune Hepatitis Group (IAHG) in its 2004 consensus statement recommended the use of HEp-2 cells 'to assess the pattern of nuclear staining'. This is to be performed after finding a positive ANA reaction on LKS screening. There is not an absolute correlation between ANA positivity found on rodent substrate and that found on the HEp-2 cell line. The protocol in our laboratory is to use both substrates at the screening point and thus avoid the problem. A possible explanation may be found in the serum dilutions used on LKS and HEp-2. A dilution in the order of 1/40 is generally used with LKS but for HEp-2 1/100 or more is the norm. Thus a weak ANA seen at 1/40 on LKS is not likely to be detected on HEp-2 at 1/100 or greater. Added to this possibility is the difference in the antigens expressed in the two substrates, one rodent and the other human. It is not beyond comprehension that they will not be identical.

Cross reference

Read Chapter 5 to find out more about anti-nuclear antibodies.

In connective tissue disorders, the detection of ANA positivity is a trigger to investigate further. This is because ANA has low disease specificity and in order to elucidate the potential disorder other investigations are required. The use of assays for nuclear related auto-antibodies such as anti-extractable nuclear antigens (ENA) and anti-double-stranded DNA are very useful in this respect. However, in AIH type 1 there appears to be no unique specificity of the ANA associated with the disease. A study by Gregorio et al. (1995) on a small paediatric population with both AIH type 1 and 2 showed 20% of the cases to have a variety of anti-ENA specificities. It is of interest that the majority of the anti-ENA positive patients belonged to the anti-LKM 1 positive group, type 2 AIH. This raises some questions, as this group were ANA negative by definition. One heretical possibility is that any ANA present would be hidden by the anti-LKM-1 in IIF if of lower titre than the anti-LKM 1. This study was performed on unfixed LKS sections and did not use HEp-2 cells.

Cross reference

You can read the consensus statement from the committee for autoimmune serology of the International Autoimmune Hepatitis Group in Vergani et al. (2004).

Anti-liver kidney microsomal antibody (LKM)

Anti-LKM was first described in 1973 by Rizzetto and colleagues. Subsequently other forms of anti-LKM have been found, having a pattern in IIF identical to that of the auto-antibody of Rizzetto's group, but having different molecular targets. A numerical postscript has been added to the descriptive 'anti-LKM' to facilitate identification. The numbering reflects chronological discovery, hence the anti-LKM of Rizzetto is designated anti-LKM 1.

The occurrence of anti-LKM 2 was associated with a hepatitis caused by the use of a diuretic agent known as tienilic acid. This was withdrawn from clinical use in 1980 and hence will not be found currently. Anti-LKM 3 has been described in a small group of hepatitis D virus (HDV) infected patients. Anti-LKM 4 may be seen in AIH type 2 associated with **APECED**.

APECED

Autoimmune polyendocrinopathy, candidiasis, ectodermal dystrophy.

Key Point

Anti-LKM 1 is not unique to AIH type 2; it is also found in some cases of hepatitis C virus infection.

CLINICAL CORRELATION 9.1

APECED

APECED is caused by a mutation of the AIRE (autoimmune regulator) gene which is located on chromosome 21q22.3. The essential features of the disorder are as given in its name. However, the endocrine disorders are primarily hypoparathyroidism and adrenal insufficiency; many other autoimmune disorders may be seen including AIH type 2 which occurs in approximately 20% of cases. APECED is also known as autoimmune polyendocrine syndrome 1 (APS1). APECED is preferred in order to avoid confusion with anti-phospholipid syndrome (APS).

Cross reference

You can read more about APECED in Chapter 7.

A further complication can arise in the case of anti-liver microsomal antibody (anti-LM). The staining pattern of anti-LM is indistinguishable in the rodent liver from anti-LKM 1. However, as the name suggests, there is no reaction seen in the kidney. This auto-antibody is found rarely; it may be seen in cases of dihydralazine induced hepatitis and there are reports of its presence in AIH. The molecular target of anti-LM is a P450 cytochrome, P450 1A2.

As can be seen in Table 9.1 many of the molecular targets of anti-LKM belong to the P450 cytochrome family. The current naming system of the P450 family as designated by the Human Cytochrome P450 (*CYP*) Allele Nomenclature Committee (Ingelman-Sundberg et al. 2000) is shown in brackets.

AIH type 2 is a rare disorder and hence its marker auto-antibody anti-LKM 1 is unlikely to be seen with great frequency in all laboratories. This does not, however, mean that any laboratory using the LKS substrate is absolved from failing to recognize the IIF pattern. Anti-LKM 1 detection forms part of the United Kingdom National External Quality Assurance Scheme (NEQAS) in General Autoimmune Serology and as such all participants must be competent in its detection. Encouragingly recent data from the scheme show a marked improvement over time of the correct identification of anti-LKM 1. The IIF pattern of anti-LKM 1 is sometimes mistaken for the more commonly seen anti-mitochondrial M2 pattern. There are several reasons for this failure which will be addressed in Section 9.3.3. The successful identification of any auto-antibody seen in IIF is obviously based on pattern recognition. It is useful to consider the individual components that constitute any particular pattern. It is by dissecting out these components that correct identification is made.

Cross reference

The report from NEQAS on reporting of anti-LKM 1 can be found at http://www.immqas.org.uk/docs/LKM%20Commentary.pdf (Davies 2008).

What are the components that signify the presence of anti-LKM 1?

Look at Figure 9.3. The cytoplasm of the hepatocytes of the rodent liver stains, usually very intensely, but the nuclei are spared. They appear as dark holes in the hepatocytes. The staining quality is an important factor and in the case of anti-LKM 1 the staining is homogenous, 'flat', and non-granular. Another striking feature is the non-staining of the hepatic portal tracts. These appear as black irregular shapes among a mass of bright green tissue. No other auto-antibody produces this pattern in the rodent liver.

TABLE 9.1 **The molecular targets of anti-LKM.**

LKM 1	P450 2D6 (CYP2D6)
LKM 2	P450 2C9 (CYP2C9)
LKM 3	UDGT (uridine diphosphate glucuronosyl transferase)
LKM 4	P450 1A2 and P450 2A6

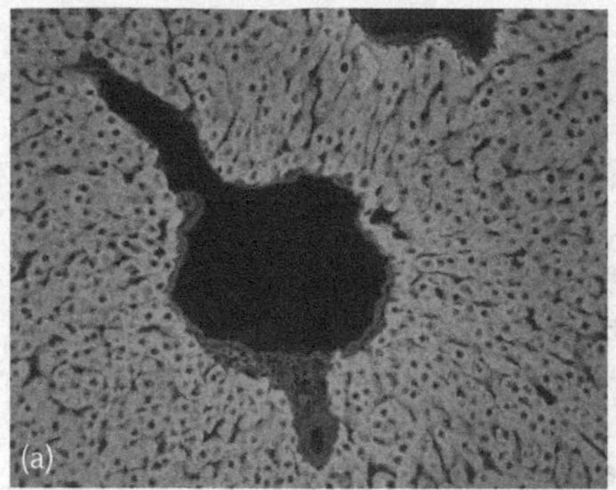
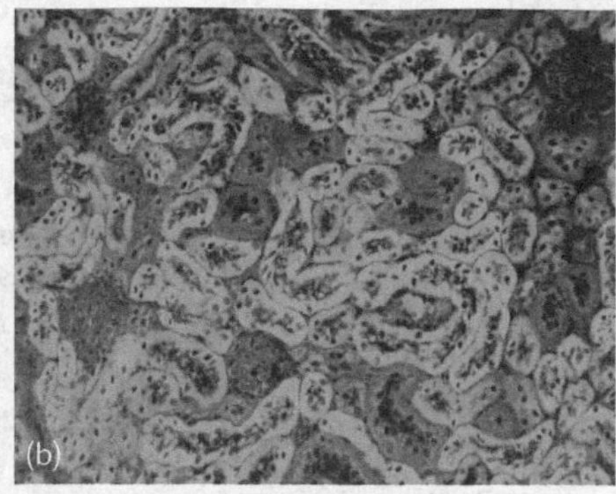

FIGURE 9.3

(a) Anti-LKM 1 on rat liver. Anti-LKM 1 stains all hepatocytes. Note the portal tract, bottom centre, is unstained, unlike anti-M2 which stains the portal tract in a granular fashion. (b) Anti-LKM 1 on rat kidney. Anti-LKM 1 preferentially stains the proximal tubules of the kidney. Also note that the glomeruli remain unstained; this is not the case in the presence of anti-M2 where they are again stained in a granular fashion.

The staining seen in the rodent kidney presents more of a problem. The proximal renal tubules are selectively stained and the distal tubules remain unstained. The differentiation of the renal tubules is difficult when seen in IIF. The appearance obviously depends on the plane of section but when the tissue is correctly orientated the proximal tubules are more elongate than the distal tubules which themselves are more circular and generally smaller. Perhaps an easier means of deciding whether or not you are seeing anti-LKM 1 is to ask the question, 'Are all the tubules stained or only some of them?' If the answer is 'only some of them', then it is more likely that you are seeing anti-LKM 1.

The third tissue of the LKS substrate is the stomach and this remains unstained by anti-LKM 1, as the name of the auto-antibody suggests. There is, however, the possibility that staining of the gastric parietal cells may occur. To reiterate, this is not due to anti-LKM 1 but to anti-gastric parietal cell antibody which may be found in some cases of type 2 AIH. In particular anti-gastric parietal cell antibody may be seen in cases of APECED associated with type 2 AIH. It is the joint incidence of the two auto-antibodies that gives rise to the confusion of the IIF pattern with that of anti-mitochondrial M2 antibody. Anti-M2 stains the gastric parietal cells because they contain the target auto-antigen.

Cross references

Mitochondrial antibodies will be discussed further in Section 9.3.

Parietal cell antibodies are discussed in more detail in Chapter 7.

Anti-liver cytosol 1 (LC 1)

Anti-LKM 1 is not the only marker of AIH type 2. Anti-LC 1 is the second marker of this disease and is less commonly found for two reasons; firstly, it is hidden by anti-LKM 1, and secondly, its appearance as the sole auto-antibody marker is rare. Also, because of its rarity it may well be overlooked. It is not the easiest of auto-antibodies to detect as its pattern may be misinterpreted as a technical artefact, especially at low titre. Anti-LC 1 is present in about 20% of anti-LKM 1 positive cases but due to its staining pattern it is overshadowed or outshone by anti-LKM 1 in IIF. The staining pattern is confined to the liver in the LKS sections. Like anti-LKM 1 this auto-antibody stains the hepatocytes, but unlike anti-LKM 1 it does not stain those hepatocytes around the centrilobular vessels. Hence the appearance in the liver is one of 'patchy' staining with both bright and dark areas visible under low to intermediate power. It is this appearance that is sometimes seen as being a technical artefact in as much as it would seem that conjugate has not been applied evenly to the whole section. The molecular target of anti-LC 1 is the enzyme formiminotransferase cyclodeaminase (FTCD). Figure 9.4 shows immunofluorescent staining of antibodies to LC 1.

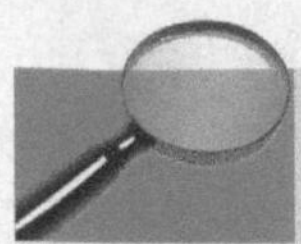

CASE STUDY 9.1 Anti-LKM 1 antibodies

Patient history

- 8-year-old female.
- GP visit 7 days previously; loss of appetite, tiredness, slight elevation of temperature.
- GP thought viral illness, patient sent home to rest.
- Mother called GP. Child very sleepy, dark urine noted.

The GP visited and on seeing the deterioration in the child called an ambulance. The child was admitted to the local hospital under the paediatricians and investigations ordered. The laboratory investigations included viral hepatitis screen, coagulation studies, liver function tests (LFTs), immunoglobulins, C3, C4, and auto-antibodies.

Results

- Hepatitis virus screen negative
- LFTs show transaminitis, AST 800 iu/L (normal range 10–50)
- IgG 57.50 g/L, IgA 0.06 g/L, IgM 1.44 g/L
- C3 0.96 g/L, C4 0.06 g/L
- INR 4.2
- Anti-LKM 1 positive 1/5120.

Significance of the results

- Negative screen for hepatitis viruses; basically removes viral infection from the diagnostic possibilities (the differential).
- AST 800 iu/L; AST (aspartate aminotransferase) is one of the components of the LFTs and elevated concentrations are indicative of hepatocyte death.
- The IgG is elevated (normal range 5.4–16.1 g/L). This is a common finding in autoimmune hepatitis, some 80% of cases present with elevated IgG.
- The IgA is decreased (normal range 0.5–2.4 g/L). A subset of patients with AIH is IgA deficient (more type 2 AIH than type 1 AIH).
- The C4 is decreased (normal range 0.15–0.58 g/L). The C4 has not been consumed by classical pathway activity, nor has the liver damage prevented its synthesis; it was never there in the first place. Again a subset of patients lacks an allele at the C4 locus and has a partial C4 deficiency.
- INR (international normalized ratio) is a coagulation parameter; ideally the INR should be 1.0. In this case the abnormal INR reflects the liver damage (clotting proteins are hepatic in origin) and rules out liver biopsy (haemorrhage would occur during such a procedure).
- The high titre anti-LKM 1 antibody is diagnostic of AIH type 2 in this case, as hepatitis virus C and B have been excluded.
- Anti-LKM 1 is not unique to AIH type 2 and may be seen in a small percentage of cases with viral hepatitis.

Subsequent to the finding of anti-LKM 1 by IIF the patient's serum was assayed by immunoblot to confirm the presence of anti-P450 2D6 (cytochrome P450 2D6 is the anti-LKM 1 molecular target). This is our normal laboratory practice for all newly found liver related auto-antibodies where a confirmatory (antigen-specific) assay exists. In this case the immunoblot also detected anti-liver cytosol 1 (anti-LC 1). This auto-antibody is also characteristic of AIH type 2 but was not seen in IIF due to its being masked by the high titre anti-LKM 1.

The patient responded well to corticosteroid therapy and when the INR returned to within normal limits a liver biopsy was performed. The histology was consistent with AIH.

Anti-soluble liver antigen (SLA)

Unlike the liver disease related auto-antibodies described earlier in this section, antibodies to SLA are not detectable by IIF on LKS substrate. The anti-SLA antibody was described in 1987 by Manns et al. and in 1993 the group of Berg (Stechemesser et al. 1993) described anti-liver pancreas (LP) antibodies. The two auto-antibodies are now known to be directed at the same target hence the term anti-SLA/LP is sometimes used. Originally the presence of anti-SLA was thought

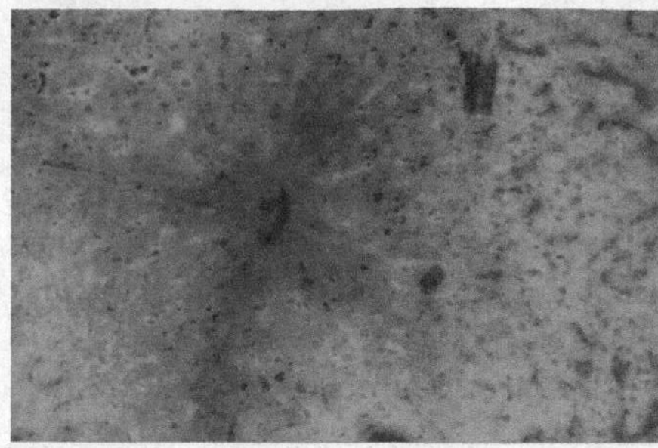

FIGURE 9.4
The molecular target of anti-LC 1 is formiminotransferase cyclodeaminase. This enzyme is found within hepatocytes, but is either absent or present in very low concentration in those hepatocytes surrounding the centrilobular vein, hence the lack of staining in these areas.

to define a third form of autoimmune hepatitis, AIH 3. This definition was based on clinical findings and the absence of the classical marker auto-antibodies for types 1 and 2 AIH. This classification has now been abandoned, as with more sensitive assay procedures anti-SLA has been found in some patients with both types 1 and 2 AIH and also in the PBC/AIH overlap syndrome.

The methodology for the detection of anti-SLA in the diagnostic setting is enzyme immunoassay or immunoblot, both of which are commercially available. In the research laboratory a radio-ligand binding assay has been described which shows more anti-SLA positivity in both forms of AIH than either of the above assays.

Key Point

Anti-soluble liver antigen (SLA) can be seen in both types of AIH.

CLINICAL CORRELATION 9.2

Liver function tests

Liver function tests mean different things to different people. Here only the 'liver enzymes' will be covered.

AST (aspartate transferase) and ALT (alanine transferase) are found within hepatocytes. When hepatocytes are damaged the enzymes are released and enter the plasma pool thereby increasing the plasma concentration. This condition is known as 'transaminitis' and is a feature of AIH.

Alkaline phosphatase is found in many tissues, one of which is bile duct epithelium. Damage to this epithelium again releases the enzyme into the plasma, raising its concentration, as may be seen in PBC.

Gamma glutamyl transpeptidase (γGT) is found in hepatocytes and biliary epithelium. Raised concentrations of γGT reflect cholestatic and ultimately hepatocyte damage. Elevated concentrations are seen in many liver diseases.

Cross reference

You can read in more detail about liver function tests in the *Clinical Biochemistry* textbook of this series.

9.2 Autoimmune sclerosing cholangitis (ASC)

ASC is a disease characterized by inflammation of both intra- and extrahepatic bile ducts and hepatitis. The ducts are replaced by fibrous tissue, hence 'sclerosing', and bile flow interrupted. Bile acids accumulate in the liver, where they are hepatotoxic. ASC may be considered an overlap syndrome as it shares many clinical and pathological features with autoimmune hepatitis and primary sclerosing cholangitis (PSC).

PSC is a disorder primarily of adults and is thought to have an autoimmune component in that a prime risk factor for the disease is a relative with the disease. Unlike most autoimmune disorders there is a male preponderance in PSC. The disease may be asymptomatic for many years, and is sometimes only discovered when investigating inflammatory bowel diseases such as ulcerative colitis and Crohn's disease. It is estimated that some 70% of PSC patients have such disorders. In childhood ASC the incidence of inflammatory bowel disease is approximately 45%.

Cholangiography
Imaging of the biliary tract.

The diagnosis of ASC relies heavily on **cholangiography** (imaging of the biliary tree). In a series reported by the group of Mieli-Vergani (Mieli-Vergani and Vergani 2008), 25% of the children had no histological evidence of bile duct pathology; it was the cholangiography that revealed the abnormalities and ultimately the diagnosis. It is largely through the work of Professor Mieli-Vergani that ASC has been recognized as a distinct disease entity.

ASC has some of the clinical and serological features of autoimmune hepatitis. Its treatment is also like that of AIH in that immunosuppression is the first line with the use of corticosteroids and azathioprine. But unlike AIH a therapeutic agent is used to address the biliary component of the disease; this is ursodeoxycholic acid. Liver transplantation is necessary in some cases.

9.2.1 Incidence

As ASC is a relatively newly recognized disorder as well as a rare one, incidence and prevalence data are not abundant. The prevalence is reported to be the same of that of AIH type 1 (Gregorio et al. 2001) in children in the UK. No doubt in time data will appear from other geographical locations.

9.2.2 Histology

As stated above, histology may not give the definitive diagnosis in all cases of ASC. The histological picture is that of interface hepatitis (as in AIH) and periductal fibrosis. In the Mieli-Vergani series (Mieli-Vergani and Vergani 2008) the pathology of the bile ducts was less severe than that seen in adult PSC.

9.2.3 Serology—the auto-antibodies

The auto-antibodies associated with ASC are ANA and SMA, as found in AIH type 1. The auto-antibody that occurs more frequently in ASC than in AIH is the perinuclear anti-neutrophil cytoplasmic antibody (P-ANCA). This P-ANCA is often referred to as 'atypical' as it does not demonstrate positivity to any single neutrophil cytoplasmic antigen. The 'typical' P-ANCA associated with the small vessel vasculitides is usually anti-myeloperoxidase (MPO). In ASC there may be positivity to MPO but there is also positivity to many other neutrophil antigens including cathepsin G and lactoferrin. This atypical P-ANCA is also seen in ulcerative colitis and other inflammatory bowel disorders which also form part of the disease spectrum of ASC.

A note of caution: the high incidence of ANA in ASC can raise problems when performing ANCA by IIF as the patterns are not totally dissimilar. Remember that ANCA and ANA are not mutually exclusive phenomena.

Other similarities exist in both ASC and AIH—elevated concentration of serum IgG (more frequent in ASC than AIH) and deranged LFTs mainly showing a transaminitis.

Key Point

ASC is clinically similar to AIH type 1 in auto-antibody profile. However, the incidence of atypical P-ANCA is far higher than in AIH type 1.

SELF-CHECK 9.2

What other important technique is used in the diagnosis of ASC and why?

Cross reference

You can read in more detail about ANCA in Chapter 6.

9.3 Primary biliary cirrhosis (PBC)

PBC is the result of the destruction of the epithelia of the small intrahepatic bile ducts. This destruction is considered to be T cell mediated. This, along with the presence of anti-mitochondrial auto-antibodies (AMA) seen in the vast majority of PBC patients, has led to the disease being designated as an autoimmune liver disease. The loss of these ducts adversely affects the normal flow of bile within the liver, known as cholestasis. The resultant accumulation of bile products is hepatotoxic and ultimately leads to the loss of hepatocytes and their subsequent replacement by fibrous tissue. If left untreated cirrhosis occurs and results in end stage liver disease. The only remedy at this stage is liver transplantation. Unlike AIH the prime treatment is not immunosuppression but is based on managing the bile acid content with the administration of ursodeoxycholic acid (less hepatotoxic than other bile acids).

9.3.1 Incidence

PBC has a relatively high incidence in Scandinavia and the northern British Isles compared with continental Europe; in USA there are pockets of high incidence. It would be interesting to know whether these pockets correspond to areas of settlement by migrants from northern Europe. Annual incidence and point prevalence vary depending on geographical location and study criteria used to gather the data (Field and Heathcote 2003). The UK appears at the top of the incidence table. Again, as with many autoimmune disorders there is a female to male preponderance; in the case of PBC this is approximately 9:1. The majority of cases present between the ages of 40 and 60 years.

9.3.2 Histopathology

The loss of intrahepatic bile ducts is a prime feature of the histology of the disease. Look at Figure 9.5. The early stage inflammatory lesion shows a mixed infiltrate of neutrophils, lymphocytes, plasma cells, and eosinophils around the duct with hyperplasia of the duct epithelia. Multinucleate giant cells and granulomas are also prominent features of the disease. The final stages of the disease are characterized by the absence of ducts and cirrhosis.

9.3.3 Serology—the auto-antibodies

The serological hallmark of PBC is the anti-mitochondrial antibody, more specifically the anti-M2 mitochondrial antibody. There are nine mitochondrial antibodies of varying clinical significance and conveniently these are designated anti-M1 to anti-M9. In cases of PBC, anti-M2 is the major auto-antibody but not the only mitochondrial antibody associated with the disease. Anti-M4 and anti-M8 are present with anti-M2 in most cases, and hence the IIF pattern seen is

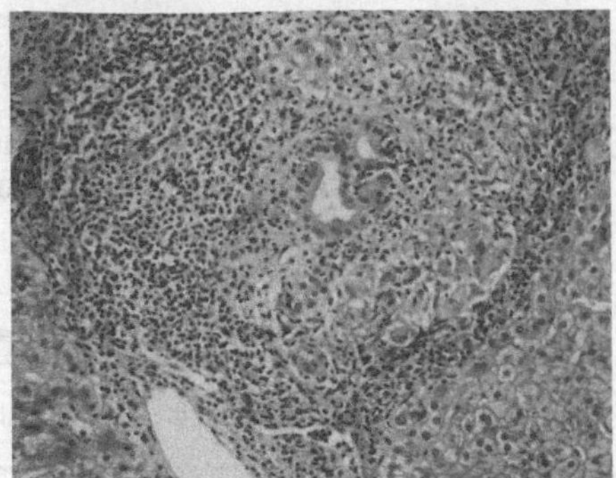

FIGURE 9.5
A case of PBC stage 1 showing mononuclear cell infiltrate (left) invading a bile duct (centre). Note eosinophils (low centre). Reproduced by kind permission of Professor Bernard Portmann.

probably a composite of all these auto-antibodies. The other significant auto-antibody is anti-M9. This auto-antibody can be found in isolation (in the absence of anti-M2) but usually is present with anti-M2. The anti-M2/M9 combination is considered to be an indicator of a less severe disease progression whereas the anti-M2/4/8 profile is indicative of a more aggressive form of the disease.

The target antigens associated with these M1-9 auto-antibodies are listed in Table 9.2 and are based on the description of Berg and Klein (1986).

The IIF patterns of the various anti-mitochondrial auto-antibodies are not dissimilar when seen in the LKS substrate. The non-PBC associated antibodies are relatively rare but when encountered may be confused with those associated with PBC. The differential staining of the LKS component tissues is the basis for determining the type of mitochondrial antibody. This, as with all IIF, is subject to many variables and may not be definitive. The IIF patterns associated with PBC are somewhat better defined.

The obvious feature of anti-M2 in IIF using LKS substrate is its granularity. Look at Figure 9.6. This is particularly well demonstrated in the liver where each hepatocyte appears to be a mass of green microdots. In contrast the staining of the liver seen in anti-LKM 1 is a smooth, homogenous pattern. Another feature which is useful to differentiate the two antibodies when looking at the liver section is the staining of the portal tracts. In the presence of anti-M2 the portal tracts are not easy to see as they blend into the general fluorescence of the hepatocytes. However, when

TABLE 9.2 Anti-mitochondrial auto-antibodies.

Antibody	Molecular target/agent	Disease association
M1	Cardiolipin	Syphilis
M2	Pyruvate dehydrogenase complex	PBC
M3	Venocuran	Drug-induced pseudo-lupus
M4	Sulphite oxidase	PBC
M5	?Cardiolipin like complex	Unclassified rheumatological disorders
M6	Iproniazid/monoamine oxidase?	Drug-induced hepatitis
M7	Sarcosine dehydrogenase	Myocarditis
M8	Outer mitochondrial membrane	PBC
M9	Glycogen phosphorylase	PBC

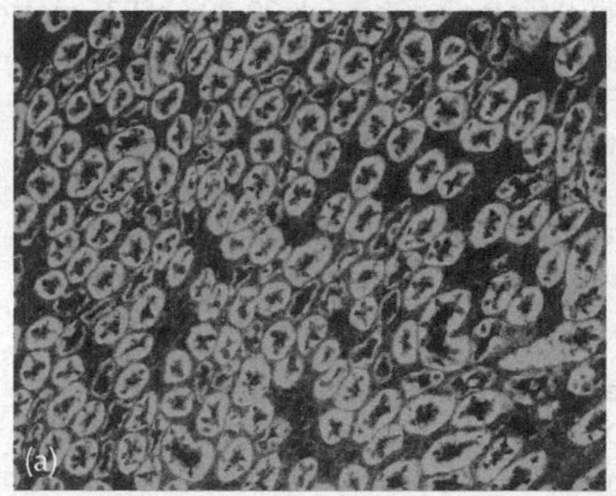

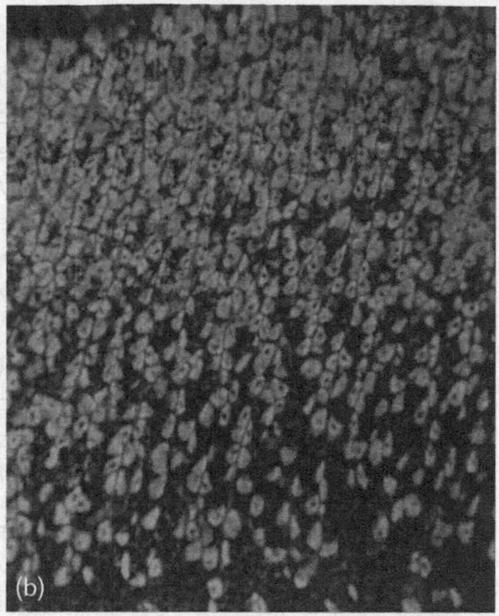

FIGURE 9.6

(a) Anti-M2 on kidney; note that all tubules stain here as this is a high titre (1/10 240) seen at screening dilution of 1/40. Also note that the two glomeruli are stained in a typical granular fashion. This is not seen in the case of anti-LKM 1. (b) Anti-M2 stains the gastric parietal cells of the rat stomach. Note the fine granularity here which is absent in anti-gastric parietal cell antibody.

the portal tracts are located, the connective tissue matrix which supports the vessels of the tract can be seen to be stained in the typical granular pattern. This same connective tissue matrix is unstained in the presence of anti-LKM 1 and appears as a black zone in the mass of fluorescence.

It is said that the distal tubules of the kidney are preferentially stained when compared to the proximal tubules. This is not obvious at the screening dilution where all tubules appear of equal intensity. The differential staining becomes clearer as the titration end point is neared. The glomeruli are another useful marker in the differentiation of anti-M2 and anti-LKM 1. Again the granularity of anti-M2 can be seen in the glomeruli, whereas in anti-LKM 1 the glomeruli remain unstained. Anti-M2 also stains the gastric parietal cells (GPC), but so does anti-GPC. Again the difference does not concern what is stained but the appearance of that staining. The cytoplasm of the GPCs is granular (the nuclei are spared in the absence of a coexistent anti-nuclear antibody).

Key Point

Anti-mitochondrial antibody M2 may be detected many years before the onset of clinical symptoms.

9.3.4 Nuclear-related auto-antibodies

Anti-M2 is sometimes accompanied by anti-nuclear antibodies in PBC. The anti-nuclear antibodies associated with PBC are the multiple nuclear dot (MND) pattern, the rim or peripheral pattern, and centromere antibodies.

Multiple nuclear dot (MND) pattern

One of the antigens responsible for the MND pattern is Sp-100, a 95–100 kDa nuclear protein which has been shown to be upregulated in cell culture in the presence of interferons. This has led to speculation concerning the role of interferons in the inflammatory process surrounding the destruction of the bile duct epithelium. While the upregulation of Sp-100 presents a 'larger' target for the autoimmune process, it does not account for the fact that only 20–30% of PBC cases are positive for anti-Sp-100. With the use of the HEp-2 cell line or one of its derivatives, the anti-Sp-100 pattern is relatively easy to detect. Look at Figure 9.7. There appears to be a consensus that the number of dots that constitute the MND pattern is around 20 per nucleus, but a definitive definition is not readily available. A similar pattern, few nuclear dots (FND), is also seen in unclassified rheumatological disorders. This pattern contains usually less than 10 dots per nucleus in the author's experience, which is too limited to be taken as definitive. It must be remembered however that anti-MND is not uniquely associated with PBC and may be seen in rheumatological disorders.

Other nuclear antigens, such as promyelocytic leukaemia (PML) antigen and small ubiquitin-like modifier proteins (SUMO), also give the MND pattern in IIF and have association with PBC. Antigen-specific assays are required to identify the molecular specificity of the auto-antibody.

Rim or peripheral pattern

The rim or peripheral ANA pattern was detectable in rodent LKS substrate before the use of HEp-2 cell lines became commonplace. However, the presence of high titre anti-M2 antibody can obscure the rim pattern in this substrate. The pattern is now known to be due to staining of the nuclear pore complex (NPC). Two major antigens have thus far been identified in the NPC as being associated with PBC: Gp 210 (a 210 kDa glycoprotein) and NUP 62 (a 62 kDa nucleoporin). The rim pattern is easily detected in most cases when using HEp-2 cells. The presence of anti-Gp 210 is associated with a more advanced stage of disease and a worsening prognosis, as evidenced by a higher Mayo risk score.

CLINICAL CORRELATION 9.3

The Mayo natural history model for PBC

This is a mathematical model for the calculation of estimated probability of survival and is based on: patient age, bilirubin concentration, albumin concentration, prothrombin time, presence of oedema (yes or no), and diuretic therapy (yes or no).

Following the computation of the above data, a risk score is derived in terms of years of survival. The calculation can be performed on the Mayo website for individual patients and is freely available: http://www.mayoclinic.org/gi-rst/mayomodel1.html

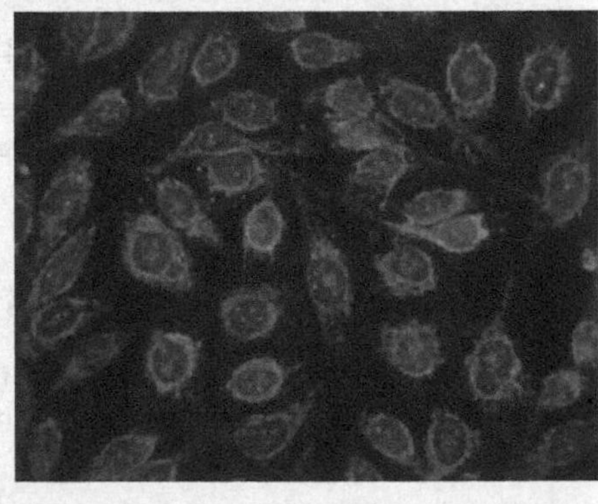

FIGURE 9.7

Anti-Sp 100 (multiple nuclear dots) on HEp-2010 cell line. Note the presence of anti-mitochondrial antibodies in the cytoplasm of the cells.

Centromere antibodies

A more probable cause of confusion is the presence of centromere antibodies which do occur in cases of PBC. The numerous dots seen in IIF of centromere antibodies can be misread for anti-Sp 100, and vice versa. The counting of individual dots is somewhat tedious and the identification of centromere antibodies relies upon the identification of the characteristic mitotic pattern seen in those cells in metaphase. The presence of anti-centromere antibody in PBC is said to be associated with a portal hypertension end point in the disease rather than a hepatic failure scenario. PBC and limited systemic sclerosis, previously known as **CREST syndrome**, should always be considered in the presence of anti-centromere antibody. The overlap syndrome of both disorders is known to exist.

CREST syndrome

A limited form of scleroderma, consisting of calcinosis, Raynaud's phenomenon, oesophageal motility, sclerodactyly, and telangiectasia.

> Key Point
>
> **Nuclear related auto-antibodies, while not diagnostic of PBC, can be of clinical significance, especially in anti-M2 negative cases.**

Cross reference

You can read more about centromere antibodies in Chapter 5.

9.3.5 Anti-mitochondrial antibody negative PBC

Not all cases of PBC have mitochondrial antibodies. The concept of AMA negative PBC is now accepted. The very high association of AMA with the disease previously led to the reasoning that in the absence of AMA there could not be PBC. The histopathological and biochemical evidence in the AMA negative PBC cases leaves little doubt that the presence of AMA is not an absolute requirement for the diagnosis of the disease.

Somewhere in the region of 95% of PBC cases are AMA positive. This statement is based on AMA positivity determined by immunofluorescence, which was once the only tool available. The discovery of the molecular nature of the antigens responsible for the immunofluorescence pattern, combined with advances in biotechnology, has made antigen-specific assays a reality. Early evidence that IIF was not the absolute arbiter of AMA positivity came from the work of Muratori et al. (2003), who demonstrated AMA positivity by immunoblot in a third of their IIF AMA negative cases. This raised the question of analytical sensitivity of IIF versus immunoblot. The antigen source used in the immunoblot was a bovine heart mitochondrial fraction and the IIF substrate was rat LKS. This may suggest that the antigen source was responsible for differences in AMA positivity. However, this group also reported that all their AMA positive cases by IIF were also AMA positive by immunoblot, indicating similarity of antigen. Hence a very small but significant percentage of once AMA negative PBC cases became AMA positive.

AMA negative PBC does not necessarily mean auto-antibody negative PBC. The nuclear related auto-antibodies described in Section 9.3.4 are strongly associated with AMA negative PBC. Original reports found the PBC related anti-nuclear antibodies were present in a higher percentage in AMA negative PBC than in AMA positive PBC. This argues well for the inclusion of HEp-2 cells in the screening of suspected autoimmune liver diseases.

More recently, Bizzaro et al. (2012) have shown that 43/100 AMA IIF negative sera were positive in a novel ELISA assay combining the recombinant triple antigen MIT3, Gp210, and Sp-100 (see Section 9.4.1). Interestingly, the ELISA and IIF for the nuclear antigens showed concordance rates greater than 90%.

It is possible to find anti-M2 in apparently well people without any overt clinical or biochemical signs of liver disease. Such a finding is considered to be evidence of disease to come and is known as a **prodrome**. It is important to report these cases as therapeutic intervention may be required. The presence of anti-M2 has been reported in women with a history of urinary tract infections. These women had no evidence of liver disease and the presence of the anti-M2 is considered to be due to molecular mimicry. Epitopes present in the causative organism of the infection, *E. coli*, are also present in the pyruvate dehydrogenase complex of the M2 antigen. (Bogdanos et al. 2004)

Prodrome
An early symptom of disease.

Key Point

A diagnosis of PBC can be made in the absence of anti-mitochondrial antibody M2.

SELF-CHECK 9.3

In what other disorders apart from those of the liver might you find anti-M2 and why?

9.4 Overlap syndromes

The term 'overlap syndromes' in respect of autoimmune liver disease refers to the coexistence of two individual disorders, one cholestatic and the other hepatitic. The most common of these overlaps is AIH/PBC, which exhibits auto-antibodies associated with both disorders. The most frequent combination is anti-M2 and anti-SLA. The rim ANA (anti-Gp210) and the multiple nuclear dot pattern (anti-Sp-100) tend to relate to PBC rather than act as marker for AIH. This overlap heralds a poorer prognosis than either of the individual disorders.

The overlap between AIH and PSC occurring in adolescents is now considered to be a separate disease entity, ASC. This disorder shares ANA/SMA of AIH and the atypical P-ANCA found in inflammatory bowel disease.
The definition of overlaps in autoimmune liver disease is not yet codified.

Key Points

- **ASC is considered to be an 'overlap syndrome' because it has features of both primary sclerosing cholangitis and AIH type 1.**
- **PBC/AIH is the most common overlap syndrome and is usually characterized by the presence of anti-M2 and anti-SLA.**

9.4.1 Alternative assays

Online Resource Centre
To see an online video demonstrating the immunoblot, log on to www.oxfordtextbooks.co.uk/orc/fbs

Anti-M2 has a characteristic cytoplasmic staining pattern on HEp-2 cells and, depending on its intensity, can mask the presence of anti-Gp 210. Antibodies to centromere and Sp-100 are not affected by such fluorescence as the antigens are situated away from the nuclear envelope. In order to overcome this particular problem, and other problems associated with

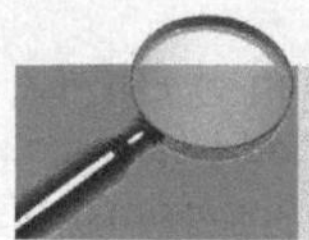

CASE STUDY 9.2 Anti-mitochondrial antibodies

Patient history

- A 47-year-old female, born in Stockholm, living in London for 20 years.
- Visits GP complaining of indigestion not responding to over the counter remedies.
- Also complaining of 'itchiness' (pruritis) from time to time on trunk and limbs; general fatigue.
- Bloods taken for investigation of possible gastric ulcer, anaemia.
- No previous medical history of note.

The results (1)

- Borderline haemoglobin and PCV
- WBC normal range
- Alkaline phosphatase 195 iu/L (NR 30–130)
- Gamma GT 67 iu/L (NR 1–55)
- Aspartate transferase 210 iu/ml (NR 10–50).

Significance of the results (1)

All the enzymes of the LFTs were abnormally high, indicating a problem with the liver. The patient gave no history of drug or alcohol abuse when questioned further by the GP. The deranged LFTs prompted the GP to order further investigations, namely auto-antibodies and immunoglobulins.

The results (2)

- IgG 25.9 g/L, IgA 3.10 g/L, IgM 5.52 g/L
- Anti-mitochondrial antibodies (AMA) positive 1/1280 by IIF.

Significance of results (2)

- IgG increased (normal range 6.34–18.11 g/L), not unusual in inflammatory liver disease of any aetiology but AIH is worth consideration.
- IgA within normal range (0.87–4.12 g/L).
- IgM increased (normal range 0.52–2.23 g/L). Raised IgM is a presenting feature of the majority of primary biliary cirrhosis (PBC) cases.
- Anti-M2 antibody at this titre is the strongest of indications of a case of PBC.

The AMA was confirmed by immunoblot as anti-M2. The immunoblot also detected anti-soluble liver antigen (SLA).

The patient underwent liver biopsy and cholangiography (imaging of the biliary tree) and was subsequently diagnosed as showing PCB/AIH overlap syndrome. The auto-antibody profile by IIF showed only the anti-M2 but the immunoblot also revealed anti-SLA. The latter is not seen on IIF, but its discovery adds to the diagnosis as this profile is typical of the overlap syndrome. The major significance being that the therapeutic regime may need to include an immunosuppressive modality, not only ursodeoxycholic acid, to manage the PBC.

subjective IIF assay, other assay systems are required. These are the antigen-specific and objective assays such as immunoblot and ELISA. Not only are these assays objective, they are also usually of greater analytical sensitivity. This was demonstrated in the cases of the AMA negative PBC, some of which become positive with a more sensitive assay. Though limited, assays for anti-Gp 210, anti-Sp 100, and anti-centromere are commercially available in either ELISA or immunoblot format.

Another approach to increase the detection rate of anti-mitochondrial antibody in PBC has been to bioengineer a recombinant antigen complex representing three of the major antigenic components of the M2 antigen. Peptides were synthesized conforming to the major epitopes of the pyruvate dehydrogenase complex (PDC-E2), 2-oxoglutarate dehydrogenase complex (OGDC-E2), and the branched chain 2-oxo-acid dehydrogenase complex (BCOAD-E2), and used in both ELISA and immunoblot. Various modifications have been made to the ELISA system over time and it has now become commercially available. Reports from two studies (Field and Heathcote 2003, Mieli-Vergani and Vergani 2008) have shown that some 60% of IIF AMA negative PBC sera were AMA positive in this test system.

The MIT3 antigen complex used in the ELISA in Section 9.3.5 is a combination of PDC-E2, OGDC-E2, and BCOAD-E2. Some immunoblots use only PDC-E2 as the mitochondrial antigen. This explains the discordance sometimes seen between IIF and immunoblot. Approximately 10% of PBC IIF positive sera show no reactivity with PDC-E2 but are reactive with one or both of the other antigens, OGDC-E2 and BCOAD-E2. Immunoblots containing the three individual components of this complex are now commercially available.

Assays for the PBC related anti-mitochondrial antibodies–anti-M4, anti-M8 (always associated with anti-M2), and anti-M9–are not commercially available in any test format.

The use of in-house Western blot or ELISA is a possible means to overcome the lack of commercial products. It must be remembered that if such assays are to be used clinically they must be subject to stringent validation within the current regulatory framework.

> **Key Point**
>
> **Antigen-specific assays such as ELISA and immunoblot are useful adjuncts to IIF and may provide information not given in IIF.**

9.5 Technical notes

The efficient demonstration of auto-antibodies by IIF consists of several stages:

- the substrate
- the patient and control sera dilutions
- the second antibody conjugate
- the fluorescence microscope
- the observer/reporter.

All of these variables must be incorporated into a suitable standard operating procedure (SOP).

> **Key Point**
>
> **Indirect immunofluorescence (IIF) is a subjective assay dependent on many components for its result.**

9.5.1 The substrate

The choice of substrate for the detection of liver disease related auto-antibodies is an important one. Historically, many laboratories prepared their own sections in house from locally available rodent tissues. However, the number of sections required in the modern laboratory to meet the current high workload makes this impossible in most cases. The advantage of such locally prepared sections was that they were unfixed and the antigenic repertoire was in its native state. It should be remembered that the patterns originally described for the majority of auto-antibodies were from such sections. There is a commercial source of unfixed rodent tissue available in the UK, but most laboratories use commercially available fixed sections. The advantage of such sections is that they have a long shelf life when stored as per manufacturer's instructions. The various fixation schedules used by commercial manufacturers do lead to some differences in the IIF pattern observed for a particular auto-antibody.

Substrate selection

The liver, kidney, and stomach (LKS) composite block is the accepted standard format for the detection of liver disease related auto-antibodies. The source is either rat or mouse and either performs well. There is a concern that the use of rat stomach may lead to the detection of **heterophile** antibodies which are of no clinical value and may be reported as anti-gastric parietal cell antibody. The pattern is readily identifiable by experienced observers but may be avoided by the use of mouse stomach.

Heterophile

An antibody against an antigen from one species that also reacts against antigens from other species. Often seen in indirect immunofluorescence.

The fixation of tissues varies from supplier to supplier and consequently the final pattern seen under the microscope may vary. The aim of fixation is to preserve the tissue in as near a life-like state as possible. This is a definition for the histologist, but for the immunologist there is another concern. Antibodies bind to specific three-dimensional structures, epitopes. The exposure of such structures to alcohols and acetone, the commonly used fixatives, may cause alteration of the epitope and thus adversely affect antibody binding. This is not in the interest of suppliers, hence the fixation schedules used by them are considered suitable for the intended purpose. The simplest approach for selection of substrate is to use a panel of known positive controls for the auto-antibodies of interest and to see how they react with the different commercial substrates. Most suppliers will be pleased to offer material for evaluation at no cost. Your laboratory SOP for the introduction of a new assay may cover this or a more specific one can be written following that format with suitable amendments.

The plane of section is of importance and should be such as to allow easy observation of the relevant tissue structures used in the identification of the auto-antibody. In the case of the liver this does not matter as the liver may be seen as a homogenous mass which appears the same regardless of plane of section. The stomach must be sectioned in a manner that allows simultaneous viewing of both the mucosa and the muscle bands and should avoid the gastro-oesophageal junction. The kidney sectional plane should reveal both cortex and medulla. This is essential in the demonstration of anti-LKM and anti-mitochondrial M2 antibodies.

9.5.2 The patient and control serum dilutions

The International Autoimmune Hepatitis Group (IAIHG) published a consensus statement on the detection of auto-antibodies in liver disease (Vergani et al. 2004). Briefly the statement advises 1/40 initial screening dilution for adults and 1/10 for paediatric cases, defined as less than 18 years old. The use of ANA, SMA, LKM 1, and AMA positive controls forms part of the recommendations. Control sera may be obtained from commercial sources or from patient samples. If using patient material there must be compliance with departmental policy and/or the local ethics committee policy. Not only does the use of positive control material conform to good practice but allows an instant reference in cases of uncertainty that may arise with patient sera.

Key Point

The use of well-characterized positive and negative control sera is essential to every successful auto-antibody assay.

9.5.3 The second antibody conjugate

Anti-human IgG fluorescein isothiocyanate (FITC) is the conjugate of choice when investigating liver disease related auto-antibodies.

The use of a chequerboard titration is the only scientific means of determining the optimum dilution of the conjugate. Manufacturers' recommendations are only suggestions but offer a central point around which to design the titration range. Again, as with all IIF the end point is subjective. The aim is to clearly visualize the auto-antibody with as little extraneous or background staining as possible. The use of counterstains to reduce backgrounds should not be necessary if the chequerboard is performed accurately.

9.5.4 The fluorescence microscope

The selection of microscopes suitable for IIF work is wide and varied. The optics and the light source are the major components of any system. Modern microscopes use dichroic mirrors in conjunction with exciter and barrier filters to achieve the desired configuration for the fluorochrome of choice. Detailed information is available on the websites of the major suppliers.

There are three main light sources: mercury vapour, xenon, and light emitting diodes (LED). The LED sources offer the advantages of longevity—up to 10 000 hours usage—compared to xenon and mercury, which are in 100s of hours. The ability to switch on and off as required with no 'warm-up' time is another advantage of the LED. There are issues of safety with high pressure lamps which are absent with the use of LED. The possibility of explosion is present and increases as the envelope ages. The escape of mercury into the local environment is another cause for concern, though any vapour readily condenses. The centring of these lamps often proves difficult and is a contributory factor in poor overall performance. The LED systems require no such centring, just an instrument-based calibration.

9.5.5 The observer/reporter

Training is a time-consuming process, perhaps even more so in the case of fluorescence microscopy. The correct identification of the relevant IIF patterns is a skill best acquired over time with the teaching of experienced colleagues. Photomicrographs from textbooks and websites are useful adjuncts to the learning process, but no substitute for regular sessions at the microscope. Because IIF is a subjective assay system it is advisable to use two observers to report. Any divergence of opinion can then be the subject of further investigation or subjected to the laboratory's SOP, which should cover such situations.

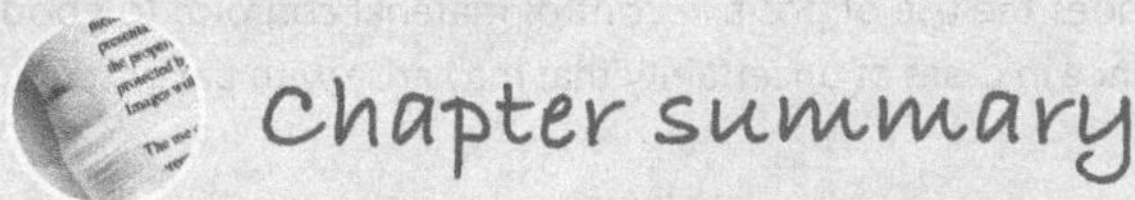

Chapter summary

- IIF is a subjective assay; antigen-specific assays are useful confirmatory tools.
- Type 1 AIH is defined by the presence of ANA and/or SMA.
- Type 2 AIH is defined by the presence of anti-LKM 1 and/or anti-LC 1.

- Anti-LKM 1also occurs in 10% of hepatitis C infection.
- Anti-liver cytosol is found in approximately 50% of type 2 AIH.
- Anti-mitochondrial antibody (M2) is the marker auto-antibody of PBC, but anti-mitochondrial antibody negative PBC exists.
- ASC is serologically like AIH type1 but also has a high incidence of atypical P-ANCA.
- Overlap syndromes exist—PBC/AIH. ASC appears to be a PSC/AIH overlap.
- Immunosuppression is the major therapeutic action, but when the biliary tree is involved a therapeutic modality is required for managing bile acids.

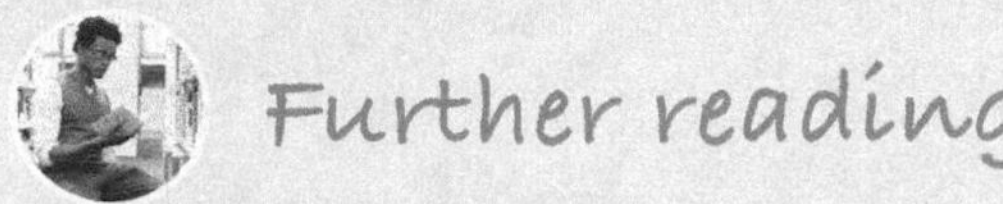

- **Davies E (2008)** ***LKM antibody–still a trap for the unwary*****. http://www.immqas.org.uk/docs/LKM%20Commentary.pdf**
- **Vergani D, Alvarez F, Bianchi F, *et al.* (2004)** ***Liver autoimmune serology: a consensus statement from the committee for autoimmune serology of the International Autoimmune Hepatitis Group*****. *J Hepatol*, 41, 677–83**

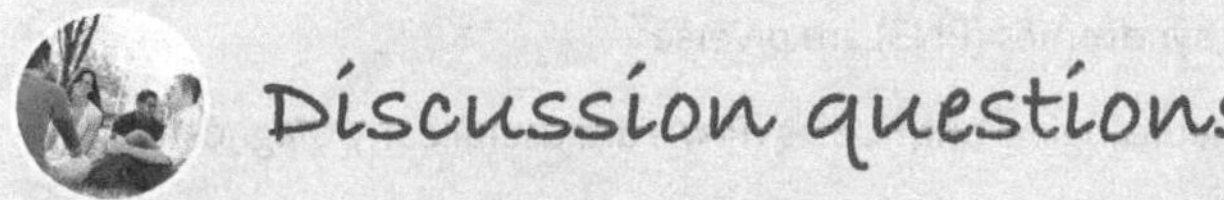

9.1 Discuss the factors influencing the result of an IIF assay for anti-LKM 1 in a child.

9.2 You receive a request for 'mitochondrial antibodies please; clinically and biochemically PBC'. Your IIF result is negative for anti-mitochondrial antibody on LKS substrate. How would you proceed?

9.3 A known PBC (anti-M2 positive) patient has transferred to your hepatology clinic. Physicians request LFTs and note a marked transaminitis along with the expected raised alkaline phosphatase. They suspect PBC/AIH overlap and subsequently request 'AIH antibodies, please'. Your IIF reveals anti-M2 to a titre of 1/640 only. How would you proceed?

Answers to self-check questions are provided in the book's Online Resource Centre.

 Visit www.oxfordtextbooks.co.uk/orc/hall2e

10

Neuroimmunology

Learning Objectives

After studying the chapter you should be able to:

- outline the immunological mechanisms involved in autoimmunity associated with paraneoplastic and non-paraneoplastic neurological syndromes
- describe why paraneoplastic syndromes (PNS) are diverse
- explain why paraneoplastic neurological antibodies (PNA) are useful early diagnostic markers of PNS
- outline with examples, why some of the antibodies are pathogenic and others unlikely to be so
- explain what the characteristics of PNS associated tumours are
- explain why there is a need for confirming specificities of PNA with more than one methodology
- explain the difference between classical and newer neurological antibodies in terms of detection, treatment, and clinical outcome.

Introduction

This chapter will provide an overview of recent developments in neuroimmunology, focusing on how clinical and laboratory investigations contribute to diagnosis leading to effective management and enhanced quality of life.

Only selected topics of interest in this specialist field will be reviewed and include a range of newer autoimmune disease markers of the nervous system that can be utilized in assisting clinical diagnosis of the neurological indisposition that may be paraneoplastic (associated with remote malignancy), non-paraneoplastic (which may be coincidently linked to cancer), or idiopathic in aetiology but differ from the inflammatory processes, demyelination (multiple sclerosis), and acute disseminated encephalomyelitis where there may be no specific biomarkers. The antibodies described in this chapter are listed in Table 10.1.

TABLE 10.1: Summary of paraneoplastic anti-neuronal antibodies, their staining patterns, associated disorders, common tumours and relevant target antigens.

(A) Well characterised PNA

Antibody	MW (kDa)	Staining pattern	PNS	Associated tumour(s)	Target antigen
Hu (ANNA1)	34–40	Nuclei of both central and peripheral neurones	PCD, PEM, SN	SCLC	HuD, PLE21/HuC, Hel-N1, 35-40 kDa nucleus and slightly cytoplasm RNA recogition motifs, translation
Yo (PCA-1)	34, 52, 62	Purkinje cell cytoplasm & axons	PCD	Ovary, breast	PCD17/CDR62 (58 kDa), cytoplasm, leucine zipper, zinc finger, transcription 34 kDa, 6 amino acid repeat
CV2/CRMP5	66	Oligodendrocytes cytoplasm	PEM/SN	SCLC, thymoma	POP66, 66 kDa, cytoplasmic in some oligodendrocytes
Ri (ANNA2)	55, 80	Nuclei of central neurones	OM, PCD, BE	Breast, SCLC, gynaecological	Nova-1 (55 kDa) and 80 kDa, nucleus and slightly cytoplasm only in CNS, RNA recognition motifs, translation
Ma2 (Ta)	41.5	Neuronal nucleoli, perikaryon	BE, LE	Testicular cancer	Unknown function
Amphiphysin	128	Central presynaptic terminals	SPS, PEM	Breast cancer, SCLC	Amphiphysin, neurophil, cytoplasm doublet bands at 125-128 kDa, synaptic vesicle-associated protein
Recoverin	23, 65	Retinal photoreceptor	Retinopathy	SCLC	Recoverin, 23 kDa, calcium binding protein
AGNA (SOX)	Predicted ~ 39	Nuclei of Bergmann glia cells	LEMS	SCLC	Transcription factor genes

(B) Partially characterised PNA

Antibody	MW(kDa)	Staining pattern	PNS	Associated tumour(s)	Target antigen
Tr (PCA-Tr)		Purkinje cell cytoplasm with "dots" in molecular layer	PCD	Hodgkin's lymphoma	Unknown function (found in the Purkinje cell cytoplasm)
ANNA-3	170	Purkinje cell cytoplasm & nucleus + glomerular podocytes	PCD, PEM, SN	SCLC	170 kDa protein found in cytoplasm of Purkinje cells and glomerular podocytes
PCA-2	280	Purkinje cell cytoplasm and other neurones	PEM, PCD. LEMS	SCLC	280 kDa Purkinje cell cytoplasmic protein
Zic4	~37	Nuclei of granular neurones, weaker on Purkinje cell nuclei	PCD	SCLC	Zinc finger protein found in cerebellum
mGluR1	~140	Purkinje cell cytoplasm, climbing fibre	PCD	Hodgkin's lymphoma	mGluR1

(continued)

TABLE 10.1: (Continued)

(C) Main pathogenic antibodies that occur with or without cancer

Antibody	Antigen	Staining pattern	Neurological disorder	Associated tumour(s)	Target antigen
AChR	Receptor	Post-synaptic neuromuscular junction	MG	Thymoma	Acetylcholine receptor or associated proteins at the neuromuscular junction
MuSK	Receptor	Post-synaptic neuromuscular junction	MG	None	Muscle specific tyrosine kinase
VGCC	Channel	Presynaptic neuromuscular junction	LEMS, PCD	SCLC	64 kDa P/Q voltage gated calcium channel, acetylcholine release
NMDAR	Glutamate receptor	Cell surface staining of transfected HEK cells	LE	Ovarian teratoma	N-terminal extracellular domain of the NR1 subunit of NMDAR
LGI1	VGKC protein	Cell surface staining of transfected HEK cells	LE with FBDS	Rare	LGI1
CASPR2	VGKC protein	Cell surface staining of transfected HEK cells	Neuromyotonia	+ / –	CASPR2
AMPAR	Receptor	Cell surface staining of transfected HEK cells	LE	+ / – Lung, breast or thymus	GluR1 and GluR2 subunits of AMPAR
$GABA_BR$	Receptor	Cell surface staining of transfected HEK cells	LE (mainly seizures)	SCLC	B1 receptor subunit of $GABA_BR$
Glycine	Receptor	Cell surface staining of transfected HEK cells	PERM	Rare	α1 receptor subunit of Glycine receptor

Abbreviations:

AChR = acetylcholine receptor, AGNA – Anti-glial nuclear antibody, AMPAR - alpha-amino-3-hydroxy-5-methyl-4-isoxazolepropionic acid receptor ANNA = antineuronal nuclear antibody, BE = brainstem encephalomyelitis, CASPR2 = contactin-associated protein-like 2, FEDS = Faciobrachial-dystonic seizures, GABA – Gamma amino butyric acid, HEK = Human Embryonic Kidney, LE = limbic encephalomyelitis, LEMS = Lambert-Eaton myasthenic syndrome, LGI1 = Leucine-rich glioma-inactivated protein 1 antibody, MG = myasthenia gravis, mGLuR1 = metabotropic glutamate receptor type 1, MuSK – muscle specific tyrosine kinase, OM= opsoclonus/myclonus, PCA = Purkinje cell cytoplasm antibody, PCD = paraneoplastic cerebellar degeneration, PEM = paraneoplastic encephalomyelitis, PERM – Progressive encephalomyelitis, with rigidity and myoclonus, PNS = paraneoplastic neurological syndrome, SCLC= small cell lung carcinoma, SN = sensory neuropathy, SOX – Sex determining region Y-box, SPS = Stiff person syndrome, VGCC = Voltage gated calcium channel, VGKC = Voltage gated potassium channel

Definitive clinical diagnosis of neurological complications affiliated with non-metastatic neurological cancer, collectively known as paraneoplastic neurological syndrome (PNS), has been assisted by the presence of a range of paraneoplastic anti-neuronal antibodies (PNA) (Table 10.1). Furthermore, identifying these antibodies in the absence of a specific aetiology alerts the clinician to carry out a thorough examination of the patient for the possible presence of an unidentified neoplasm. In most cases, early diagnosis of the tumour is essential as it provides an opportunity for effective treatment.

Recently there has been substantial growth in neuronal antibodies associated with the subgroups of paraneoplastic encephalitic syndrome which show remarkable response to immunomodulation (Table 10.1c). These auto-antibodies have been identified to exert their effects by interfering with the cell-to-cell communication during neuronal signal transmission process and have been classified as acting extracellularly, in contrast to the previously described paraneoplastic neurological antibodies which have their target located often in the intracellular compartment.

In this chapter the characteristic elements of neurological disorder, neoplasm, and classical neurological antibodies, together with a range of newer antibodies, will be discussed.

10.1 Terminology

The terms used in this chapter are unlikely to be found in other chapters and are different to those describing other disease processes. Furthermore, nomenclature used in the naming of these antibodies has not been standardized; consequently an antibody maybe referred to by different names, leading to confusion. A brief description of the terms most commonly used in this review has also been included here.

10.2 Epidemiology

Malignancy-related neurological disorders are rare and their relative rarity makes it difficult to carry out extensive clinical, epidemiological, and experimental studies in individual laboratories. The few studies that have addressed the incidence and prevalence of PNS in the overall cancer population have found an estimated frequency of around 0.01% (1/10 000), whereas in a recent UK survey conducted amongst physicians, about 50 PNS were reported in one year, which approximates to an incidence of 0.0001% (Rees 2004). Such low incidences are likely to reflect under-reporting of PNS. Others studies have focused on either the association of certain cancers with PNS or on the specific PNAs, their neurological syndrome, and associated neoplasm. It is worth noting that neuromuscular abnormalities like **Lambert-Eaton myasthenic syndrome (LEMS)** can occur in up to 3% of patients with small-cell lung cancer. Conversely 50–70% of patients with LEMS have an underlying cancer. A study by Pittock et al. (2005) looked at the detection of PNA in 120 000 samples received over a 15-year period from patients suspected of neurological disorders. They found low detection frequencies of PNA, with the highest frequency of 0.4% assigned to an antibody known as ANNA1. These data are summarized in Table 10.2. More recent studies by Dalmau et al. (2008) suggest that if serological screening is targeted as per the clinical context, 25% of patients may have an appropriate antibody.

Lambert-Eaton myasthenic syndrome (LEMS)
Muscle weakness, fatigue, difficulty swallowing, and autonomic symptoms.

As regards to the age, the patient group affected by PNS, particularly paraneoplastic cerebellar degeneration (PCD), tends to be in their latter part of life with several studies quoting median range above 60 years.

TABLE 10.2 Detection frequency of PNA from 120 000 patients suspected of paraneoplastic neurological syndrome (adapted from Pittock et al, 2005).

PNA	Frequency (%)
ANNA1	0.4
CRMP5/CV2	0.4
PCA-1	0.2
PCA-2	0.1
Amphiphysin	0.06
ANNA2	0.02
ANNA3	0.001
PCA-Tr (Tr)	0.002

10.3 Clinical features of paraneoplastic syndromes

Paraneoplastic syndromes refer to a collection of clinical disorders that occur at remote sites from a tumour or its metastases and can be of a nervous, cutaneous, endocrine, gastrointestinal, haematological, renal, or rheumatological origin/nature. When the nervous system is involved (central or peripheral, including the neuromuscular junction and muscle), it is known as paraneoplastic neurological syndrome (PNS) and can affect any level of the nervous system. PNS are rare, debilitating, immune-mediated neurological disorders diagnosed when other cancer-related specific aetiologies such as metastases, vascular, infectious, metabolic, or treatment-related causes have been ruled out. It has been known since the eighteenth century that certain neurological illnesses, termed 'classical syndrome' almost always accompany a neoplasm, whilst neurological deficits less commonly associated with malignancies were nominated as 'non-classical PNS'. These are shown in Table 10.3. Clinically, PNS can be defined as 'definite' or 'possible', based on combined evidence arising from neurological examination (classical or non-classical syndrome), the involvement of cancer, and the presence of well-characterized PNA (Graus et al. 2004). The criteria for the definitive or possible diagnosis of PNS are shown

TABLE 10.3 Classic and non-classic neurological disorders associated with cancer.

	Classic–strong cancer link	Non-classic–weak cancer link
Central nervous system	Encephalomyelitis Limbic encephalitis Subacute cerebellar degeneration Opsoclonus–myoclonus	Brainstem encephalitis Stiff-person syndrome Paraneoplastic visual syndromes Motor neuron syndromes
Peripheral nervous system	Subacute sensory neuronopathy	Acute sensorimotor neuropathy Chronic sensorimotor neuropathy Subacute autonomic neuropathy Paraneoplastic peripheral nerve vasculitis
Neuromuscular junction & muscle	Lambert–Eaton myasthenic syndrome Dermatomyositis	Myasthenia gravis Neuromyotonia Acute necrotizing myopathy Cachectic myopathy

TABLE 10.4 Diagnosis of PNS.

Neurological syndrome	Antibody	Cancer
Any	Well characterised	None
Classic syndrome	None	Develop within 5 years
Non-classic syndrome	Any paraneoplastic Ab	Develop within 5 years
Non-classic syndrome	+/– antibody	Cured after cancer treatment
Neurological syndrome	**Antibody**	**Cancer**
Any	Partially characterised	None
Classic syndrome	None	None; but at high risk
Non-classic syndrome	None	Develop within 2 years

in Table 10.4. These rare neurological illnesses (classical syndrome), when present in a patient implies a very high clinical index of suspicion of a PNS. A brief description of these conditions follow, together with antibodies associated with such ailments as LEMS, **myasthenia gravis**, **neuromyotonia**, and other relevant disorders.

Myasthenia gravis
Weakness and rapid fatigue of voluntary muscles.

Neuromyotonia
Abnormal nerve impulses from peripheral motor neurons causing twitching, stiffness, cramps, and slowed movement.

Key Point

Autoimmune neurological syndromes may or may not be associated with an underlying cancer.

SELF-CHECK 10.1

What is meant by classical neurological syndrome?

10.3.1 Signs and symptoms

The most common signs and symptoms of PNS include difficulty in walking, maintaining balance, swallowing, loss of muscle tone and fine motor coordination, slurred speech, memory loss, vision problems, dizziness, sleep disturbances, dementia, seizures, numbness, and tingling in the limbs. The specific syndromes will be explored in slightly more detail in Sections 10.3.2–10.3.11.

Limbic encephalitis
Inflammation of the brain leading to memory loss, drowsiness, confusion, disorientation, and seizures.

Encephalomyelitis
Inflammation of both brain (encephalitis) and spinal cord (myelitis).

Cerebellar degeneration
Damage to the cerebellum, with loss of muscle control and balance.

Key Point

The common neuroimmunological syndromes associated with well-recognized antibodies are myasthenia gravis, LEMS, limbic encephalitis, encephalomyelitis, and cerebellar degeneration.

SELF-CHECK 10.2

Define paraneoplastic neurological syndrome (PNS).

10.3.2 Paraneoplastic encephalomyelitis (PEM)

Encephalomyelitis (EM) is a generalized term used for inflammation of brain and spinal cord. In about 10%, EM is paraneoplastic where multiple areas of the brain are affected by neuronal loss and inflammatory infiltrates. The term PEM alone provides limited information on the main clinical picture and therefore should not be used in isolation especially if a single predominant area of the CNS is affected (Graus et al. 2004). Depending on the predominant area of central nervous system involvement, patients may be classified under different semiologies which are discussed in Sections 10.3.3–10.3.11. 9% of PEM patients have limbic encephalitis (affecting the hippocampus and limbic system), 10.5% have subacute cerebellar degeneration, 6% have brainstem encephalitis, and some patients have autonomic **neuropathy**. 54% of patients have dorsal root ganglia involvement causing subacute sensory neuronopathy. The spectrum of neurological symptoms can vary from numbness to respiratory failure (Graus et al. 2001). A single abnormality may manifest clinically in 30% of the cases.

Neuropathy
Disorder of peripheral nervous system involving motor, sensory, and/or autonomic nerves.

10.3.3 Paraneoplastic cerebellar degeneration (PCD)

PCD, the most commonly occurring PNS, is a disorder of the cerebellum and occurs at a frequency of 37% in patients with PNA. The cerebellum consists of white and grey matter; the latter is subdivided into molecular and granular layers (containing densely packed granular cells). The Purkinje cells, which can be easily identified by their large size and location at the border of the granular layer facing the molecular layer, comprise a mere 0.3% of the human cerebellum. Figure 10.1 shows the location of the cerebellum and Figure 10.2 its cellular structure.

Post mortem studies on subjects with PCD revealed an almost complete absence of cerebellar Purkinje cells, an observation that might explain the reason behind the rapid onset of symptoms (weeks to a few months). Functionally, the cerebellum is responsible for sensory (information) perception, coordination, and motor control. Lack of coordination is termed as ataxia. Fifty percent of cerebellar ataxia is of a paraneoplastic origin.

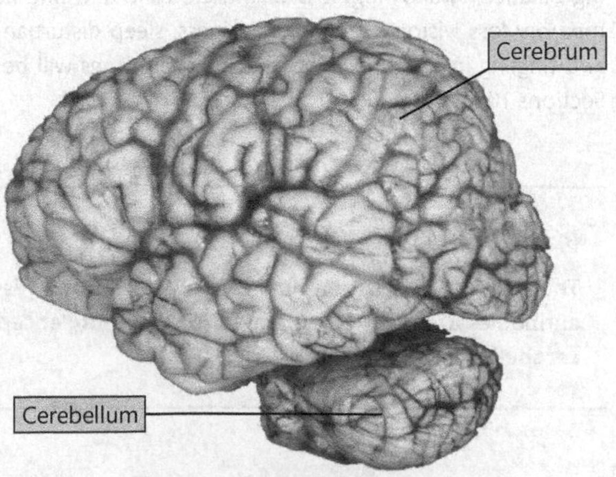

FIGURE 10.1
Human brain showing the location of cerebellum (Latin: 'little brain'), which is located in the inferior posterior region of the head and is made up of two hemispheres.

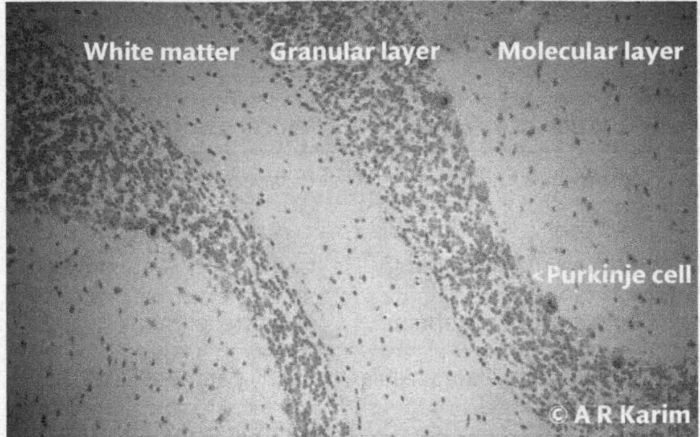

FIGURE 10.2
Haematoxylin- and eosin-stained section of primate cerebellum showing the white matter and the granular and molecular layers. Large Purkinje cells are located at the border of the granular and the molecular layer.

Clinically, the characteristic signs of cerebellar involvement are obvious: the patient walks with a wide-legged, unsteady, lurching gait and can have jerky limb movements on volitional activity. These acute symptoms are accompanied by nausea, vomiting, dizziness, and uncoordinated movement which usually progress to a severe stage where simple tasks like walking, sitting, and eating cannot be performed without assistance. Patients can also suffer from inability to communicate verbally (due to slow and slurred speech) or ataxia (owing to nystagmus and double vision coupled with unsteady hands).

10.3.4 Paraneoplastic limbic encephalitis (PLE)

A recent UK-based prospective study of encephalitis has divided its causes into three major categories with the largest being infection (42%) where the offending pathogen in most cases is herpes simplex virus. For the next largest group, the cause is idiopathic (37%), and the third group comprises 21% with the aetiology due to an acute immune-mediated process (Granerod et al. 2010), which includes post-viral infection. It is entirely possible that a good proportion of the so-called "idiopathic" encephalitis could well be due to as yet unidentified immune mechanisms.

LE is attributed to a disturbance in the limbic system (located at the base of the brain) and represents changes in the individual's personality, rapid loss of short-term memory, drowsiness, confusion, disorientation, depression, irritability, and seizures (Gultekin et al. 2000, Dalmau and Bataller 2006). Many clinical features are common amongst both types of LE (paraneoplastic and non-paraneoplastic) and not all symptoms/signs may be present in every patient.

In 64% of cases, MRI findings show brain abnormalities. These symptoms are not confined solely to PLE but can also occur in association with other ailments such as brain metastases, toxic therapy, or herpes infection, thus complicating the diagnosis. The onset of the symptoms can be acute or subacute and the paraneoplastic form of LE is often associated with small-cell lung carcinoma (40%), testicular germ cell tumours (20%), breast cancer (8%), Hodgkin's disease, and thymoma, but in the last few years this condition has been recognized as also being non-paraneoplastic and usually responsive to immunotherapy, availing a greater opportunity for treatment and recovery.

LE can be accompanied by a range of newer autoimmune disease markers that supplement the already existing list of classical paraneoplastic neurological antibodies such as Hu, Ma, CV2, and amphiphysin (see Table 10.5).

TABLE 10.5 Encephalitic antibodies, their relationship with antigen location, and cancer association.

Antibody in encephalitis	Location of target antigen	Cancer association
Hu (ANNA1), CV2 (CRMP5), Amphiphysin, Ma2 (Ta)	Intracellular	Paraneoplastic
AMPAR, $GABA_{B1}R$, mGluR5	Extracellular/membrane	Commonly paraneoplastic
NMDAR, CASPR2, Contactin 2	Extracellular/membrane	± Paraneoplastic
LGI1, GAD, Glycine	Intracellular & extracellular/ membrane	Rarely paraneoplastic

NMDA = N-methyl-D-aspartate; AMPAR = α-amino-3-hydroxy-5-methyl-4-isoxazolepropionic acid receptor, $GABA_{B1}R$ = Gamma-AminoButyric Acid receptor type B1, LGI1 = Leucine-rich glioma inactivated protein 1, CASPR2 = Contactin-associated protein 2, mGLuR1 = metabotropic glutamate receptor type 1, GAD = glutamic acid decarboxylase.

10.3.5 Opsoclonus-myoclonus (OM)

Opsoclonus-myoclonus (OM)

Rapid, irregular eye movements (opsoclonus) coupled with quick, involuntary muscle jerks (myoclonus).

Opsoclonus-myoclonus (OM) is also known as Kinsbourne or 'dancing-eyes-dancing-feet' syndrome and is defined by the presence of rapid, irregular eye movements (opsoclonus) in either vertical or horizontal direction, coupled with quick involuntary muscle jerks (myoclonus) of the limbs and trunk. Symptoms of cerebellar dysfunction are also frequent with this disorder (Rossiñol and Graus 2008). Paraneoplastic OM (POM) is seen in 50% of children with neuroblastoma and about 20% of adults with OM have underlying malignancy of lung (SCLC), breast, or gynaecological origin. In some adults, POM can occur in conjunction with SCLC but without a related antibody. Reports of other neoplasms exist in the literature.

10.3.6 Stiff person syndrome (SPS)

Stiff person syndrome (SPS)

Progressive, severe muscle stiffness or rigidity, mainly in spine and legs.

Stiff person syndrome (SPS) is considered as a CNS syndrome and belongs to the non-classical category of PNS. SPS is a rare form of autoimmune neurological disorder featuring symmetrical progressive and severe muscle stiffness or rigidity, mainly in the spine, and intense painful muscle spasms may be triggered by sensory stimuli. Muscle rigidity can vary during the day and may reduce in intensity with sleep. Muscle spasm, which may be accompanied by intense pain, can immobilize the limbs so that walking becomes slow and difficult. Severe spasms have been known to inflict femoral fractures or abdominal hernia. In about 20% of cases, a paraneoplastic variation of SPS can also exist in patients with breast, colon, or lung cancer, Hodgkin's disease, or thymoma.

Cross reference

You can find a fuller account of stiff person syndrome in the review by Meinck and Thompson. (2002).

SPS is thought to occur because of lack of inhibition of the spinal cord reflexes. These reflexes are usually under the control of neurons secreting gamma-aminobutyric acid (GABA). GABA can be produced by the enzyme glutamic acid decarboxylase (GAD) and antibodies against GAD are seen in approximately 50% of SPS patients. In fact, SPS used to be described as 'spinal interneuronitis' for a long time. SPS associated with anti-amphiphysin antibodies are often paraneoplastic in origin. Some patients may only have either an arm or leg involved and are termed to have 'stiff limb syndrome'.

10.3.7 Paraneoplastic sensory neuronopathy (PSN)

The term neuronopathy was coined to describe neurological syndromes arising from damage to the cell body of the neurons of the peripheral nervous system observed in patients with tumours of lung origin, usually SCLC (70–80%), but can also be identified with neoplasms of ovary, breast, or Hodgkin's disease (Graus et al. 2001). Approximately 20% of neuronopathies are of paraneoplastic origin. The main clinical complaints are subacute numbness and paraesthesia (pins and needles), which can be asymmetrical and patchy, usually starting with the upper limbs and rapidly progressing to a state where the patient becomes wheelchair- or bed-bound with disability. The syndrome is often painful (shooting, burning sensations) and when large sensory fibres are involved, sensory ataxia (unsteadiness due to reduced sensation) may also be present. Sensory loss can affect the face, chest, and abdomen. Patients may also present with gastrointestinal pseudo-obstruction (constipation and vomiting), due to the involvement of the neurons of the myenteric plexus.

10.3.8 Myasthenia gravis (MG)

MG is an autoimmune disorder of the peripheral nervous system affecting the neuromuscular junction (NMJ) and occurs at an approximate rate of 0.2% (1/5000). Clinically, it can be referred to either as ocular MG where only the eyelids and extra-ocular muscles are weak or as generalized MG in which subnormal muscle strength can be observed in other muscles. The weakness is variable, painless, and can fluctuate from day to day, and muscles are typically fatiguable (i.e. aggravated with exercise or activity).

Ocular MG causes fatiguable weakness of the eyelids or eye movement. Ptosis (drooping of the eyelid) is usually bilateral, can be asymmetrical and is generally made worse with persistent up-gaze; consequently, patients may have difficulties with reading and watching television, because of double vision.

A generalized form of MG can affect a variety of muscles, leading to unstable or waddling gait, weakness in arms, hands, fingers, legs, and neck, difficulty in swallowing, shortness of breath, and impaired speech. Many patients may appear to be depressed due to an expressionless face (sometimes referred to as 'myasthenic snarl'), resulting from fatigued facial muscles (Juel and Massey 2007).

10.3.9 Lambert–Eaton myasthenic syndrome (LEMS)

This is another disorder of the NMJ, which has a predilection to a different group of muscles to those involved in myasthenia gravis (respiratory, ocular, or the bulbar muscles that control swallowing, breathing, and speech). In LEMS, trunk and leg muscles are more prominently involved. In over 90% of patients, muscle weakness starts in the legs proximally and then spreads to other muscles resulting in fatigue and difficulty in swallowing (Vedeler et al. 2006). Autonomic symptoms are frequent features of LEMS, comprising of dry eyes and mouth, blurred vision, impotence, constipation, sweating, and orthostatic hypotension (Vincent 2008).

LEMS can be divided into two groups; one without and the other with cancer–the latter is termed as paraneoplastic LEMS. Both conditions are indistinguishable in terms of clinical expression or neurophysiology (the test used to confirm LEMS). In about 50–70% of patients with LEMS, the disorder is paraneoplastic, usually caused by small-cell lung cancer (SCLC). LEMS can also coexist with other PNS.

10.3.10 Neuromyotonia (NMT)

NMT (undulating myokymia or Isaac's syndrome), often described as peripheral nerve hyperexcitability (PNH), is an autoimmune disorder commonly found to have impact on the limbs and trunk. NMT is manifested as spontaneous and continuous muscle fibre hyperactivity of the peripheral motor neurons, causing muscle stiffness, twitching (myokymia), painful cramps, and slowed movement. Muscle cramps in NMT are indistinguishable from other normal cramps but the hyperactivity of muscle continues even during sleep. One of the frequent autonomic complaints by the patient is excessive sweating. NMT is not a fatal condition, but it can also exist with thymoma (20%), and on occasions may coexist with CNS symptoms (known as Morvan's syndrome).

Paraneoplastic neuromyotonia has been reported with SCLC, thymoma, and Hodgkin's disease, predating the cancer by up to 4 years.

Key Points

- **Well-defined neurological syndromes such as myasthenia gravis, LEMS, limbic encephalitis, and neuromyotonia are more likely to be associated with specific antibodies and may or may not be associated with an underlying cancer.**
- **PNS and antibodies may precede the detection of tumours by several months or even longer.**

10.3.11 Dermatomyositis

Dermatomyositis is characterized by painful muscle weakness, raised muscle enzyme levels, and skin changes including papules over the knuckles, photosensitive skin rashes, and periorbital violaceous inflammation. Patients may have periungual erythema which is painful to touch. Up to 25–30% of patients with dermatomyositis may have an underlying tumour. The chance of finding an underlying tumour reduces after the first 3 years; common tumours are those affecting lung, breast, gastrointestinal tract, or ovaries. Antibodies against Transcriptional Intermediary Factor 1 γ (TIF1γ, anti-p155) are seen in 25% of patients by using ELISA or immunoblotting and can be a marker of underlying cancer. Other antibodies implicated in autoimmune dermatomyositis include those against a nuclear helicase protein, Mi 2, and a nuclear matrix protein, p140.

10.3.12 Treatment of PNS

Treatment and management of PNS is tailored to individual needs, as determined by clinical investigation, confirming subtypes of PNS, presence or absence of tumour, and detection and type of PNA. These factors will determine the course of the disease, which varies from patient to patient. PNS is considered as an autoimmune disorder, therefore it is logical to consider immunomodulatory therapies (steroids, plasma exchange, or IVIG) for these patients. Such intervention has been of little or no value in some subtypes of PNS, for example PLE, SSN, and PCD, where there has been irreversible neurological damage. Generally, early detection and treatment of the underlying tumour is by far the best current approach for stabilizing neurological symptoms, curtailing further permanent neurological damage, and providing symptomatic therapy in an attempt to improve the quality of life.

Immunotherapy has been beneficial in patients with functional abnormalities, such as MG, LEMS, and NMT, where improvement has been seen, and may be of some benefit to children with OM but not adults. These recommendations were made by The European Federation of Neurological Societies (EFNS) task force (Vedeler et al. 2006). The newer autoimmune neurological syndromes like LE respond very well to immunotherapy and in some cases would need aggressive treatment with IVIg, plasma exchange, steroids, Rituximab or other immunosuppressive agents.

10.4 Malignancies commonly associated with PNS

With the exception of brain tumours, PNS can correlate with almost any type of malignant cancer, but commonly those affecting the lung, ovaries, breast, testes, or lymphoid tissue (Hodgkin's disease). Pathologically, cancers associated with a PNS resemble any other non-PNS cancer except for being relatively smaller in size and infiltrated by immune mediators such as lymphocytes and plasma cells. The fundamental role of the immune system in the control of growth and metastasis is supported by literature reports: in rare cases, there has been spontaneous remission of cancer in patients harbouring PNAs, and in 20% of PNS cases the cancer is never found even at post mortem examination.

In the majority of cases, the cancer can be detected up to 24 months after diagnosis of PNS. It is believed that the longer the cancer is undetectable, the less likely it will appear in the future. Unlike solid tumours, PNS associated with lymphomas often arise at an advanced stage of the neoplasia. LE and PCD are more common in Hodgkin's disease, whereas sensorimotor neuropathy and dermatomyositis are more common in non-Hodgkin's lymphoma patients.

Detection of cancer should be thorough using multiple imaging modalities like CT, MRI or PET, according to local protocols and regular review of the patient is advisable in order to search for a possible underlying malignancy, especially in patients with high risk (e.g. smokers). Monitoring should continue for up to 4 years (Vedeler et al. 2006). Specific screening protocols may be used using risk-stratification scores like DELTA-P for LEMS, and is beyond the scope of this chapter.

> Key Point
>
> **Neurological syndromes can be associated with any neoplasm, but the commonly occurring ones are SCLC, Hodgkin's lymphoma, ovarian, testicular, and breast cancers.**

10.5 Paraneoplastic neurological antibodies (PNA)

Paraneoplastic neurological anti-neuronal antibodies are perhaps the most important early diagnostic markers of PNS. Typically, the symptoms frequently precede the detection of the associated tumour by up to 2 years (Gultekin et al. 2000).

A relationship between neurological disorder and systemic tumours has been known for decades, with immunological involvement first being hypothesized in the early 1950s by Russell Brain et al. (1951). The involvement of the immune system against cancer has been the subject of debate for many years. Over this period, evidence has accumulated from various models supporting the concept of natural immunity to cancer. For example, it is well known that there is a higher risk of cancer developing in patients who are immunocompromised, irrespective of whether the immunodeficiency is primary or caused by human immunodeficiency virus (HIV) infection or immunosuppressive therapy for organ transplantation (Swann and Smyth 2007, Grulich et al. 2007). This concept is further supported by the observation that in immunodeficient mouse models there is an increased incidence of cancers. Human disorders like PNS also provide additional valuable circumstantial evidence for immune system involvement (see Table 10.1). Pathological studies on post mortem brains from paraneoplastic cerebellar degeneration (PCD) have demonstrated a general loss of neurons in the affected areas of the central nervous system (CNS) together with infiltration by B cells, $CD4^+$ T helper and cytotoxic $CD8^+$ T cells. Immune-mediated processes such as intrathecal IgG (oligoclonal bands) were also evident in the cerebrospinal fluid (CSF) of patients with PNS. A conclusive breakthrough in this field came in the 1980s when evidence for immunological involvement in neurological disorders due to systemic neoplasm was provided by Posner and colleagues (Graus et al. 1985).

These workers found specific ANNA1 (Hu) antibodies in the serum of a patient with PNS and small-cell lung carcinoma (SCLC). These antibodies were shown to bind not only to the patient's tumour but also to neuronal cells of the central nervous system. This discovery provided concrete scientific support for the autoimmune basis of paraneoplastic neurological disorders. The commonly accepted hypothesis for the pathogenesis of PNS is that the immune response is initially triggered by brain antigens expressed by the tumour (also known as onconeuronal antigens), seemingly in an attempt to eradicate the cancer. Consequently, the antigen-specific cytotoxic T and B cells gain access to both the tumour and the brain tissue, thereby targeting cells that are expressing onconeuronal proteins. Such an autoimmune response against neuronal antigens is thought to be responsible for neuronal destruction and hence the clinical condition. The symptoms exhibited are dependent on the area of the brain affected. Despite the important role of immunological factors in the pathogenesis of PNS, the direct pathogenic role of these antibodies (with the exception of few) has yet to be proven. The immune attack is directed against intracellular (cytoplasmic or nuclear) antigens which have an important role in neuronal development and function. These groups of antibodies are probably an epiphenomenon or a marker for autoimmune disease processes rather than being directly involved in causing neuronal damage. For this reason, patients rarely respond to treatments that diminish the levels of these antibodies. Conversely, epitopes exposed on the extracellular surface can be accessible to auto-antibody attack thus characterizing them both as pathogenic and as diagnostically important disease specific biomarkers. Consequently, treatment with immunomodulation therapy in patients harbouring such cell surface antibodies has seen greater success.

In the last two decades the list of anti-neuronal antibody specificities identified in patients with PNS has expanded at a steady rate. With this expansion, a consensus was initiated that aimed to provide clear guidelines for detection and classification of paraneoplastic anti-neuronal specific antibodies (Moll et al. 1995) for greater uniformity in laboratory screening of PNAs.

Despite these positive developments, a degree of confusion remains because a single antibody specificity may be found associated with more than one neurological disorder, and individual syndromes can be associated with different antibody specificities. A further compounding factor is that less than 50% of patients with PNS will harbour PNAs and in 30% more than one PNA is likely to be detected (Pittock et al. 2004). For this reason screening is preferable rather than testing for specific PNA. It is also important to bear in mind that PNA can be found in up to 16% of cancer patients who are neurologically asymptomatic, whilst up to 11% of subjects with PNA and neurological symptoms may not have a detectable neoplasm. To address this a study was supported by the European Union to define standards for the diagnosis and classification of PNS.

Cross reference

These guidelines (Graus et al. 2004) are referred to in the section on the use of PNAs in diagnosis.

Key Point

PNAs are not always tumour- or syndrome-specific, but there are well-recognized associations. Hence screening for a broad range of antibodies (e.g. using indirect immunofluorescence with primate cerebellar sections) may be preferable in neurological syndromes that are not so well defined.

10.5.1 Auto-antigens

There are a multitude of antigens which are recognized by their respective PNA. There is heterogeneity in both function and cellular location of the antigens. Despite this, in most cases the antigens responsible for the paraneoplastic syndromes have been identified and the respective genes have been cloned and sequenced. Not all tumours of a particular type express the antigens. Most antigens are nervous system restricted. A number of the antigens are expressed by neuronal cells of both the peripheral and central nervous system, whilst some are specific to the central nervous system, and a proportion are particular to the Purkinje cells of the cerebellum. These onconeuronal antigens responsible for PNS have since been identified and the genes involved cloned to produce recombinant proteins for both testing and research purposes.

10.5.2 PNA detection in the laboratory

'Neuro-oncoantigens' found in the cerebellar tissue are in their native environment, with structure and epitopes preserved. This provides an ideal environment for visualizing the antigen-antibody interaction, both specific and novel. The only drawback is co-localization of other non-neuronal antigens which may exhibit reactivities similar to those of specific antibodies. To overcome this, it is desirable to confirm any positive reaction with an alternative method, e.g. Western blotting, recombinant proteins, ELISA, or competitive assay.

Indirect immunofluorescence

In our hands the method of choice of screening for PNAs is by indirect immunofluorescence (IIF) using primate cerebellar cryosections, as this is rapid, reliable, and reproducible, and is used by 90% of laboratories who provide this service. Although rodent cerebellar sections can suffice and are frequently used, monkey tissues are preferable for reasons of antigenic similarity.

Cross reference

Full details of the methodology are given elsewhere (Karim et al. 2005); it is based on the guidelines published by Moll et al. (1995).

All positive sera are subjected to alternative methods of confirmation of reactivity for the reasons mentioned. There are exceptions to this rule and these will be dealt with under the appropriate antibody section.

Confirmation of reactivity

Various test kits are available commercially that provide a qualitative assay for human IgG antibodies to highly purified antigens or recombinant as coated parallel lines on strips. In addition to the usually six characterized (see Section 10.6) onconeuronal antigens on a strip, there is also a control band to indicate the correct performance of the incubation step.

METHOD 10.1 Detection of PNA by indirect immunofluorescence (IIF)

- **Frozen sections of monkey cerebellum are incubated with test sera at a dilution of 1/50 to allow specific antibody-antigen binding to take place.**
- **Unbound immunoglobulins are removed by a wash step.**
- **The bound human immunoglobulins (IgG class) are visualized using sheep anti-human IgG (monkey absorbed) conjugated to fluorescein.**

Immunoblots

Commercial preparations of immunoblots painted with recombinant proteins of the most common antigens and control bands are also available. In addition to verifying the specificity of PNAs, these blots are very useful for determining co-localization of more than one antigen. The new generation of immunoblots, which are costly but have a wide range of specificities, include amphiphysin, CV2, Ma-2, Ri, Yo, Hu, recoverin, SOX1, titin, Zic4, GAD 65, and Tr.

A sample is considered positive when it binds to a specific recombinant protein that is consistent with the cerebellar pattern.

Key Point

If the screening tests for PNA are positive, further specific tests should be performed using immunoreactive strips or immunoblots.

Quality assurance for neurological antibodies

There are only a few neurological antibodies which have an external quality control scheme operated by the United Kingdom National External Quality Assurance Service (UKNEQAS). Two are fully accredited schemes: acetylcholine receptor and paraneoplastic neurological antibodies. The latter has over 100 participants worldwide and samples are sent out six times annually. There are also two other schemes operating in pilot phase (ganglioside and glutamic acid decarboxylase antibodies) and pending full accreditation in the near future. UKNEQAS are looking into starting pilot schemes for other newer antibodies.

Internal controls

The situation with regards to the internal quality control for routine screening still poses a major problem as there are limited stocks available to share. Understandably, these being rare antibodies, most centres have limited supply of controls. Regardless of this more and more centres are screening for paraneoplastic neurological antibodies, but only a few centres provide a full and comprehensive service for the detection of a wide range of PNAs.

SELF-CHECK 10.3

What is the rationale for confirming antibody reactivity with an alternative methodology?

10.5.3 Role of PNA in diagnosis of PNS

The recommended guidelines for the use of PNAs to complement diagnosis can be divided into three categories. The first category is the *well-characterized antibodies*, which are strongly associated with both the neoplasm and well-defined neurological disorder (Figure 10.3). The second type are known as *partially characterized antibodies*, which have an unidentified target antigen; the experience with this class of antibodies is often confined to one laboratory and/or reported in only a few patients (Figure 10.4). Lastly, the third category of PNAs comprises those antibodies that occur with a specific disorder but do not differentiate between PNS and non-PNS cases (Figure 10.5). Below are given three scenarios where the combination of clinical tests can be utilized to diagnose PNS with particular emphasis on the involvement of PNA (Graus et al. 2004).

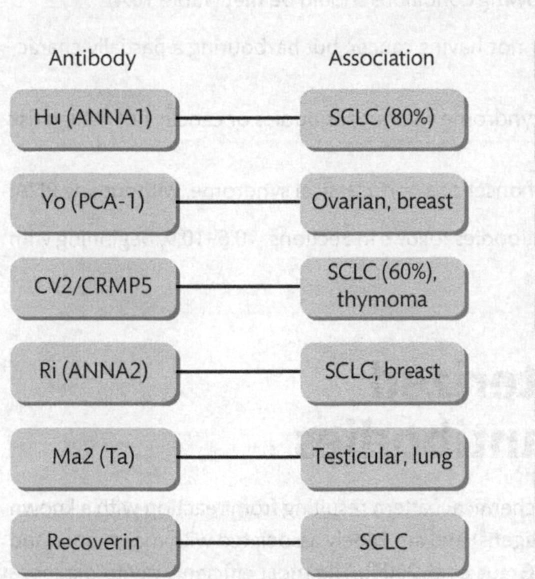

FIGURE 10.3
Defined PNAs and their commonly associated malignancies. SCLC, small-cell lung cancer.

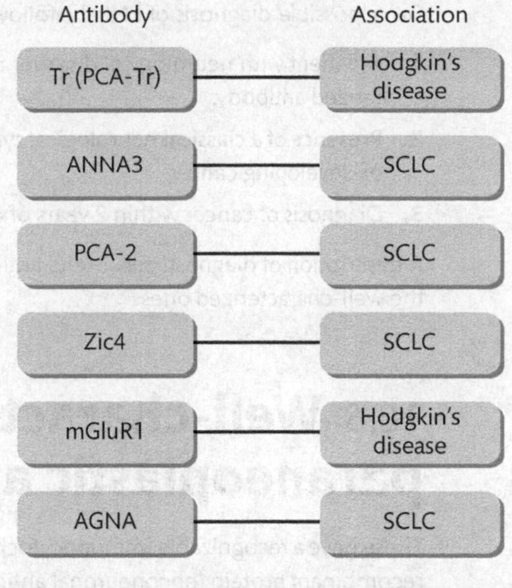

FIGURE 10.4
Partially defined PNAs that have been reported in a limited number of patients and often by a single group of workers. SCLC, small-cell lung cancer.

PNAs can assist in a 'definitive' diagnosis of PNS (Table 10.4) in cases of:

1. A patient with neurological disorder not having cancer but harbouring a well characterized antibody.
2. A patient with non-classical PNS harbouring any PNA developing a cancer within 5 years of diagnosis of the neurological disorder.
3. A classical neurological syndrome with the diagnosis of cancer within 5 years of the neurological symptom onset.
4. A non-classical neurological syndrome which resolves on treatment of the cancer without any concomitant immunotherapy.

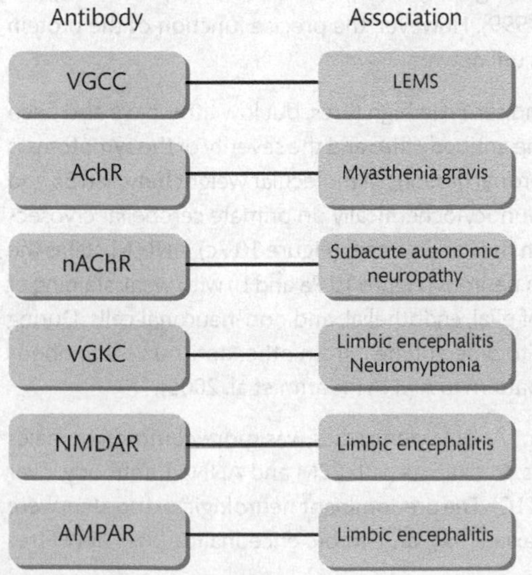

FIGURE 10.5
Antibodies that can be detected irrespective of the presence of cancer and are often pathogenic. LEMS, Lambert–Eaton myasthenic syndrome.

For a 'possible' diagnosis of PNS the following conditions should be met (Table 10.4):

1. A patient with neurological disorder not having cancer, but harbouring a partially characterized antibody.
2. Presence of a classical neurological syndrome without antibodies or cancer, but at high risk of developing cancer.
3. Diagnosis of cancer within 2 years of onset of a non-classical syndrome, without any PNA.

A description of diagnostically useful antibodies follows in Sections 10.6–10.9, beginning with the well-characterized ones.

10.6 Well-characterized paraneoplastic antibodies

These have a recognizable immunocytochemical pattern resulting from reaction with a known recombinant protein (onconeuronal antigens) and are widely associated with malignancy and a well-defined neurological syndrome (Graus et al. 2004). The most efficient way to diagnose PNS is to identify one of the PNAs in this category as they have a high specificity (>90%) for PNS. Anti-neuronal antibodies belonging to this category include (in descending order of occurrence): Hu > Yo > CV2 > Ri > Ma2 > amphiphysin.

10.6.1 Anti-neuronal nuclear antibody type 1 (ANNA1, Hu)

ANNA1, also known as Hu antibody, is the most commonly occurring and widely investigated PNA. The antigen associated with this antibody is HuD (Shams'ili et al. 2003) which is comprised of a family of neuronal nuclear proteins (HuD, HuC/ple21, Hel-N1, and Hel-N2) that differ by alternative splicing of their mRNAs. It is an intranuclear RNA-binding antigen with three RNA recognition motifs. The antigen's expression is normally restricted to the central and peripheral neurons and is thought to regulate the cell cycle, specifically in early neuronal development and maintenance. In addition to its expression in neuronal tissue, HuD is also expressed in the patient's own tumour and in small-cell lung carcinomas, neuroblastomas, sarcomas, and prostate carcinomas (Dalmau and Posner 1999). However, the precise function of the protein in both its native location and in tumours is unknown.

ANNA1 is usually present in both the CSF and serum in high titres, but low titres have also been found. However, any correlation between the antibody titre and the severity of the symptoms is uncertain. ANNA1 antibody reacts with neuronal proteins of molecular weight between 35 and 40 kDa (Figure 10.6a) and when tested immunocytochemically on primate cerebellar cryosections the staining is particularly prominent in the Purkinje cells (Figure 10.7c). ANNA1 stains the nuclei of both central and peripheral system neurons (Figure 10.7a and b) with weak staining of the cytoplasm, and is absent in the nuclei of glial, endothelial, and non-neuronal cells. During detection and identification, it is important to differentiate it from other anti-nuclear antibodies as these can have a similar distribution pattern to ANNA1 (Karim et al. 2005).

In a series of 200 patients, the occurrence of ANNA1 antibodies was more common in males with a median age of onset around 62 years. In patients with PEM and ANNA1 antibody, over 85% had lung cancer (of which 77% were SCLC). The predominant neurological disorders were sensory neuronopathy (54%), cerebellar ataxia (10%), and limbic encephalitis (9%). Low titres

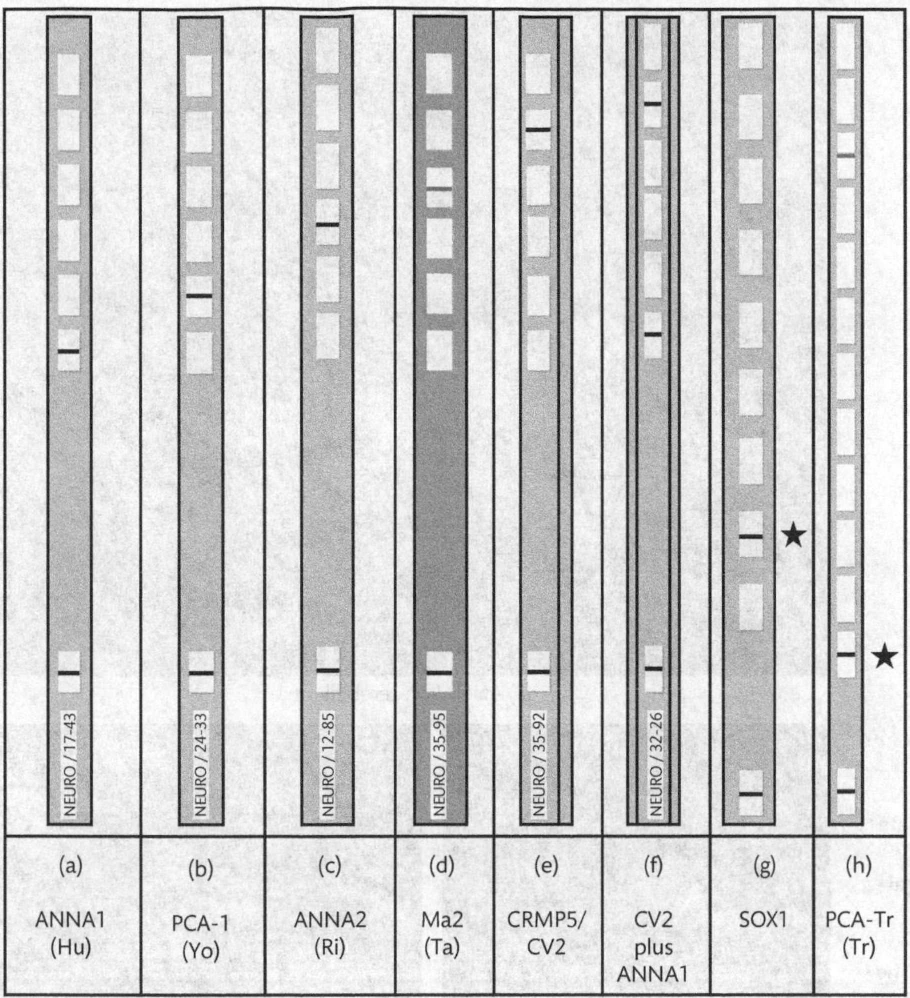

FIGURE 10.6

Strip coated with specific paraneoplastic antigens from the top down: amphiphysin, CRMP-5/CV-2, Ma2, ANNA2, PCA-1, and ANNA1, incubated with serum to confirm specificity against ANNA1 (a); PCA-1 (b); ANNA2 (c); Ma2 (d); CRMP-5/CV-2 (e); SOX1 (g); and Tr (h). Asterisks mark the antigen–antibody reaction. Also an example of specificity of ANNA1 coexisting with CRMP-5/CV-2 antibodies (f).

of anti-ANNA1 are found in 16% of SCLC patients who do not have neurological symptoms (Graus et al. 2001).

The prognosis for patients harbouring this antibody is very poor with no improvement of neurological function after treatment of the cancer, but the symptoms may be stabilized and further progression limited. Death occurs from PEM (60%) and tumour-related complications (40%).

Other ANNA1 associated tumours include neuroblastoma, prostate tumours, rhabdosarcoma, seminoma, and adenocarcinoma of the gall bladder. Like most PNS, the tumour may only become clinically apparent many months after the onset of the neurological symptoms.

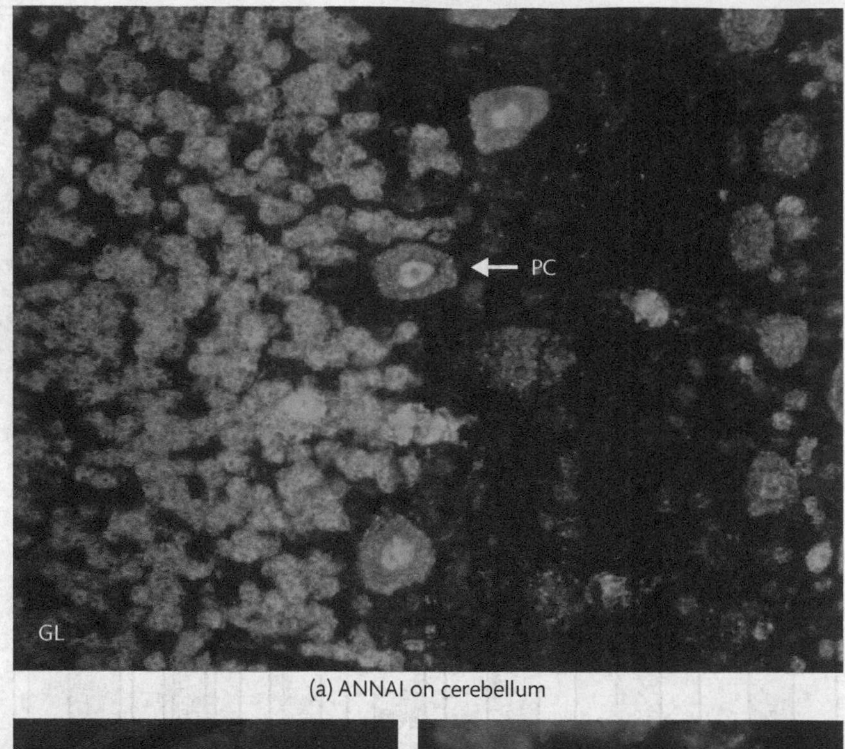

(a) ANNAI on cerebellum

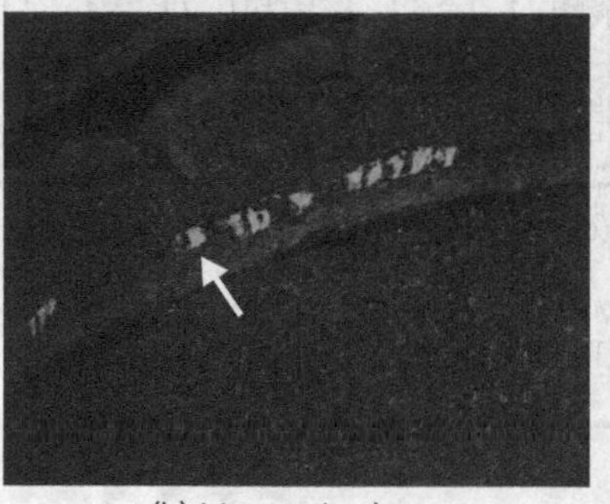

(b) Myenteric plexus

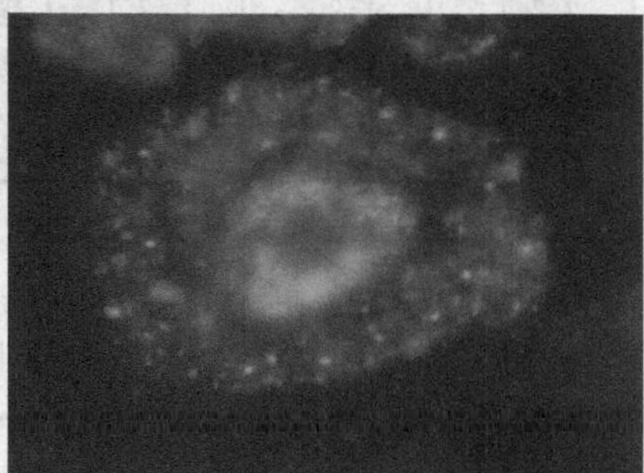

(c) Purkinje cell showing ANNAI staining

FIGURE 10.7
ANNA1 antibody reactivity on primate cerebellum showing in (a): nuclear and cytoplasmic staining of all central (granular layer (GL) and Purkinje cells (PC)); and in (b) peripheral neurones (of the stomach (arrow)). The predominantly nuclear staining of the Purkinje cell (PC) is more clearly visible at the higher magnification (c).

10.6.2 Purkinje cell antibody 1 (PCA-1, Yo)

PCA-1 antibody recognizes three types of Yo proteins, also known as Cerebellar Degeneration Related proteins: CDR34, CDR52 (CDR1), and CDR62 (CDR2) representing 34, 52, and 62 kDa proteins respectively (Dalmau and Posner 1999). These antigens are the second most common amongst onconeuronal antigens to have been reported and are highly expressed in the cerebellar Purkinje cell cytoplasm, testes, and some neuroectodermal cell lineages. CDR2 onconeuronal antigens are also expressed in tumours (such as ovarian and breast cancers) of patients with the PCA-1 antibody.

CDR1 is a 223-amino acid polypeptide containing 34 tandem repeats of six amino acids and a leucine zipper motif (Giometto et al. 1999). The polypeptide CDR2 comprises 510 amino acid residues with the leucine-zipper domain. This is the major epitope for the antibody. The antigen is expressed in the cerebellum, brain stem, intestinal mucosa, small-cell lung carcinoma, squamous-cell lung cancer, and secondary tumours of adenocarcinoma of the colon. CDR2, an intracellular antigen, binds to myc and can be expressed in cancers found in neurologically normal individuals (Roberts and Darnell 2004).

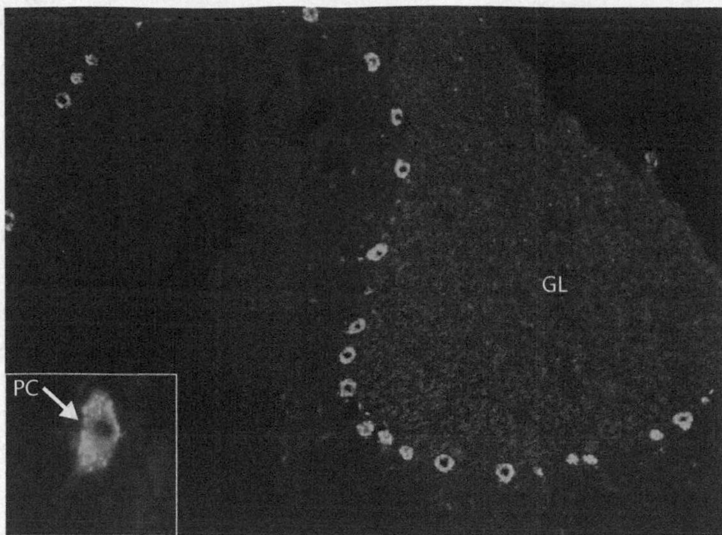

FIGURE 10.8
PCA-1 (Yo) staining on cerebellum can give an appearance of a 'pearl necklace' around the granular layer (GL) and is characterized by coarse speckling in the cytoplasm of Purkinje cells (PC, see insert).

PCA-1 is a polyclonal complement-fixing antibody, restricted to the IgG1 subclass, which to date has not been found to coexist with any other PNA. On cerebellar cryosections, coarse granular staining in the cytoplasm of Purkinje cell neurons with sparing of the nucleus is observed (Figure 10.8) (Karim et al. 2007). Immuno-electron microscopy has shown that the antibody binds to ribosomes, the granular endoplasmic reticulum, and the Golgi complex vesicles of Purkinje cells. Western blot analysis usually shows bands at 34, 52, and 62 kDa. Injection of antibody into mice has not shed any light on its function except that it does not cause disease or disrupt the blood–brain barrier. Figure 10.6b shows an example of blot confirming antigen recognized by anti-PCA-1 antibody.

This antibody is more frequently detected in female patients (60–65 years of age); very few cases have been reported in males. Patients suffer from cerebellar ataxia leading to rapid and progressive deterioration of speech, nystagmus, impaired coordination, and ataxic gait, leaving them severely incapacitated within 3 months of diagnosis. Death occurs in 30% from the debilitating neurological condition and from tumour progression in over 50% of the patients.

The incidence of PCD is about 40% in PCA-1 patients, and 80% of these are likely to be associated with treatable gynaecological, breast, or ovarian malignancies. On treatment, however, there is no improvement in the neurological function and most patients remain neurologically disabled.

10.6.3 Anti-CRMP5/CV2 antibody

The molecular target of CV2/CRMP5 antibodies involves a family of proteins, called Collapsin Response-Mediator brain Proteins (molecular mass of 62–66 kDa), which comprises five cytosolic phosphoproteins (CRMP1, CRMP2, CRMP3, CRMP4, and CRMP5). The dominant antigen is CRMP5 and its specificity rests predominantly in the N-terminal epitopes; it exists as a tetramer in the adult brain and the gene responsible is located on human chromosome 2. CRMP5 has a relatively low sequence homology with the other four members of the CRMP family but is expressed in the developing nervous system in a similar distribution pattern to that of CRMP2.

In the adult rat, the immunocytochemical distribution of anti-CV2/CRMP5 antibody is restricted to the cytoplasm and processes of a subpopulation of oligodendrocytes in the white matter (Honnorat et al. 1996), where it recognizes a neuronal cytoplasmic antigen known as CRMP5 (Yu et al. 2001).

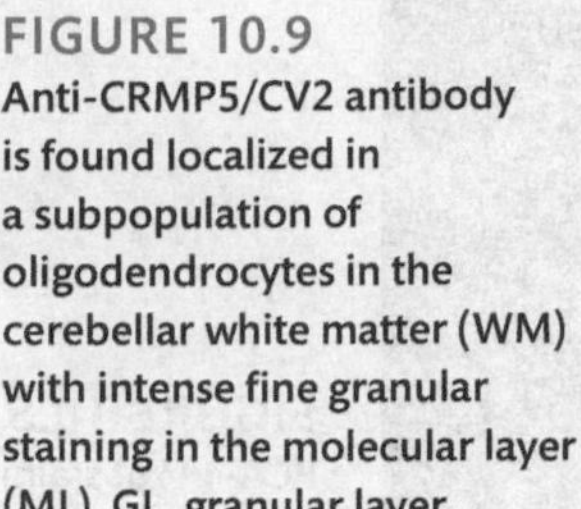

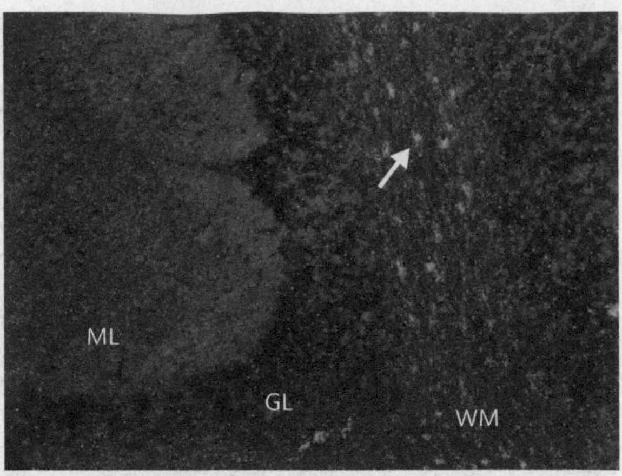

FIGURE 10.9
Anti-CRMP5/CV2 antibody is found localized in a subpopulation of oligodendrocytes in the cerebellar white matter (WM) with intense fine granular staining in the molecular layer (ML). GL, granular layer.

Figure 10.9 shows the staining of anti-CRMP5/CV2. This type of staining is distinct from anti-ANNA1 staining, which is confined to the neuronal nuclei, and when tested on cerebellar extract a protein of molecular size 62 to 66 kDa is recognized. The anti-CV2/CRMP5 can coexist with other PNAs such as ANNA1 or anti-amphiphysin antibody. Figure 10.6e shows anti-CRMP5/CV2 alone, and you can see it coexisting with ANNA1 in Figure 10.6f.

In the clinical setting, patients with this PNA tend to be males (70%), having an average age of about 62 years. This antibody is associated with peripheral neuropathy (47%), autonomic neuropathy (31%), cerebellar ataxia (26%), subacute dementia (25%), and NMJ disorders (12%). Patients with this antibody most frequently have SCLC (77%) and thymoma (6%). Other malignancies have been reported with CRMP5/CV2 reactivity. The mean survival time for patients with SCLC and CRMP5/CV2 antibody is more than twice that of patients with the same tumour and similar symptoms but different PNA.

10.6.4 Anti-neuronal nuclear antibody type 2 (ANNA2, Ri)

ANNA2 antigens, also known as Ri, are highly conserved neuron-specific RNA binding proteins encoded by the Nova-1 and Nova-2 genes. Nova-1 contains three RNA recognition motifs, which are homologous to the KH motifs of the hnRNP K protein. The third KH motif of Nova-1 is a target for the anti-ANNA2 antibody; binding of the auto-antibody results in inhibition of Nova-1 binding to RNA. An extensive study by Graus et al. (1993) revealed that all the areas of the central nervous system tested harboured the ANNA2 antigen, with the exception of the Gasserian, dorsal root, sympathetic ganglia and the myenteric plexus. All non-neuronal tissue lacked the ANNA2 antigen except for the pituitary gland.

ANNA2 is a rare antibody and reacts with the target antigen in the nuclei and to a lesser extent in the cytoplasm of neurons of the central nervous system with an immunocytochemical pattern resembling that of anti-ANNA1. In contrast to ANNA1, ANNA2 does not react with the peripheral nervous system such as the myenteric neuron. On Western blots of cerebellar extract, anti-ANNA2 IgG recognizes two bands with relative molecular weight 55 and 80 kDa. Anti-ANNA2 antibody specificity can be confirmed by the recombinant protein; look at Figure 10.6c to see this. It is important to note that ANNA2 can coexist with various other PNAs such as ANNA1, CV2/CRMP5, ANNA3, and VGCC.

Clinically the mean age of onset is around 65 years and 71% of the patients are smokers presenting with a broad range of neurological signs and symptoms. Adult patients mostly harbour

ANNA2 antibody (Pittock et al. 2003) with neurological disorders affecting the brainstem (71%), cerebellum (50%), and peripheral nerves (25%). The predominant clinical features are ataxia and ocular movement disorders (opsoclonus/myoclonus). Opsoclonus can exist alone or with myoclonus hence it is described as either paraneoplastic opsoclonus ataxia or paraneoplastic opsoclonus myoclonus ataxia. There is a higher incidence of this antibody seen in females (ratio of 2:1), and underlying malignancy of breast or small-cell lung carcinomas is found in 75% of cases. Less frequent cases of ovarian, fallopian tube, bladder, and cervical cancer have been reported. The presence of antibodies has been reported in some cases of ovarian carcinomas without manifesting paraneoplastic neurological syndromes. The detection of anti-ANNA2 antibodies should prompt a careful search for an underlying tumour, especially breast cancer or small-cell lung carcinoma. Occasionally a tumour may not be found, although the presence of an occult tumour cannot be ruled out, and this makes close follow-up advisable. Disability is severe—within a month of onset of neurological symptoms, 32% of patients are usually confined to a wheelchair (Pittock et al. 2003).

10.6.5 Anti-Ma2 (Ta) antibody

The three Ma antigens were identified by probing cDNA libraries with patient sera; all three share significant sequence homology. Voltz et al. (1999) reported two onconeuronal proteins (Ma1 and Ma2, also known as Ma and Ta respectively) associated with PNS. Like other paraneoplastic antigens, they are expressed in both tumours and immuno-privileged sites (neuronal tissue and testis). The distribution of Ma1 mRNA is highly restricted to the brain and testis. Ma1 is located on chromosome 14 and it expresses a peptide of 330 amino acids and molecular weight 37 kDa, whereas Ma2 is located on chromosome 8, has a predicted molecular weight of 40 kDa (Figure 10.6d) and is expressed in the brain only (Rosenfeld et al. 2001). Ma2 displays (a) unique epitope(s) in that it is recognized by all patients' sera studied. The existence of a new family member, Ma3, was reported in the literature (Rosenfeld et al. 2001). The gene for Ma3 is located on chromosome X and its mRNA is expressed in brain, testis, and several systemic tissues (kidney and trachea). The function of the Ma proteins is currently unknown (Voltz et al. 1999).

The predominant member of the Ma family is Ma2, an IgG polyclonal antibody found in the serum and cerebrospinal fluid of patients with paraneoplastic disorder, that reacts with nucleoli, but less so with the nucleus and cytoplasm of central nervous system neurons (Figure 10.10). There is no reactivity against glial cells. Ma1 reacts with both the brain and testicular germ cells, whilst Ma2 antibody reacts with systemic tissue as well.

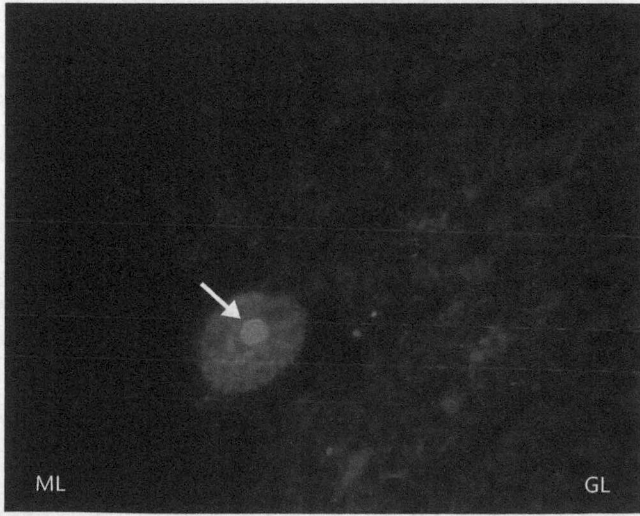

FIGURE 10.10 **The nucleolus (arrow) of the Purkinje cell is predominantly stained with anti-Ma2 antibody. GL, granular layer; ML, molecular layer.**

In over 50% of patients with Ma reactivity, both Ma1 and Ma2 antibodies were present together and no evidence is available for the coexistence of any other PNA. Anti-Ma2 patients tend to be predominantly male (median age of 23 years) with symptoms of short-term memory loss, seizures, confusion, excessive daytime sleepiness (32%), eye movement abnormalities (92%), and vertical gaze paralysis (60%), all of which develop from dysfunction of limbic, brainstem, or diencephalic system, alone or in combination. Ataxia can be found in 38% of the Ma-patients. Ma2 associated encephalitis is different from the classical PLE or brainstem encephalitis. In 53% of such cases germ cell tumours of the testis are found in these patients (Dalmau et al. 2004).

Immunity to Ma antigens appears unique in that 50% of the patients with testicular cancer who respond well to treatment achieve complete remission of the tumour with accompanying improvement or stabilization in neurological deficit. As yet the reason for this is unclear.

In a study by Rosenfeld et al. (2001), Ma1 and Ma3 specificities were more common in older patients, who tended to develop a wider range of cerebellar symptoms with more intense dysfunction; a high proportion (82%) have non-germ cell neoplasms, including lung (large cell), parotid, breast, and colon.

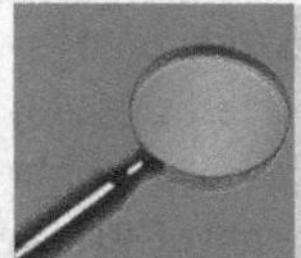

CASE STUDY 10.1 Ma antibody associated with mesothelioma

SM was a 62-year-old man with a history of right-sided pleural effusion. He smoked 20 cigarettes a day, then changed habit to daily pipe smoking. He complained of double vision.

Neurological examination

Mostly normal except for:

- **broad-based ataxic gait veering to both sides**
- **nystagmus on lateral gaze**
- **significant wasting of quadriceps**
- **no weakness or sensory symptoms.**

Laboratory and other investigations

All biochemical and immunological parameters were normal except for:

- **iron, which was low**
- **immunoglobulin (IgG was 24.91 and IgA was 5.01 g/L)**
- **raised complement C3 (2.07)**
- **paraneoplastic neurological screen was positive for Ma2 antibody (please see Figure 10.10, which exemplifies the distribution seen on the cerebellum)**
- **Ma2 reactivity was confirmed on recombinant blot (look at the example given in Figure 10.6d)**
- **MRI of the head and spinal cord were normal**
- **pleural biopsy showed mesothelioma.**

Outcome

One year later, patient died.

Post mortem examination

Tumour metastasized to lymph node with mediastinum, chest wall, right adrenal gland, and liver.

Of the three Ma antibodies (Ma1, Ma2, and Ma3), Ma2 antibody is more commonly identified and usually found in association with testicular tumour in younger men who frequently have limbic encephalitis, but can be associated with other cancer in older patients. This is a rare antibody and about 50 cases have been reported around the world.

The case described in Case Study 10.1 illustrates that although antibodies may have been initially described with one type of tumour and neurological syndrome (testicular cancer and limbic encephalitis), they may frequently be identified in other types of tumours and neurological signs (mesothelioma and cerebellar degeneration).

10.6.6 Anti-amphiphysin antibody

Amphiphysin, with its two isoforms, I and II, is a neuronal protein that is highly concentrated in the synaptic vesicles and that has a molecular weight of 128 kDa. It plays a role in clathrin-mediated endocytosis and forms a dimer that binds to dynamin and synaptojanin through carboxy-terminal Src-homologous (SH3) domains. It has been proposed to have a role in intracellular signalling and is essential for synaptic vesicle recycling in neurons. Amphiphysin is also expressed in certain types of endocrine cells (e.g. adrenal and pituitary), retina, and spermatocytes.

Anti-amphiphysin antibody is found in paraneoplastic SPS with malignancies of breast and lung (SCLC) as well as in patients with encephalomyelitis or sensory neuropathy, especially when the cancer involved is SCLC.

Serum positive for this antibody reacts with the neuropil of human and rodent frontal cortex, hippocampus, cerebellum, and spinal cord. In the cerebellum, there is intense diffuse staining of the neuropil in the cerebellar cortical molecular layer whilst intense granular staining in the periphery of perikarya and the granular cell layer, but little or no immunoreactivity in the Purkinje cell cytoplasm (Figure 10.11), nor any other neuronal cell body. This characteristic staining can easily be confused with anti-mitochondrial or anti-glutamic acid decarboxylase (GAD). In 74% of the patients, amphiphysin can coexist with other PNAs such as ANNA1, CRMP5/CV2, and PCA-2, thus complicating the identification; therefore the specificity of the antibody may need to be confirmed by other methodologies, such as Western blotting, which should reveal a protein of molecular size of around 128 kDa.

Neurological disorders accompanying amphiphysin reactivity are diverse; this may be due to the pathology associated with the presence of other PNAs. The onset of symptoms is subacute, occurs around the age of 64 years and leads to 40% of patients being confined to a wheelchair within 6 months. Symptoms include sensory neuropathy, encephalopathy, myelopathy (spinal cord involvements), cerebellar syndrome, and paraneoplastic SPS. Paraneoplastic amphiphysin-associated SPS is more common in females (39%) than males (12%).

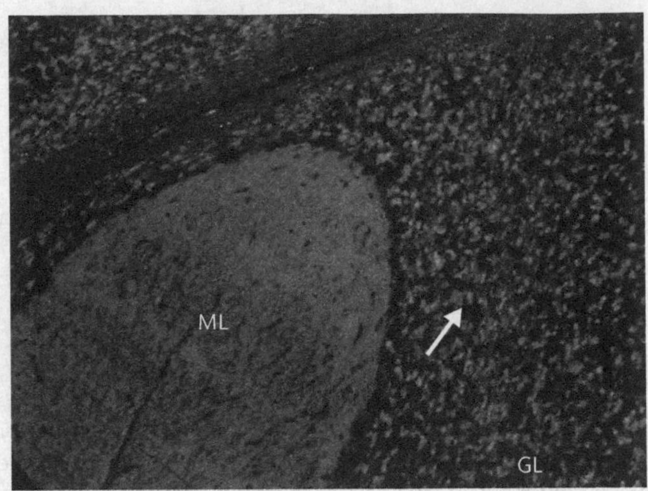

FIGURE 10.11
On cerebellum anti-amphiphysin antibody reacts intensely with the neuropils in the granular layer (GL) but not with the granular cells, which are visible as 'black holes' (arrow). The molecular layer (ML) is often uniformly stained.

A malignant neoplasm is found in 79% of patients, the most common being SCLC and breast tumour. Other less frequent cancers, e.g. non-SCLC lung cancer and melanoma, have also been reported. Pittock et al. (2005) found that treatment had no significant effect on survival rate in patients with cancer.

Cross reference

A selection of typical and atypical immunofluorescence patterns seen on cerebellum can be found on the University of Birmingham clinical immunology website: http://www.ii.bham.ac.uk/clinicalimmunology/Neuroimmunology/.

Key Point

Certain PNAs have well-characterized antigens, with Hu (ANNA1), Yo (PCA-1), and CRMP-5/CV-2 antibodies being the most commonly detected.

10.7 Partially characterized paraneoplastic antibodies

The partially characterized PNAs lack clearly identified target antigens and are often reported by a single group of investigators and/or in a few patients. The most frequent of the PNAs are: Tr > ANNA3 > PCA-2 > Zic4 > mGluR1.

10.7.1 Anti-PCA-Tr (Tr) antibody

Tr antigen is found in the cytoplasm of central neurons and it is widely expressed in the developing rodent brain. Abolition of anti-Tr immunoreactivity by preincubation of the tissue with pepsin suggests that the antigen is a protein. Until recently it was thought that the inability to detect common proteins on Western blots may not be due to a low concentration of the antigen but to the antibody being directed against conformational epitopes which may have become modified during preparation (Graus et al. 1997). Now there is a commercially available immunoblot which is coated with the antigen for Tr.

IgG1 and IgG3 are the major subclasses of anti-Tr antibody found in the serum and CSF of patient with Hodgkin's disease. In about 7% of patients, this antibody is only found in the CSF. Immunohistochemically, the staining pattern on the cerebellum resembles PCA-1 distribution.

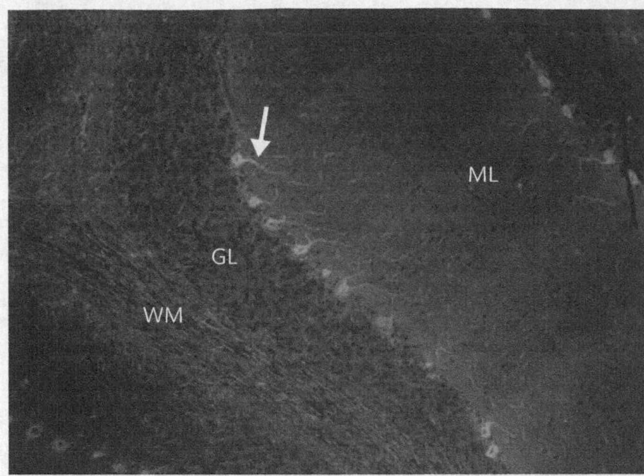

FIGURE 10.12
The Purkinje cell body and its dendrites (arrow) react with anti-PCA-Tr antibody. This fine-speckled (uniform) staining is distinct from that of the coarse speckles seen with PCA-1 (Yo). GL, granular layer; ML, molecular layer; WM, white matter.

The fine speckled staining of the cytoplasm and proximal dendrites of Purkinje cells is, however, distinct from that of Yo (Figure 10.12). Previously, the identification of anti-Tr reactivity was strictly based on immunocytochemical criteria where the Purkinje cell cytoplasmic staining is combined with a characteristic punctuate (dots) staining in the molecular layer of the cerebellum (not seen with Yo antibody), and is suggestive of immunoreactivity against dendritic spines of the Purkinje cells. The immunoreactivity is confined to central neurons and the antibody rarely stains the neoplasm. The specificity of Tr antibody can be confirmed using immunoblots. Recent studies have confirmed that the antigenic target is delta/notch-like epidermal growth factor-related receptor (DNER) (Greene et al. 2014).

In the clinical setting anti-Tr reactivity is found predominantly in the male population with mean age of onset around 61 years, and there is a tight correlation between acute onset of symptoms, usually PCD and Hodgkin's disease (Bernal et al. 2003). Clinical improvements are seen in 14% of younger patients after treatment of the disease; the antibodies are known to disappear spontaneously, and also after successful treatment for Hodgkin's disease.

10.7.2 Anti-ANNA3 antibody

This antibody is very rare, being described in only 11 patients with PNS, the majority of which are afflicted with SCLC (Chan et al. 2001). Immunocytochemically, the staining of the cerebellum is distinct from that of ANNA1 and ANNA2, and the nucleoli are spared in all three. ANNA3 staining is specifically nuclear. Purkinje cell nuclei are most prominently stained with much lower reactivity in the nuclei of molecular layer neurons. No staining is seen in the neurons of the granular layer or in the cytoplasm of other cerebellar neurons. Its unique reactivity is not only confined to the CNS antigen (molecular size 170 kDa) but also extends to the nuclei of the kidney podocytes (but not the cytoplasm). ANNA3 has been reported to coexist with other PNAs (anti-CV2/CRMP5 (20%) and ANNA1).

The precise function of the antibody is unclear, but the theory is that it can have an effective anti-tumour response through the activation of $CD4^+$ T helper lymphocytes.

Due to the rarity of ANNA3, information on its prognostic utility is quite limited. In addition to SCLC, it has been found in patients with adenocarcinoma. ANNA3 appears to be a specific marker for tobacco-related airway cancer.

The onset of symptoms in the adult is around 64 years, with approximately equal frequency in both genders. Like other PNA, ANNA3 symptoms are also acute and diverse, usually multifocal, and may include cerebellar ataxia, sensorimotor neuropathies, myelopathy, and brainstem and limbic encephalopathy.

10.7.3 Anti-Purkinje cell antibody type-2 (PCA-2)

Experience with this antibody is also limited and confined to only ten patients. PCA-2 reacts in reticular fashion with cerebellar Purkinje cell cytoplasm and dendritic processes together with the cytoplasm of dentate nucleus neurons (Vernino and Lennon 2000). In contrast to PCA-1 and PCA-Tr, additional reactivity can be found in the nerves innervating the renal arterioles. The molecular size of both the tumour and cerebellar antigen is approximately 270 kDa.

PCA-2 can coexist with other neuronal auto-antibodies, e.g. voltage-gated calcium channels, CV2/CRMP, or acetylcholine receptor antibodies, and its function and pathological role is yet to be determined.

The onset of neurological symptoms is subacute and occurs predominantly in females (~2:1) around the age of 60 years. The underlying neoplasm is SCLC in 80% of patients, who are mostly smokers, and the presenting symptoms are limbic encephalitis (50%), cerebellar ataxia (30%), autonomic neuropathy (10%), and motor or sensory neuropathy (10%).

10.7.4 Anti-Zic4 antibody

Zic4 antibody is another addition to the panel of existing PNAs but the experience with this antibody is confined to one laboratory (Bataller et al. 2004). It has been identified in both the serum and the CSF of patients with paraneoplastic neurological disorder and neoplasm of the lung (SCLC, 92%).

Zic proteins are thought to have an important role in the development of the nervous system. Mutations of Zic genes have been linked to cerebellar malformation, spina bifida, and/or sensorimotor gait.

Zic4 antibody can be screened on the brain showing binding predominantly to the neuronal nuclei of the cerebellar granular layer and with less intense staining in other neurons, including Purkinje cells and brainstem. Detection of Zic4 may be complicated by its frequent coexistence with other onconeuronal antibodies (ANNA1, ANNA2, or CV2/CRMP5). On cerebellar Western blots, Zic4 recognizes many proteins including a 37 kDa band which is considered to be the Zic4 antigen. For definitive identification, confirmation by recombinant Zic4 should be utilized and now commercial immunoblots are also available for the detection of Zic4.

The onset of symptoms in Zic4 patients occurs at around 66 years. Only 18% of patients have Zic4 antibodies alone and these developed cerebellar syndrome (88% of males), increasing to 52% in the presence of coexisting SCLC-related PNAs (ANNA1 and/or CRMP5). As a result, 82% of these patients develop additional symptoms including paraneoplastic encephalomyelitis. Paraneoplastic disorder was absent in 16% of the patients despite harbouring an SCLC and Zic4 antibody.

10.7.5 Anti-metabotropic glutamate receptor 1 (mGluR1) antibody

This antibody, directed against metabotropic glutamate neurotransmitter receptors, is believed to modulate excitatory synaptic transmission in the central nervous system and is thought to have a role in neural plasticity, learning, and memory function. Anti-mGluR1 associated with paraneoplastic cerebellar ataxia recognizes a membrane neurotransmitter receptor of molecular weight 140 kDa, located on the dendritic spines of the Purkinje cell. Ataxia can be induced by blocking the mGluR1 receptor with anti-mGluR1 antibodies.

Anti-mGluR1 antibodies are an IgG class that bind to the Purkinje cell bodies and dendritic spines, the latter staining appearing as intense punctate staining in the molecular layer.

These antibodies are found in Hodgkin's disease associated cerebellar ataxia, often occurring during remission of the disease. The published data is reported in just two patients with anti-mGluR1 antibodies and PCD. Both subjects were females and after treatment one showed clinical improvement coupled with diminished serum antibodies, whilst the other was bedridden and showed no improvement in the ataxia despite being in complete remission (Sillevis Smitt et al. 2000).

10.7.6 Other metabotropic glutamate receptor antibodies

Other metabotropic glutamate receptor antibodies described include those against mGluR3 (schizophrenia) and mGluR5 (limbic encephalitis with Hodgkin's disease, also known as Ophelia syndrome). Immunohistochemistry using brain tissue and cultured hippocampal neurons is used to recognize the antibody. As with most of the newer antibodies, HEK cells transfected with mGluR5 can be used to identify the antibody using immunofluorescence.

10.7.7 Anti-glial nuclear antibody (AGNA)

AGNA (also known as SOX1, after its antigenic protein), is a relatively recent addition to the list of neurological antibodies. These antibodies are directed against the Bergmann glia found in the Purkinje cell layer of cerebellum and have been described in patients with PNS (usually Lambert–Eaton myasthenic syndrome) associated with SCLC (Graus et al. 2005). SOX antibodies are highly specific for SCLC and may help in distinguishing SCLC-associated LEMS from the non-paraneoplastic form (Titulaer et al. 2009).

Screening for the candidate antigen for AGNA using a foetal brain library revealed SOX1 protein (Sabater et al. 2008), which belongs to the Sry-like high mobility group superfamily, which are DNA-binding transcriptional factors with more than 20 proteins identified. SOX1 and SOX2 have an important role in neurogenesis and are both thought to be targets for the AGNA, with higher positivity seen against SOX1. Immunohistochemistry or immunofluorescence using rat cerebellum shows characteristic staining of the nuclei of Bergmann glia (Figure 10.13) that can be confirmed with a newer generation of commercial immunoblots against SOX1 (Figure 10.6h).

Key Point

More and more new antibodies and their clinical associations are being recognized.

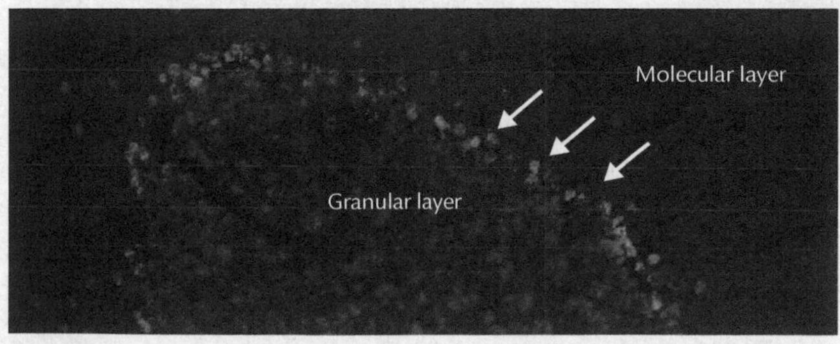

FIGURE 10.13

SOX1 antibody on cerebellum. Bergmann glia cells (arrows) are found in the Purkinje cells layer which is on the border of the granular and molecular layer.

10.8 Pathogenic antibodies with or without cancer

The classical early biomarkers mentioned in the previous sections of this chapter are considered non-pathogenic, and with their target binding sites located inside the cells are referred to as 'intracellular acting'. They are thought to exert their destructive effects on the neurons through cytotoxic T cell intervention. These biomarkers are very specific for diseases of the nervous system and usually indicate the presence of an underlying peripheral malignancy which may not be detectable at the time of presentation. Table 10.5 shows the relationship between antigen location, type of antibody, and possible cancer association.

In contrast, the mode of action of the newer markers differs from that of the classical paraneoplastic neurological antibodies in that they are pathogenic and have their antigens located on the cell surface membrane of the pre- or post-synaptic junctions. The antigenic sites are exposed to the extracellular environment for easy access to both the autoimmune system and, consequently, therapeutic intervention. During the interaction of the auto-antibodies with these extracellular antigens, the propagation of signal transmission along the nerve fibre is impaired, serving to precipitate abnormal neuropsychiatric function requiring urgent and accurate diagnosis to prevent significant morbidity and mortality. The antibody titres correlate with the improvement in the disease state and can often be used as a marker for treatment response.

The remainder of the chapter will focus on syndromes in which the immune attack is directed against surface antigens, i.e. where the auto-antibodies are believed to be pathogenic. This group of antibodies includes disorders which may also be of non-paraneoplastic or paraneoplastic (cancer associated) origin and involves the peripheral nervous system (chiefly, neuromuscular transmission). These can be broadly classified into antibodies at the NMJ and other CNS antibodies, now more commonly known as neuronal surface antibodies (NSA).

10.8.1 Neuromuscular transmission and NMJ antibodies

Messages are transmitted by the brain from nerve to nerve and/or from nerves to muscles as electrical signals (nerve impulses). On the arrival of the signal at the junction, whether it is neuron to neuron (synapse) or nerve to muscle (neuromuscular junction, NMJ), it is converted into chemical signals for transmission across the gap (synaptic gap). At these junctions there are several transmembrane proteins vulnerable to antibody mediated autoimmune attack. Of interest are a few proteins, two of which are located on the pre-synaptic motor nerve terminal, i.e. the voltage-gated calcium channels (VGCC) and the voltage-gated potassium channels (VGKC), and another two being the acetylcholine receptor and the muscle specific kinase (MuSK), which are present on the post-junctional folds of the muscle. VGKC have now been shown to be complexed with other proteins and are more widely distributed in the nervous system. The VGKC-complex antibodies will be described in detail with the NSAs (see Section 10.82).

Briefly, the electrical impulse opens the VGCC to allow influx of extracellular calcium into the nerve terminal. The increase in intracellular calcium triggers the release of a neurotransmitter (acetylcholine (ACh)) into the synaptic gap, activating the muscle membrane and prompting the opening of the sodium and potassium channels. The movement of the ions that follows creates an electrochemical gradient across the plasma membrane (more sodium moves in than potassium out), producing a local depolarization of the motor end plate, known as an end-plate potential, which spreads across the surface of the muscle fibres, thus initiating muscle contraction.

The transmembrane receptors and their associated proteins located at the junction have been direct targets for autoimmune attack by pathogenic auto-antibodies causing peripheral nervous system disorders. They include antibodies to P/Q-type VGCC in patients with Lambert-Eaton myasthenic syndrome (LEMS), muscle acetylcholine receptor (AChR) or muscle specific kinase (MuSK) in patients with myasthenia gravis (MG), voltage-gated potassium channels (VGKC) in some patients with peripheral nerve hyperexcitability (neuromyotonia), and ganglionic acetylcholine receptor in some patients with autonomic neuropathy.

Acetylcholine receptor (AChR) antibody

The acetylcholine receptor, an integral transmembrane protein, is classified according to its pharmacological property of relative affinity and sensitivity to nicotine and muscarine. Depending on the pharmacological response to these drugs, the receptors can be designated as either nicotinic or muscarinic. Antibody against the former receptor (nictonic) present at the neuromuscular junction causes the loss of receptor function and/or receptor density and leads to myasthenia gravis. These high affinity antibodies, when injected into an animal model, tend to produce many of the symptoms seen with MG and therefore are considered to have a pathogenic role.

The AChR antibodies are IgG1 and IgG3 with high specificity and confirm clinical suspicion of MG. Anti-AChR antibodies can be measured by either radioimmunoprecipitation assay (RIA) or commercially available non-isotopic ELISA utilizing high affinity α-bungarotoxin (snake venom from banded krait, *Bungarus multicinctus*). Low affinity antibodies against clustered AChR can be detected using an immunocytofluorescence technique utilizing transfected cells, where AChR is clustered using rapsyn (Leite et al. 2008). These are seen in up to 50% of patients with ocular and generalized myasthenia, who do not harbour either AChR or MuSK antibodies (Jacob et al. 2012).

MG is a rare disorder but occurs in a bimodal distribution affecting predominantly young (less than 40 years) females (F:M ratio is 7:3) or older men (Juel and Massey 2007). Anti-AChR antibodies are found in 80% of patients with generalized MG and 55% of those affected with ocular MG. Approximately 10% of the patients with MG will have tumour of the thymus gland (Vincent 2008), which upon resection leads to clinical improvement.

The muscle AChR is a pentameric transmembrane protein consisting of two α1 subunits and one each of β, δ, and ε subunits in the adult NMJ. By contrast, the neuronal nicotinic AChRs have α3 subunits, and these are essential for the function of autonomic ganglia. Ganglionic/neuronal AChR antibodies are seen in about 50% of patients with autoimmune autonomic gangliopathy, characterized by rapid onset of autonomic failure, gastrointestinal dysmotility, postural drop in blood pressure, lack of sweating, dry mouth, and bladder dysfunction (Vernino et al. 2009). The antibodies are detected using radioimmunoprecipitation assay, similar to the muscle AChR assay. However, radiolabelled epibatidine is used instead of bungarotoxin.

Muscle specific kinase (MuSK) antibody

Approximately 15% of MG patients are seronegative for AChR antibody but harbour instead antibodies to Muscle Specific Kinase (MuSK) which is found in and is required for the development of the NMJ (Hoch et al. 2001). This antibody is present in about 70% AChR seronegative patients (5–8% of all generalized MG patients). MuSK antibodies tend to be of IgG4 subclass and do not appear to stimulate the complement cascade. However, their pathogenic role has been proven with both active and passive transfer models (Viegas et al. 2012). Patients tends to have more prominent ocular and bulbar (respiratory/swallowing etc.) weakness and are usually more resistant to immunomodulatory therapy. Thymus enlargement is not seen with MuSK-MG.

Low-density lipoprotein-receptor related protein 4 (LRP4) antibody

LRP4 is an agrin receptor critical for forming the NMJ junction. LRP4 antibody has been seen in up to 10% of patients with myasthenia who do not have AChR or MuSK antibodies (Zhang et al. 2012). As with many of the newer antibodies, detection is by using immunocytofluorescence techniques using transfected cells. Both active and passive transfer models have confirmed the pathogenicity of these antibodies (Shen et al. 2013).

Very recently a new antibody against a clustering protein of AChR, known as contactin, has been found in otherwise seronegative myasthenia patients using an ELISA technique. (Gallardo et al. 2014).

Voltage-gated calcium channel (VGCC) antibody

VGCC is a transmembrane protein, a pore-forming moiety that is exposed to the surface, designated to at least five categories (L, N, P/Q, R, and T) based on electrophysiological and pharmacological properties of its α1 subunit. The P/Q type VGCC is highly expressed in the cerebellum and is sensitive to conotoxin, a neurotoxin from the marine cone snail. The P/Q type channels are the most frequent targets in autoimmune LEMS and the associated antibodies (anti-VGCC) have been shown to reduce acetylcholine release when injected into animals. It is this process that is involved in the pathology of LEMS.

The preferred method for routine quantification of anti-VGCC antibodies is by radioimmunoassay (see Method 10.2).

Anti-(P/Q)-VGCC antibody is associated with Lambert–Eaton myasthenic syndrome, most commonly in patients with small-cell lung carcinoma (60%); less common cancers have also been reported. There is a very high correlation between anti-VGCC antibody and LEMS (91%). LEMS is a disorder of neuromuscular transmission characterized by weakness of proximal muscle, depressed tendon reflexes, post-tetanic potentiation, and autonomic changes (Vedeler et al. 2006). Initially, the aetiology resembles myasthenia gravis (MG), although the course of the two diseases is distinct.

In the paraneoplastic form, almost all patients with LEMS and SCLC have VGCC antibody, usually against type P/Q channels. They also develop neurological signs and symptoms indicative of cerebellar involvement together with clinical features of LEMS.

10.8.2 Neuronal cell surface antibodies

Several antibodies have now been discovered which target antigens present on the neuronal cell surface. These are often referred to as autoimmune encephalitis or limbic encephalitis (LE) antibodies. The full repertoire of these auto-antibodies is currently available routinely in only a few specialist centres and consists of glutamate type (N-methyl-D-aspartate (NMDAR)), alpha-amino-3-hydroxy-5-methyl-4-isoxazolepropionic acid (AMPAR type 1 & 2)), voltage-gated potassium channel associated proteins (leucine-rich glioma inactivated protein 1 (LGI1) and contactin-associated protein 2 (CASPR2)), and gamma-aminobutyric acid receptor type B1 ($GABA_{B1}R$).

NMDAR antibody

Anti-N-methyl D-aspartate (NMDA) receptor is composed of four NR units; each subunit has a molecular size of about 100 kDa and together they form an ion channel/receptor. The two NR1 units make up a binding site for glycine while the other two NR2 (A, B, C, or D) subunits bind glutamate. Activation of the NMDA receptors facilitates an increase in intracellular Ca^{2+} ion, initiating a cascade of cellular events. It has been suggested that NMDAR antibodies inhibit the receptors on the pre-synaptic GABAergic interneurons resulting in reduction of GABA release, thereby diminishing inhibition of the post-synaptic glutamatinergic transmission. Furthermore, reduction in receptor density has been observed, resulting from internalization of the receptor–antibody complex. This is the basis for the pathogenic effects of this antibody, which can be reversed by modulating the levels of the NMDAR antibody in the patient. Cellular distribution of the NMDAR antibodies can be ascertained on non-permeabilized hippocampal neurons or cerebellum where the NMDAR antibody binds to the neuropils in both the molecular layer of the hippocampus and the granular layer of the cerebellum. The NMDAR antibodies can also be determined with much higher sensitivity and specificity using NR1 transfected HEK cells (Figure 10.14a). These cells are now commercially available for detecting NMDAR antibodies.

Recently, autoimmunity to the NR1 subunit of the NMDA receptor has been identified in more than 500 patients with severe but treatment-responsive limbic encephalitis with prominent psychiatric presentation, involuntary movements, autonomic symptoms, and respiratory depression. This syndrome was initially described in young women over the age of 18 years with ovarian teratoma (56%) but has also been reported at a lower frequency (9%) in girls under the age of 14 years. Most recent observations suggest that the spectrum of the disease is expanding to include non-neoplastic cases and it is no longer confined to the female gender. Furthermore, varying levels of NMDAR antibodies are found in different subsets of patients. For instance, the levels of NMDAR antibody in the non-paraneoplastic patients are significantly lower than those found in the paraneoplastic syndrome. There appear to be two phases of the disease—the early one is linked to CSF lymphocytosis and the latter phase seen with the appearance of CSF oligoclonal bands—but in any case the treatment appears to be more effective in the early stages, whether it is immunotherapy or tumour removal (Titulaer et al. 2013).

Voltage-gated potassium channel complex (VGKC) antibodies

VGKC is also a transmembrane protein, its α-subunit forming the actual channels specific for potassium movement and having a crucial role in returning the depolarized cell to a resting state. VGKC belongs to the Shaker (*Drosophila* carrying mutant gene for VGKC) family of potassium channels. The three important isotypes of the α-subunit (KV1.1, KV1.2, and KV1.6) present in both the CNS and the peripheral nervous system have very high affinity for the neurotoxin (α-dendrotoxin) found in the venom of green mamba snakes (*Dendroaspis* spp.). It was thought that this property of the α-subunit was utilized for measuring all the anti-VGKC antibodies.

Anti-VGKC antibodies were originally tested on rat cerebellum where they stained the molecular layer but not Purkinje cells. Reactivity was also found in the neurons of the hippocampus. Routinely, these antibodies are measured using radioimmunoassay (see Method 10.2).

Until recently all the VGKC antibodies were thought to be directed towards the VGK channels but evidence suggests otherwise. It has now been established that most of these antibodies are directed against proteins associated with VGKC. Two main proteins have been identified as targets for some VGKC antibodies: leucine-rich glioma inactivated protein 1 (LGI1), which is more common, and contactin-associated protein 2 (CASPR2). The significance of VGKC antibodies detected by RIA, in the absence of a classical syndrome (LE or neuromyotonia, NMT—see later in this section) or the more specific antibody subtypes (e.g. LGI1 or CASPR2) is currently unknown.

The specific antibodies directed against the proteins associated with the VGKC are detected using a highly sensitive and specific cell-based assay (transfected HEK cells).

Leucine-rich glioma-inactivated protein 1 (LGI1) antibody

LGI1 is a secreted neuronal protein which links to disintegrin and metalloproteinase-containing proteins (ADAM22 and ADAM23) in the brain, forming a trans-synaptic protein complex which includes pre-synaptic potassium channels and post-synaptic AMPA receptors. Blockage of LGI1 reduces AMPAR mediated synaptic transmission in the hippocampus leading to the neurological syndrome. A distinct seizure semiology involving movements of the face and arm, known as faciobrachial dystonic seizures, has been described in patients with LGI1 antibodies. As opposed to CASPR2 antibodies described later in this section, the vast majority of patients with LGI1 antibodies have a central nervous system disease, notably limbic encephalitis, neuro-cognitive dysfunction, and seizures. Hyponatremia (low sodium levels) is seen in a good proportion of patients and MRI may show medial temporal lobe signal changes.

Immunocytofluorescence using HEK293 cells transfected with LGI1 (Figure 10.14b) is the most common method for detection of these antibodies and commercial kits are available with a panel of antibodies.

Contactin-associated protein 2 (CASPR2) antibody

Neuromyotonia is the most common form of peripheral nerve hyperexcitability, caused by auto-antibodies to VGKC, resulting in an increase in the release of acetylcholine into the synaptic cleft and thus prolonging the action potential.

The onset of symptoms is either acute or subacute, affecting both genders with equal frequencies, and occurs at a median age of 65 years.

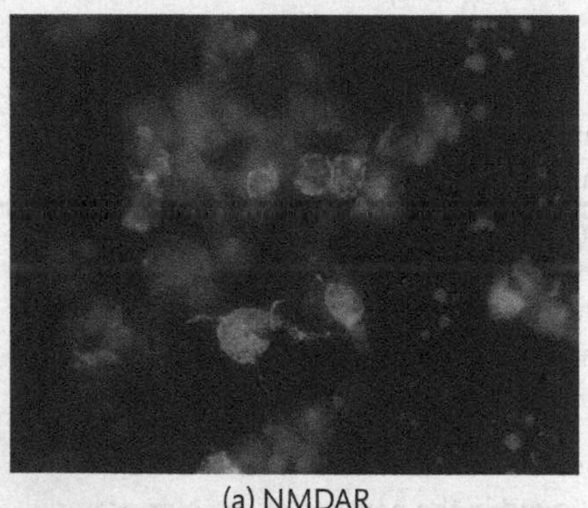

(a) NMDAR

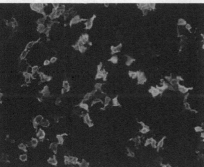

(c) CASPR2

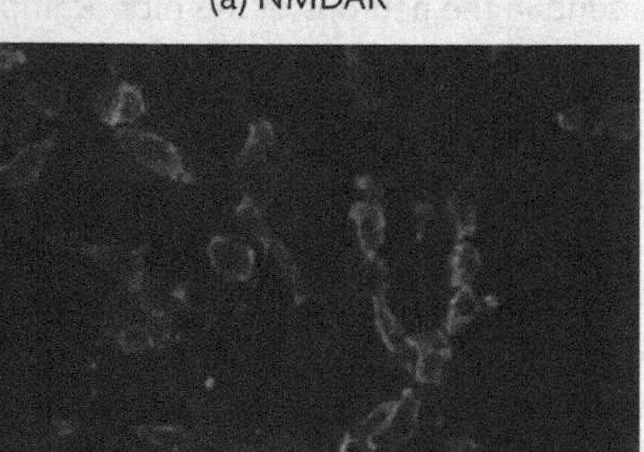

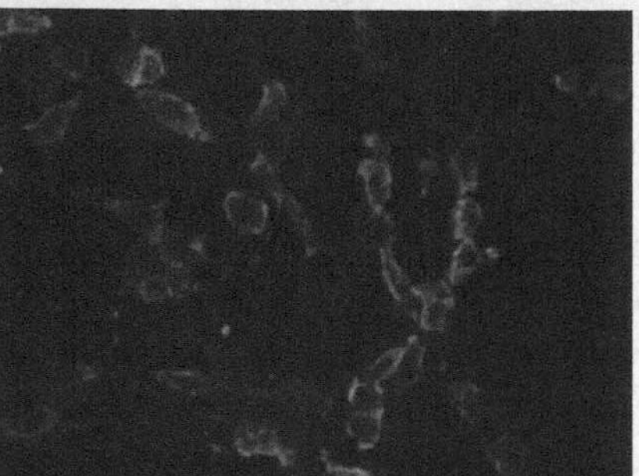

(b) LGI1

FIGURE 10.14

Human serum from patients with autoimmune encephalitis showing expression of relevant cytoplasmic proteins in HEK cells transfected with (a) NMDAR, (b) LGI1, and (c) CASPR2. As you can see the transfection is not 100%, thus providing an inbuilt negative control.

CASPR2 helps in clustering of VGKC at the juxtaparanode and, given the large extracellular sequence, is an ideal target for autoimmunity. Even though the clinical spectrum can be very similar to those having LGI1 antibodies, peripheral symptoms like neuromyotonia, neuropathic pain, and autonomic dysfunction are relatively more common with CASPR2 antibodies.

It is suggested that in patients with a high clinical suspicion of autoimmune limbic encephalitis, if the immunofluorescence using LGI1/CASPR2 transfected cells are negative, neuronal cultures and immunohistochemistry on hippocampal sections may help in identifying patients who may respond to immunotherapy.

Recent studies carried out by the Mayo Clinic, also using commercial transfected cells, have demonstrated that CASPR2 (Figure 10.14c) is less common than LGI1; they further concluded that both antibodies are associated with a diverse neurological presentation which often overlap, but these antibodies occur in a minority of patients suggesting that there are yet undiscovered targets (Klein et al. 2013).

AMPAR antibodies

Antibodies to AMPAR (alpha-amino-3-hydroxy-5-methyl-4-isoxazolepropionic acid receptor), a glutamate receptor, have been described in a few patients with autoimmune limbic encephalitis, the majority having an underlying malignancy. Antibodies reacting against neuronal cell surface antigens were found to be reacting against the GluR1 and GluR2 subunits of AMPAR by immunoprecipitation. Similar to the NMDAR assay, HEK293 cells expressing GluR1/GluR2 receptors have been used for diagnostic testing of these antibodies in the sera or CSF (Lai et al. 2009). These antibodies are thought to reduce the GluR2-AMPAR clustering at the synapse thereby causing the neurological syndrome. Presence of this antibody should lead to a hunt for any underlying neoplasm, most commonly lung, breast, or thymus.

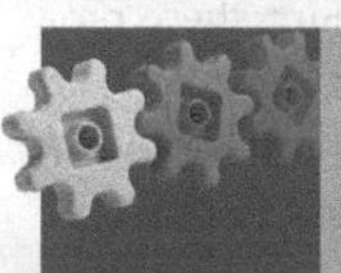

METHOD 10.2 Anti-VGCC and anti-VGKC measured by radioimmunoassay

Measuring antibodies to VGCC

Immunoprecipitation is a quantitative method that uses antigen-antibody reaction complexes to identify proteins that react specifically with an antibody in mixtures of proteins.

Briefly, a radiolabelled synthetic peptide, ω-conotoxin MVIIC (which has a high affinity for the P/Q subunit), is used to label the solubilized P/Q type VGCC extracted from cerebellum. This indirectly radiolabelled P/Q-VGCC is incubated with the test serum and will form a complex with the anti-VGCC IgG. The radioactivity in the precipitated complex is proportional to the concentration of the antibody.

Measuring antibodies to VGKC

Essentially the principle is the same as VGCC except that the protein extract comes from the cerebral cortex and the high affinity radio-ligand is α-dendrotoxin. This assay measures antibodies to VGKC subtypes KV1.1, KV1.2. and KV1.6.

Gamma-aminobutyric acid (GABA)$_B$ receptor 1 (GABA$_{B1}$R) antibody

Inhibitory GABA receptors and other synaptic proteins play an important part in modulating memory and other cognitive functions. G-protein coupled GABA$_B$ receptors are highly localized in the hippocampus, thalamus, and cerebellum. Four main clinical syndromes are associated with GABA$_{B1}$R antibodies—limbic encephalitis and seizures, status epilepticus, ataxia, and opsoclonus–myoclonus syndrome. Seizures are often prominent and consistent with extracellular localization of these antibodies; treatment response to immunotherapy is often very satisfactory. Antibodies may or may not be linked to SCLC, but have not been found in the absence of the neurological syndrome (Höftberger et al. 2013). In contrast to NMDAR antibodies, GABA$_B$R antibodies alter synaptic function without altering the synaptic levels of receptors.

Gamma-aminobutyric acid (GABA)$_A$ receptor (GABA$_A$R) antibody

Unlike the metabotropic G-protein coupled GABA$_B$R, GABA$_A$R is a ligand-gated ion channel which inhibits synaptic transmission in the brain. GABA$_A$R is a pentamer and the antibodies are often directed against the α1 subunit, detected using immunostaining of HEK293 cells expressing the α1/β3 subunits of the receptor. Currently high titre GABA$_A$R antibodies have been described in patients with severe and refractory epilepsy or status epilepticus. Low titre antibodies may coexist with intracellular GAD65 and thyroid peroxidase antibodies and its pathogenic role is currently under evaluation.

Dipeptidyl-peptidase-like protein 6 (DPPX) antibody

Neuropsychiatric symptoms, often with a preceding history of diarrhoea, have been linked to a cell surface auxiliary subunit of the Kv4.2 potassium channels. These potassium channels belong to the mammalian Shal K^+ family and are distinct to the VGKCs (Shaker, Kv1) described earlier. In addition to the strong expression in the hippocampus and cerebellum, these proteins are strongly expressed in the myenteric plexus (and hence the potential relevance of the preceding gastrointestinal illness). Immunocytochemistry on HEK 293 cells transfected with DPPX-S (short cytoplasmic domain containing 32 amino acids), and DPPX-L (long cytoplasmic domain with 88 amino acids) is often used for diagnosis.

Glycine receptor antibody

Glycine receptors (GlyR) are ligand-gated pentameric transmembrane ion channels which mediate inhibitory neurotransmission in the brainstem and spinal cord by modulating the chloride currents. IgG1 complement-fixing antibodies have been identified using α-1 GlyR transfected cells in patients with progressive encephalomyelitis, rigidity, and myoclonus (PERM). Patients often have painful muscle spasms triggered by sensory stimuli, frequent falls, excessive startle response (hyperekplexia), autonomic dysfunction, and eye movement disorders (Carvajal-Gonzalez et al. 2014).

Dopamine 2 receptor (D2R) antibody

A subtype of encephalitis patients have prominent involuntary movements similar to Parkinsonism, dystonia, and chorea, and are thought to have basal ganglia involvement. Elevated dopamine 2 receptor IgG has been found using immunocytochemistry on D2R transfected HEK cells (Dale et al. 2012).

10.9 Miscellaneous antibodies

10.9.1 Glutamic acid decarboxylase (GAD) antibody

GAD enzyme converts glutamic acid to gamma-aminobutyric acid (GABA), an inhibitory neurotransmitter in the brain and a putative paracrine hormone found in pancreatic islet cells. GAD exists as two isoforms (65 and 67 kDa), which share 64% sequence homology and are expressed in the central nervous system, pancreatic islet cells, testis, oviduct, and ovary. GAD65 is a membrane-anchored protein responsible for vesicular GABA production. GAD67, on the other hand, is a cytoplasmic protein involved in the formation of cytoplasmic GABA. In the pancreas, GAD65 (found in beta cells) is 200 times more abundant than GAD67 (alpha cells). Naturally, there are two anti-GAD antibodies, one involved in diabetes mellitus (GAD65) and the other associated with stiff person syndrome (GAD67).

Cross reference

Read Chapter 7 for more information on autoimmune type 1 diabetes.

Immunocytochemical detection of GAD67 antibodies utilizing cerebellum produces a characteristic staining pattern revealing peripheral GABAergic nerve terminals of the cerebellar glomeruli, which you can see in Figure 10.15a. GAD65 is best visualized on the pancreas where it stains β cells (Figure 10.15b). These antibodies can also be detected by other methods (blot, ELISA, and radioimmunoassay).

Very high titres of GAD antibody are usually found in patients with neurological disorder, including SPS (36%), cerebellar ataxia (28%), and other CNS disorders (18%). Interestingly, few

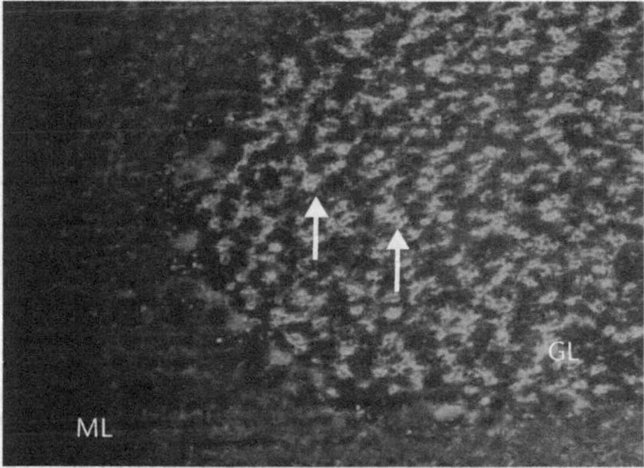

(a) GAD antibody on cerebellum

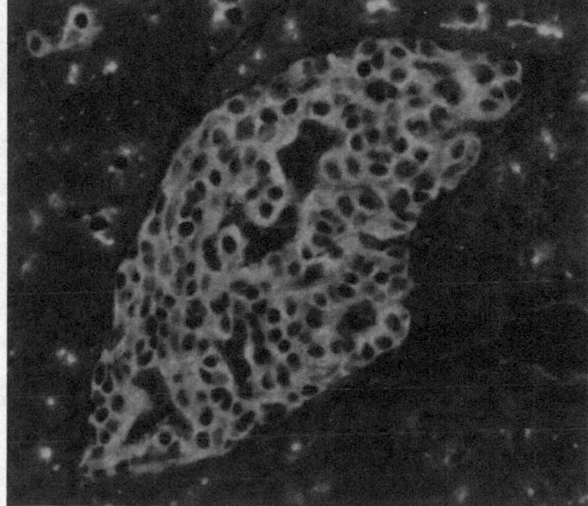

(b) GAD antibody: pancreatic islet cells

FIGURE 10.15
Anti-GAD antibody showing reactivity in the granular layer (GL) of the cerebellum (a). Note the staining of the γ-aminobutyric acid nerve terminals (arrows), which is of a similar distribution to amphiphysin. Unlike amphiphysin there is no staining of the molecular layer (ML) with GAD antibody. Primate pancreas can express antigens for the GAD antibody in the cytoplasm of the β cells (b).

cases of epilepsy in association with GAD antibodies exist. Patients with SPS and ataxia were predominantly females (over 86%) with a mean age of about 60 years and half of them developed diabetes mellitus (Saiz et al. 2008). In a few cases, SPS and ataxia can coexist. The majority of patients have no underlying malignancy. Intrathecal synthesis of GAD antibodies leads to high CSF/serum GAD index (i.e. $\frac{\text{CSF GAD}}{\text{Serum GAD}} \div \frac{\text{CSF Albumin}}{\text{Serum Albumin}}$ higher than 1), which is often a marker of the neurological syndrome.

Four cases of paraneoplastic origin harbouring GAD antibodies have been reported without diabetes in males with mean age of 67 years but with classical syndrome of LE, PEM, and PCD (Saiz et al. 2008). All four patients had underlying malignancy of the lung (SCLS and non-SCLC), pancreas, and thymus.

10.9.2 Anti-ganglioside antibodies (AGA)

Anti-ganglioside antibodies (AGA) are markers of immune mediated neuropathies; their target antigens (gangliosides) are located in the myelin sheath. Gangliosides share a common epitope and are compounds composed of a glycosphingolipid consisting of a hydrophobic ceramide and a hydrophilic oligosaccharide chain with one or more N-acetylneuraminic acid (sialic acid) residues linked to the sugar chain. They are found widely distributed throughout the cell membrane with the two hydrocarbon chains of the ceramide moiety embedded in the plasma membrane and the oligosaccharide on the extracellular surface. Gangliosides are abundant in the myelin sheath (Schwann cells of the peripheral nervous system) and oligodendrocytes of the CNS. The fact that the onset often occurs after infections with *Campylobacter jejuni*, cytomegalovirus, Epstein-Barr virus, mycoplasma pneumoniae, or haemophilus influenza suggests that the pathogenesis may be due to antibodies against microbial ganglioside-like structures that may cross-react with gangliosides in the myelin sheath and induce inflammatory processes, thereby causing demyelination.

Gangliosides are named in shorthand using the Svennerholm system as G (ganglio) followed by the number of sialic acids (A = 0, M = 1, D = 2, T = 3, Q = 4, P = 5, H = 6, S = 7) and the numbers 1, 2, 3 etc., which refer to the order of migration in thin layer liquid chromatography. Variation in the basic structure is further sub-classified to a, b, c etc. Measurements of clinically relevant AGAs (usually IgG and IgM) are widely available in many centres and include GM1, GM2, GD1a, GD1b, and GQ1b. This range of antigens will capture almost all neuropathy related antibodies (see Table 10.6). AGA are routinely measured by ELISA or screened by immunodot/line blots assay. In the latter case quantification relies on visual examination of the colour of the dots/line followed by assigning the reaction as negative, weak positive, or positive. With some commercial dot blots, scanner and software are provided to assist with the interpretation, thus removing operator bias.

In the clinical setting, neuropathies (pain, numbness, paraesthesia, or weakness in the limbs) associated with AGA comprise acute inflammatory demyelinating polyneuropathy (AIDP), which can be subdivided into Guillain-Barré syndrome (GBS), acute motor axonal neuropathy (AMAN), and Miller-Fisher Syndrome (MFS) (Figure 10.16).

In 1916, Guillain-Barré syndrome was first described in two soldiers as a potentially fatal disorder with rapidly progressive paralysis. GBS is an acute predominantly motor neuropathy that may be precipitated by infection and follows a monophasic course. GBS occurs at a frequency of 1 to 2 per 100 000 with a slight male predominance, and in a third of the patients AGA can also be found. Several clinical subtypes of GBS can exist and are given below:

- In acute motor axonal neuropathy (AMAN), neurological deficit is entirely confined to motor neurons, often leading to respiratory failure but with normal sensation. The disease may be seasonal (summer epidemics) due to outbreaks of bacterial enteritis contaminating water supplies.

TABLE 10.6 Neuropathies associated with anti-ganglioside antibodies and their cross reactions with other gangliosides due to shared epitopes. These antibodies are often associated with neuropathies but not always detected.

Neuropathies	Class	Ganglioside	Other antigens with shared epitope
Acute motor axonal neuropathy (GBS)	IgG	GM1	GD1b
Multifocal motor neuropathy	IgM		
Chronic inflammatory demyelinating polyneuropathy	IgM	GM2	–
Acute motor neuropathy	IgG	GD1a	GM1, GM2, GT1a, GT1b
Acute ataxic sensory neuropathy	IgG	GD1b	GT1b, GQ1b
Chronic ataxic sensory neuropathy	IgM		
Miller-Fisher syndrome	IgG	GQ1b	GT1a, GD1b

- Acute motor sensory axonal neuropathy (AMSAN), a subtype of AMAN where both the motor and sensory fibres involved cause severe axonal damage. Like AMAN, it is likely due to an autoimmune response against the axoplasm of peripheral nerves. Recovery is slow and often incomplete. AIDP, AMAN, and AMSAN usually affect all four limbs and can involve cranial nerves and respiration.
- Miller-Fisher Syndrome (MFS) is a rare variant of GBS and was described in 1956 as an acute triad of ophthalmoplegia (paralysis of the extraocular muscles due to cranial nerve involvement), ataxia, and areflexia (absence of reflex).

Treatment of GBS consists of good intensive care, recognizing respiratory failure and providing respiratory support as and when required. Plasma exchange and intravenous immunoglobulin have proved equally effective.

10.9.3 Myelin associated glycoprotein (MAG) antibody

MAG, a glycoprotein component of myelin of both the CNS and the peripheral nervous system, has a similar epitope to that found on other glycolipids such as sulphated glucuronyl lactosaminyl paragloboside and sulphated 3-glucuronyl paragloboside. This glycoprotein, an integral membrane protein of molecular size 100 kDa, can be found in oligodendrocytes and Schwann cells. It is located in the periaxonal region of the myelin and may function in cell interactions and myelination.

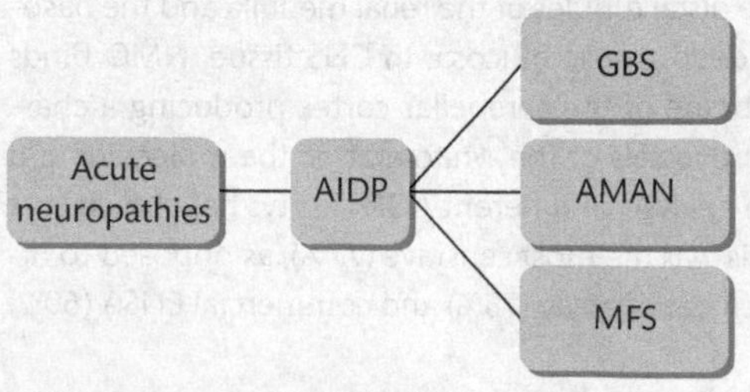

FIGURE 10.16
Antiganglioside antibodies can be associated with acute inflammatory demyelinating polyneuropathy (AIDP), which can be subdivided into Guillain-Barré syndrome (GBS), acute motor axonal neuropathy (AMAN), and Miller-Fisher Syndrome (MFS).

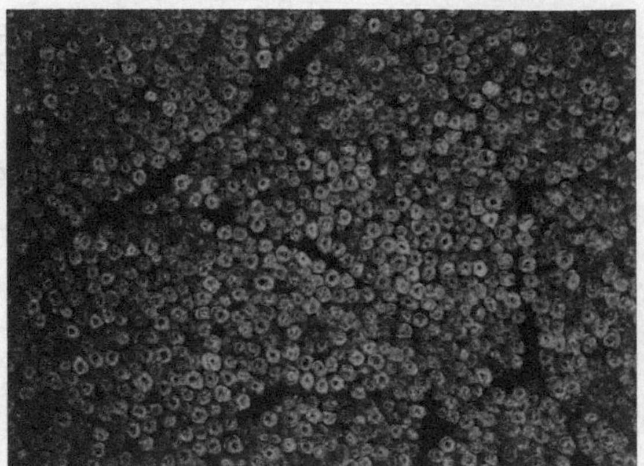

FIGURE 10.17
Transverse section of primate sciatic nerve axons showing staining of the inner and outer myelin sheath with IgM anti-myelin-associated glycoprotein antibody.

High titres of anti-MAG antibodies are found in 50% of patients with IgM paraproteinaemic demyelinating neuropathy. The IgM antibodies are considered to be responsible for demyelination seen in neuropathy. This type of IgM paraproteinaemia can be associated with Waldenström's macroglobulinaemia and multiple myeloma. Anti-MAG paraproteins show cross-reactivity with gangliosides, such as GD1b, GT1b, GQ1b, and sulphatides. These antibodies tend to be IgM kappa, and can be detected by immunofluorescence using peripheral nerve (Figure 10.17) or quantified by ELISA.

Cross reference

For further information on anti-MAG antibodies the reader is referred to a recent article by the European Federation of Neurological Societies (2006).

Clinically, the syndrome associated with MAG antibody is chronic senorimotor demyelinating neuropathy often with tremor. Anti-MAG (IgM) antibodies are considered as pathogenic and therapeutic strategy is directed at reducing circulating antibodies by plasma exchange, inhibition by intravenous immunoglobulin infusion, or reduction of synthesis by steroids administration.

10.9.4 Aquaporin 4 (AQP4) or NMO antibody

Neuromyelitis optica (NMO), also known as Devic's disease, is an immune-mediated inflammatory demyelinating disorder affecting the optic nerve and spinal cord. In the initial stages of the disease, NMO resembles multiple sclerosis (MS) and since neither disorder had a specific marker, 30% of patients with NMO can be misdiagnosed as MS. It is important to distinguish NMO from MS as the former's outcome is worse. The treatment of each condition is also different. With the recent discovery of a specific antibody marker, NMO-IgG (for neuromyelitis optica), the issues highlighted have become less problematic.

The antigen for the anti-NMO antibody is a water channel protein known as aquaporin 4 (AQP4), found in both CNS and non-CNS tissue. It is an integral protein of the plasma membrane and is the predominant water channel in the CNS responsible for a pathological role in brain oedema. Damage to astrocytes in particular by AQP4 has been implicated as the cause of neuromyelitis optica.

Anti-NMO recognizes antigens present in the distal tubules of the renal medulla and the basolateral membranes of epithelial cells in the deep gastric mucosa. In CNS tissue, NMO binds predominantly to the juxtaposed pial membrane of the cerebellar cortex producing a characteristic linear staining, and also to the microvessels of the white matter, the molecular and granular layers (Figure 10.18). A multi-centre analysis of different AQP4 assays has shown that flow cytometry of IgG bound transfected cells was the most sensitive (77%), as opposed to direct cytofluorescence visualization using a cell based assay (73%) and commercial ELISA (60%) (Waters et al. 2012).

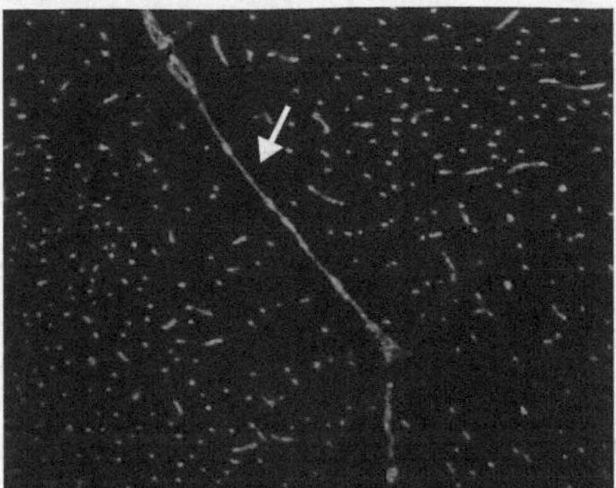

(a) Molecular layer: juxtaposed pial membrane and microvessels

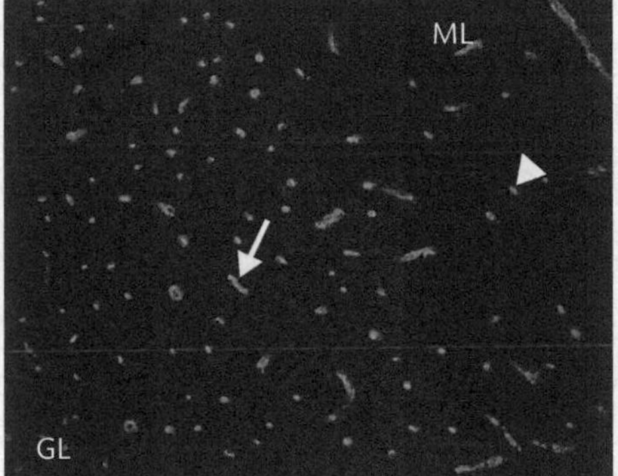

(b) Granular layer: microvessels

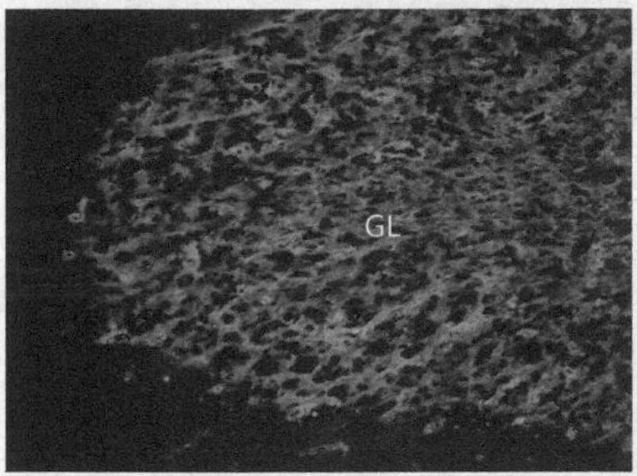

(c) Granular layer

FIGURE 10.18
Aquaporin 4 antibodies (AQP4) bind to the juxtaposed pial membrane of the cerebellum producing linear staining (a, arrow). The red colour in (b) is ethidium bromide staining the nucleus of the granular layer (GL) cells interlaced with microvessels (arrow) expressing the AQP4. Arrow head shows microvessels in the molecular layer (ML). Often the AQP4 sera can also be associated with other intense staining in the granular layer (c).

AQP4 is found in 73% of the patients with clinical NMO and in 46% of the patients at high risk of developing NMO. Females with a median age of 41 years are predominantly affected (> 5:1). Clinical features of bilateral optic neuritis are present in 67% of the patients, with 71% suffering from severe attack-related weakness. Spinal cord inflammation which spreads over more than three vertebral segments (longitudinally extensive transverse myelitis) is quite suggestive of NMO. Within 5 years, there is loss of vision in at least one eye or an inability to walk independently. In 84% of the patients the brain MRI is different from MS. Immunological studies of the CSF show these patients do not usually have oligoclonal bands or abnormal CSF levels of IgG.

In contrast to MS, NMO patients derive benefit from plasmaphoresis and immunosuppression while in MS immunomodulation is currently the treatment of choice.

Cross reference

For further information on anti-AQP4, the reader is referred to articles by Lennon et al. (2004) and Wingerchuk and Weinshenker (2014).

NMO antibody is a welcome addition to the range of disease specific markers and discriminates NMO from other optic neuritis, or myelitis, with high sensitivity (73%) and specificity (91%). With such specificity and sensitivity, the patient can benefit from early diagnosis and treatment. Furthermore, this can also provide valuable information on monitoring treatment and disease progression.

10.9.5 Myelin oligodendrocyte glycoprotein (MOG) antibody

The myelin-oligodendrocyte glycoprotein (MOG) is localized to the outer surfaces of the myelin sheath and oligodendrocytes. It is considered as an auto-antigen responsible for demyelinating disorders of the central nervous system including optic neuritis (ON), which can be part of acute disseminated encephalomyelitis (ADEM), MS, and NMO manifestations. Recent studies suggest that anti-MOG antibodies may also play a role in NMO and other studies have reported the coexistence of MOG and NMO antibody in patients with ON. Testing for both antibodies in ON appears to improve the sensitivity, although almost half the patients remain seronegative. MOG antibody positive NMO patients are thought to have fewer attacks and better recovery than those harbouring AQP4 antibodies.

These antibodies can be measured using enzyme-linked immunosorbent assay.

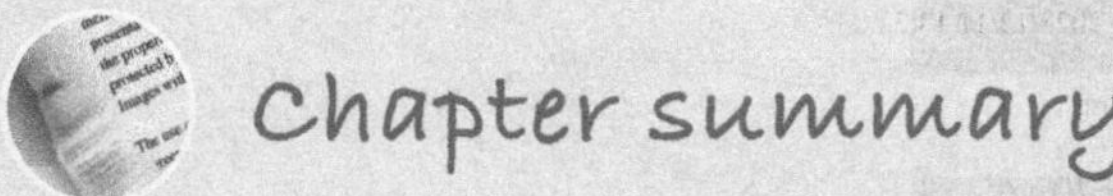

- The immune-mediated processes involved in curtailment of a neoplasm are diverse and complex and have devastating effects on the nervous system.
- The discovery of highly specific anti-neuronal antibodies (an early diagnostic marker of PNS) may provide an invaluable adjunct for diagnosing PNS and alerting clinicians to search for an underlying tumour.
- Often, the specificity of the antibody can predict the likely location of the cancer.
- The association of these antibodies with rapidly deteriorating and devastating neurological symptoms that frequently lead to morbidity and mortality necessitates an early and rapid diagnosis followed by prompt treatment.
- There is then a greater chance of stabilizing the condition and preventing further neuronal cell death and permanent disability.

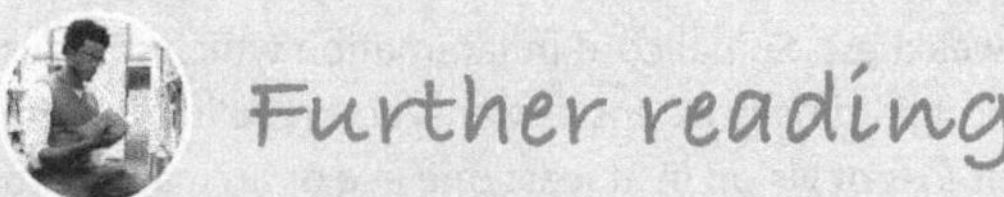

- **European Federation of Neurological Societies/Peripheral Nerve Society (2006) *Guideline on management of paraproteinemic demyelinating neuropathies. Report of a joint task force of the European Federation of Neurological Societies and the Peripheral Nerve Society*. *J Peripher Nerv Syst*, 11, 9–19.**

- Graus F, Delattre JY, Antoine JC, *et al.* (2004) *Recommended diagnostic criteria for paraneoplastic neurological syndromes*. *J Neurol Neurosurg Psychiat*, **75**, 1135–40.
- Karim AR, Hughes RC, Winer JB, Williams AC, Bradwell AR, (2005) *Paraneoplastic neurological antibodies: A laboratory experience*. *Ann N Y Acad Sci*, **1050**, 274–85.
- Lennon VA, Wingerchuk DM, Kryzer TJ, *et al.* (2004) *A serum autoantibody marker of neuromyelitis optica: Distinction from multiple sclerosis*. *Lancet*, **364**, 2106–12.
- Meinck HM, Thompson PD, (2002) *Stiff man syndrome and related conditions*. *Mov Disord*, **17**, 853–66.
- Moll JWB, Antoine JC, Brashear HR, *et al.* (1995) *Guidelines on the detection of paraneoplastic anti-neuronal-specific antibodies: Report from the Workshop to the Fourth Meeting of the International Society of Neuro-Immunology on paraneoplastic neurological disease*, held October 22-23, 1994, in Rotterdam, The Netherlands. *Neurology*, **45**, 1937–41
- Wingerchuk DM, Weinshenker BG (2014) *Chapter 26–Neuromyelitis optica (Devic's syndrome)*. *Handb Clin Neurol*, 122, 581–99.

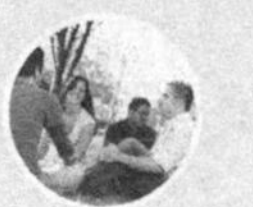

Discussion questions

10.1 What evidence is there for the autoimmune basis of PNS?

10.2 Explain how a remote neoplasm can cause neurological deficit.

10.3 Explain how well-characterized paraneoplastic neurological antibodies can be used in the clinical setting.

10.4 What are the likely outcomes in patients with PNS?

Answers to self-check questions are provided in the book's Online Resource Centre.

 Visit www.oxfordtextbooks.co.uk/orc/hall2e

11

Flow cytometry and primary immunodeficiency

Learning Objectives

After studying this chapter you should be able to:

- describe a number of well-defined immunodeficiencies
- explain the clinical features of these immunodeficiencies
- outline the expected findings by flow cytometry
- discuss the limitations of flow cytometry in the diagnosis of immunodeficiency and other techniques available
- describe the current treatment options.

Introduction

Our knowledge of the immune system has increased greatly over the last decade. The discovery of many new types of primary immunodeficiency and the study of these have played a huge part in unravelling the complexities of the immune system. This process is ongoing and it is difficult to keep up to date in this fast moving field. Techniques for measuring the immune system and its function are relatively crude. Flow cytometry has proved to be a very useful tool for detecting abnormalities in the cells of the immune system. This chapter introduces some of the better-described primary immunodeficiencies for which flow cytometry plays a role in their diagnosis.

A healthy immune system has three main functions.

- To protect the body from infection and damage from foreign pathogens.
- To protect against abnormalities of self that occur in malignancy.
- To maintain tolerance of self, which depends on an intact immune system.

Immunodeficiency refers to defects in the immune system resulting in gaps in the body's defence against pathogens. This presents with recurrent, uncommonly severe, or unusual infections. The type and site of infection will depend on which part of the immune system is defective. In many immunodeficiencies, autoimmunity and malignancy can also be seen. Primary immunodeficiency is present at birth and is caused by genetic mutations, which can be inherited, or that occur spontaneously. Causes of acquired immunodeficiency include infections and side effects from therapeutic treatments such as certain drugs and radiation therapy.

Immunodeficiency
Defects in the immune system resulting in gaps in the body's defence against pathogens.

Cross reference
Secondary or acquired immunodeficiency is caused by external factors such as viral infection; the classic example is HIV. This is discussed in Chapter 12.

Depending on severity, primary immunodeficiencies can present in the first few weeks of life, as in severe combined immunodeficiency (SCID), or they can manifest much later, presenting in adulthood such as combined variable immunodeficiency (CVID). Immunodeficiency should be suspected if a patient has either recurrent or persistent infections, severe infections requiring hospital treatment, or unusual or so-called opportunist infections not normally seen in the healthy population. To be involved in the investigation of a possible immunodeficiency is the chance to play detective. Factors such as type, site of infection, and age of onset all provide important clues. Knowledge of how the immune system deals with different types of pathogens will allow investigations to be targeted appropriately. For example, phagocytic cells clear extracellular pathogens, such as encapsulated bacteria. They do this by targeting organisms that have first been opsonized (coated) with complement and specific antibodies. To investigate a patient suffering from recurrent bacterial infections, it may be necessary to investigate the presence and function of the phagocytes, the specific antibodies, complement components, and the ability to opsonize the bacteria.

A family history can be invaluable in the investigation of PIDs. Information about early infant deaths, sex of the patient, affected relatives, and consanguinity can all be used to identify possible modes of inheritance. Knowing if the condition appears X-linked or autosomal recessive (AR), can suggest certain PIDs.

An initial screen would normally consist of a full blood count, immunoglobulins, and, if indicated, lymphocyte subsets.

It is becoming increasingly recognized that a number of hypomorphic mutations in genes known to cause PID occur. With a hypomorphic mutation there is reduced function of the gene product and the outcome is often very different to previously described, e.g. missense mutations or deletions where there is no gene product. These disorders may have less severe features and can present much later in life and provide monogenic answers to some disorders previously thought to be polygenic in origin.

It is not within the scope of this book to give a complete list of primary immunodeficiencies. This chapter is an introduction to some well-described immunodeficiencies for which flow cytometry is useful in the diagnosis (Table 11.1). This is by no means a comprehensive list and other texts should to be referred to (e.g. Ochs et al. 2013).

11.1 Lymphocyte subsets

The availability of **monoclonal antibodies** has greatly increased our ability to study and define the cells of the immune system. When monoclonal antibodies started to be produced in increasing numbers an international nomenclature system was adopted. **Clusters of differentiation (CD)** numbers were allocated to define the specificities of the various clones. Antibodies specific for structures on the surface of cells can be used to define cell types, as in lymphocyte subsets, the stage of maturation, as in leukaemia typing, and also the status of the mature cell, i.e. naïve or activated.

Monoclonal antibodies
Antibodies produced from a single clone of cells, consisting of identical molecules.

Clusters of differentiation (CD)
Cell surface molecules on lymphocytes that are recognized by monoclonal antibodies to allow identification of the cell by flow cytometry.

All cells in peripheral blood are derived from haematopoietic pluripotent stem cells, which are found in the bone marrow. White blood cells all play a role in the immune system and can be

TABLE 11.1 **Examples of types of infections and associations with particular immunodeficiencies.**

Site of infection/clinical presentation	Type of infection	Possible immunodeficiency
Upper airways, sinus/chest, and ear infections	Bacterial infections: pneumococcus, *Staph aureus*/streptococci, and meningococcus	B cell/antibody defects
Severe pneumonias, gut infections leading to diarrhoea, and failure to thrive. Unusual opportunistic infections	Viruses (CMV, VZV, adenovirus, molluscum contagiosum), fungi (candida, *Pneumocystis jirovecii*), and cryptosporidium	T cell deficiencies
Recurrent pyogenic infections. Abscesses of skin and internal organs. Granulomatous	Bacterial infections: *Staph. aureus*, burkholderia. Invasive fungal infection, aspergillus	Neutrophil defect
Recurrent infections with the same type of pathogen	Neisseria	Complement
Invasive pneumococcal infection	*Streptococcus pneumoniae* or pneumococcus	IRAK4

Cross reference

You can read in more detail about white blood cells in the *Haematology* textbook of this series.

identified by light microscopy using differences in their size, shape of nucleus, and the presence or absence of granules in the cytoplasm.

There are three main populations of white blood cell found in peripheral blood.

- Neutrophils, eosinophils, and basophils, have multiple or bi-lobed nuclei and granules in their cytoplasm and are collectively known as **granulocytes**.
- Monocytes and the smaller lymphocytes generally have a clear cytoplasm and a large single nucleus and are referred to collectively as **mononuclear cells**.
- **Lymphocytes** can be further broken down into three major subsets: T, B, and NK cells, which all appear similar when viewed by light microscopy. T cells can be further defined as helper T cells or cytotoxic T cells.

Granulocytes

White blood cells filled with granules containing enzymes which enable digestion of micro-organisms and production of inflammatory responses. Includes neutrophils, eosinophils, and basophils.

Mononuclear cells

White blood cells with only one nucleus. Includes monocytes and lymphocytes.

Lymphocytes

A type of white blood cell of which there are three subtypes: B cells, which give rise to humoral immunity; T cells, which give rise to cellular immunity; and natural killer cells.

The identification and quantitation of the basic lymphocyte subsets by flow cytometry is an essential part of the diagnosis of many immunodeficiencies. Absent, decreased or even increased populations of the various lymphocyte subsets can be useful in the diagnosis and monitoring of immunodeficiency.

By using a flow cytometer the size (forward scatter) and granularity/complexity of the cytoplasm (side scatter) of a cell can be determined enabling differentiation of the white blood cells, but in addition the amount of fluorescence associated with the cell can also be detected. By using monoclonal antibodies conjugated to a fluorescent molecule and specific to different structures on the surface of lymphocytes, the various subsets can be identified. Different combinations of antibodies against various specificities can be combined. Antibodies are generally conjugated to a fluorescent molecule; if not, additional staining steps are required. If the antibodies are conjugated to different fluorochromes they can be used simultaneously as flow cytometers have a number of detectors, to which light from different parts of the spectrum can be directed.

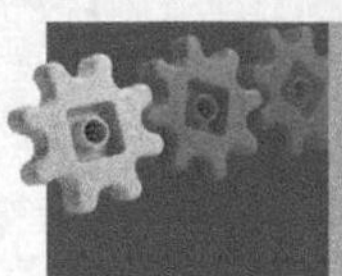

METHOD 11.1 Preparation of sample for flow cytometry

To stain a sample, antibodies are mixed with whole blood and allowed to bind, usually at room temperature for 15 minutes (time and temperature at which incubations should be carried out may differ—manufacturers' data sheets should always be referred to).

A lysing solution (there are many commercial varieties available) is added to remove the red blood cells—again incubation times may vary.

The sample may now require washing in phosphate buffered saline to remove unbound antibodies and red cell debris.

If the presence of a fluorescent antibody, and not cell size and granularity, is to be used to identify populations of cells samples may not require washing.

Online Resource Centre

To see an online video demonstrating flow cytometry, log on to www.oxfordtextbooks.co.uk/orc/fbs

A number of tubes containing different antibody combinations may be required to identify all the populations of interest. This is generally referred to as a panel. The basic panel should enable a pure lymphocyte gate to be set (CD45 versus side scatter) and all major lymphocyte subsets to be identified. This can be seen in Figure 11.1. The inclusion of beads of known concentration into the tube will enable absolute counts to be calculated. This is now standard practice in most Clinical Immunology laboratories. It allows an accurate measurement of the number of cells present in the sample using a single platform. Lymphocyte subsets are now routinely reported as both an absolute count (cells/μl) and as a percentage of lymphocytes.

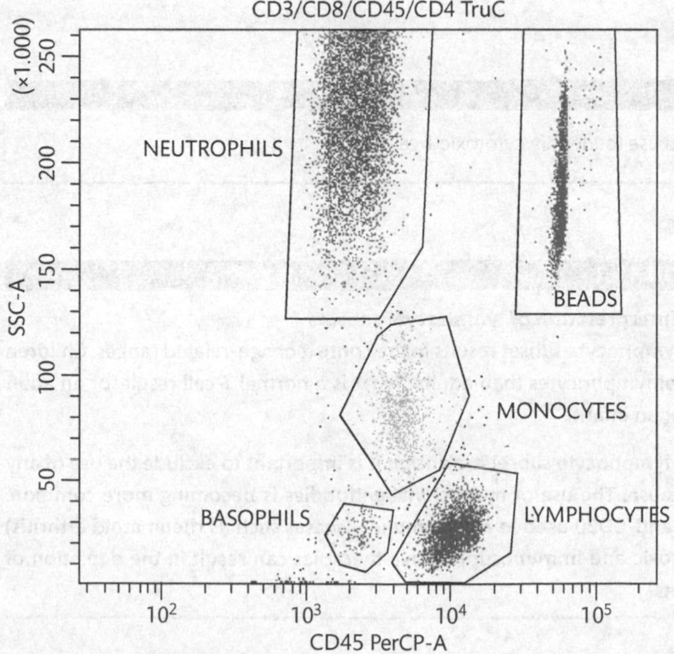

FIGURE 11.1
CD45 versus side-scatter lymphocyte gating. The plot shows an example of normal whole blood stained with an antibody to CD45, a pan white cell marker that is found at a higher density on lymphocytes than granulocytes. Red blood cells have been removed by lysis and the remaining cells run through a flow cytometer. The *x*-axis shows the amount of CD45 (the more CD45 antigen on the surface of the cell the more fluorescent conjugated anti-CD45 antibody will bind and the greater the fluorescent signal detected by the flow cytometer). The *y*-axis denotes the amount of light the cells side-scattered when they passed in front of the laser and relates to the granules in a cell's cytoplasm. Neutrophils have a large number of granules in their cytoplasm and so have a high side-scatter signal. By plotting CD45 expression against granularity, four distinct populations appear. Beads are incorporated into the tube to enable an absolute count to be calculated.

TABLE 11.2 Antibodies used in basic lymphocyte subset panel.

Antibody specificity	Population identified in peripheral blood
CD3	T cells
CD19	B cells
CD16+/ CD56	NK cells (CD3 negative), CD16 also on neutrophils. CD56 is also on a subpopulation of T cells
CD4	Helper T cells ($CD3^+$), also monocytes
CD8	Cytotoxic T cells ($CD3^+$), also some NK cells
CD45	Panleukocyte marker
HLA-DR	B cells, monocytes, activated T cells

When constructing a panel for the first time it is essential to be aware of which markers are lineage-specific, i.e. CD3 is only expressed on T cells, and which are expressed on more than one cell type, i.e. CD4 is expressed on both helper T cells and monocytes. Table 11.2 shows which antibodies are used in the basic lymphocyte subset panel and which cell populations they can identify.

Fluorochromes
A fluorescent chemical that emits a specific colour when illuminated by light.

It is also important to consider the amount of antigen present on the cell. **Fluorochromes** are different in strength, in that the number of molecules of phycoerythrin (PE) that need to be present on a cell before they can be seen above background is much fewer than a weaker fluorochrome such as fluorescein isothiocyanate (FITC). The brightest fluorochrome should ideally be chosen for the weakest antigen.

Commercial antibody cocktails are available. If constructing in-house combinations extensive validation is required. A useful document to refer to is the BCSH guidelines for multicolour flow cytometry.

SELF-CHECK 11.1

What antibodies would you use to identify cytotoxic T cells?

CLINICAL CORRELATION 11.1

Important factors in the interpretation of lymphocyte subsets

It is essential to interpret lymphocyte subset results in the context of age-related ranges. Children have much higher levels of lymphocytes than adults. What is a normal T cell result for an adult may be profoundly low for an infant.

When cells of a particular lymphocyte subset are absent it is important to exclude the use of any treatments as being the cause. The use of monoclonal antibodies is becoming more common. Some, such as rituximab (anti-CD20 used in autoimmune diseases such as rheumatoid arthritis) target B cells. Other cytotoxic and immunosuppressive therapies can result in the depletion of various lymphocyte subsets.

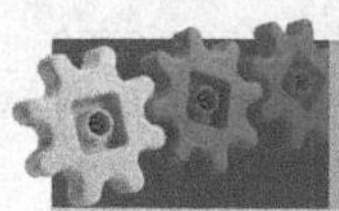

METHOD 11.2 Quality assurance in flow cytometry

Settings

It is important to ensure the flow cytometer is correctly set up. It is possible to place a population anywhere on a plot by decreasing or increasing the power to a detector. Detectors are normally set using negative populations. There is also the problem of spectral overlap between the emission spectra of the various fluorescent molecules used. This will result in the signal being measured in more than one detector requiring that 'compensation' be applied to correct for this.

Instrument quality control

Various types of beads are used extensively to enable software to automatically set up suitable settings, including compensation, as well as to ensure the flow cytometer is working optimally.

Samples

Cells are fairly labile and the age of samples and how they are stored can affect results. This may vary for different assays but in general testing within 24 hours is preferable. Clots in samples will affect results and adequate mixing of whole blood samples is essential if accurate absolute counts are required.

Once samples have been processed and stained they should be acquired on the flow cytometer as soon as possible or kept at 4 °C in the dark–this varies depending on the technique. Fluorochromes are sensitive to bright light.

Isotype controls

Each monoclonal antibody should bind to its specific antigen only. Structures on the surface of a cell may bind to the protein or fluorochrome. Antibodies with a specificity that should not be present in the assay can be used to determine any non-specific binding. These antibodies should be of the same isotype (i.e. IgG1) and conjugated to the same fluorochrome as the primary antibody. Ideally the isotype control should also be from the same manufacturer as different companies use different protein levels.

There is some debate as to when isotype controls should be used. Where distinct stained and unstained populations are expected to be present, isotype controls are considered to be unnecessary. Naturally occurring negative populations that are present are preferably used. Fluoresence minus one (FMO),where one antibody is left out, of in-house cocktails can be helpful. The behaviour of an isotype control cannot always be assumed to be exactly the same as the antibody of interest. Assays that require stimulation or other manipulation of the sample before staining may increase non-specific staining by upregulation of various receptors, and isotype controls can be helpful.

Lymphocyte subsets

The percentages of T, B, and NK cells found in a lymphocyte gate when added together, the so-called 'lymphosum', should be 100% ± 5%. Failure of this may indicate the gate is not set correctly. NB it is vital that the gate includes all populations of interest or they will not be counted.

Where multiple tubes are set up in a panel on the same patient, any antigens measured more than once should be reproducible between tubes. Percentages would be expected to be within 3% and absolute counts within 10%.

$CD4^+$ and $CD8^+$ T cells when added together should be close to the $CD3^+$ total. If not then double negative populations should be considered, or the presence of gamma delta T cells.

Stabilized whole blood controls are available with target values, although these can be quite generous. These are whole process controls but as antibodies are used they can work out to be very expensive. There is no real consensus as to how often these should be run.

When measuring absolute counts using reference bead populations, accurate pipetting is critical. Process should be in place to monitor the accuracy of pipettes and any automated sample preparation instruments used.

It can be useful to check lymphocyte counts against those obtained from a full blood count as this will pick up any sample-specific pipetting errors such as the presence of small clots.

The next three sections (11.2–11.4) describe the three main types of lymphocytes. Knowledge of how cells develop, their functions, and interactions with other cells is critical to understanding the underlying defects that cause immunodeficiency. Possible causes of abnormal findings in the measurement of these different types of lymphocytes are also discussed.

Cross reference

Suitable immunology textbooks include Murphy (2011), Male et al. (2012), or Owen et al. (2013).

Previous knowledge of the immune system structure and function is assumed in order to aid the understanding of this section. There are a number of good immunology texts that will support the following sections.

11.2 T cells

11.2.1 Development

T cells, like all cells found in peripheral blood, are derived from pluripotent haematopoietic stem cells, initially from foetal liver and then subsequently bone marrow. T cells differ from other blood cells in that they mature in the thymus. Stem cells seed the thymus, where they are provided with growth factors such as interleukin (IL)-7 and cell-to-cell interactions essential for development. Progenitor T cells first appear in the cortex of the thymus and do not express CD4 or CD8 and are therefore referred to as double negative (DN).

To fulfil their function T and B cells require an immensely diverse repertoire of receptors enabling them to recognize all potential pathogens. Each mature T or B cell will have a unique receptor. Diversity is generated by DNA rearrangement of a relatively small set of germ line genes: variable (V), joining (J), and in T cell receptor (TCR) β and δ chains only, diversity (D), so VDJ. For example, when you throw one dice, you have the possibility of throwing six possible numbers. If you have two dice, this increases to 36. In TCR generation you have three dice (the V, D, and J genes). Despite having a relatively small number of each of these genes, by breaking them, resorting them randomly, and then rejoining them, a large number of different receptors can be generated. In addition, where these different segments join, nucleotides can be added or removed increasing the diversity even more. This process is an adaptation of the normal DNA repair mechanisms, which exist to maintain the integrity of DNA when accidental damage from factors such as ionizing radiation occurs.

During this process several proteins have been shown to play a role. The products of the recombination activating genes (RAG-1 and RAG-2) are important in initiating the break but are not part of normal DNA repair. Other important factors such as Artemis, cernunnos, and DNA ligase IV also have a critical role in normal DNA repair.

Mature TCRs consist of two chains, either α and β or γ and δ. Some DN cells will remain DN and rearrange and express a γδ receptor. The majority of T cells rearrange the TCR β chain first, which is then expressed on the surface as a pre T cell receptor complex in association with the CD3 molecule. If the gene rearrangement is unproductive this receptor will not be formed and the cell will die from apoptosis. The TCR α chain gene rearrangement now occurs and cells express both CD4 and CD8 and are termed double positive (DP).

Major histocompatibility complex (MHC)

A group of genes that code for cell-surface histocompatibility antigens and are the principal determinants of tissue type and transplant compatibility.

Positive selection

The survival of a T cell through the TCR binding to MHC with weak affinity, ensuring T cells can recognize self and are non-reactive.

Negative selection

T cell recognition of self-antigen in the thymus resulting in deletion by apoptosis.

The likelihood of these rearrangements resulting in receptors recognizing self is high, so a process of selection now occurs during which > 95% of thymocytes are eliminated. The survival of the T cell depends on interactions through the TCR. To survive, the TCR needs to bind with weak affinity to the **major histocompatibility complex (MHC)** expressed by thymic epithelial cells. No recognition results in cell death. This is referred to as **positive selection** and ensures T cells will recognize foreign antigen only in the context of self-MHC.

Cells that recognize self-antigens and therefore bind with high affinity are deleted by apoptosis. This is called **negative selection**. Ubiquitous self-antigens are presented mainly by dendritic cells. The autoimmune regulator (AIRE) gene activated in thymic epithelial cells enables organ specific antigens to be expressed, which might otherwise not be presented to the immature T cells. Cells with TCR recognizing MHC class I become $CD8^+$ and those recognizing MHC class II, $CD4^+$ T cells.

11.2.2 Function

Because of this selection process T cells will only react with antigens in the context of MHC. This enables T cells to recognize antigens that originate from inside the cell. These antigens can be synthesized from within the cell, as in a viral infection, or taken up by **endocytosis**, as occurs in antigen presenting cells (APC) such as macrophages, dendritic cells, and B cells. The antigens are processed and presented by MHC molecules, the binding sites of which hold the antigenic peptides and can therefore determine which part of the antigen is presented to the T cell. This may explain why MHC haplotype can affect susceptibility or resistance to autoimmunity and infection.

Endocytosis

The process by which a cell ingests material with the formation of vesicles. Includes phagocytosis and pinocytosis.

APC are found mainly in the secondary lymphoid organs. Here helper $CD4^+$ T cells interact with the APCs, which provide co-stimulatory signals necessary for naïve T cell activation. Using chemical messages such as cytokines or direct cell-to-cell contact, the activated $CD4^+$ T cell sends a message back to the presenting cell. Interaction with a $CD4^+$ T cell enables B cells to switch from their default of making IgM to other isotypes such as IgG, and macrophages to activate and destroy intercellular and extracelluar antigens.

Cytotoxic $CD8^+$ T cells with help from $CD4^+$ T cells can secrete molecules capable of killing cells infected with virus. It is important therefore that MHC class I is expressed on most nucleated cells in the body, as a viral infection may occur anywhere.

11.2.3 Absent T cells

Severe combined immunodeficiency (SCID)

Complete absence of T cells can be seen in SCID. Even if B cells are present their function is severely impaired in the absence of help from $CD4^+$ T cells.

SCID is very rare, with an incidence of approximately 1 in 500 000, and is more common in boys than girls. Infants present within the first few months of life with poor growth, failure to thrive (FTT), and often a persistent low lymphocyte count. They have recurrent infections, often in the respiratory tract and gut, are unable to clear viruses, and are susceptible to opportunistic infections such as *Candida* and *Pneumocystis carinii* pneumonia (PCP). The diagnosis of SCID is a paediatric emergency. It is essential that the child be referred immediately to a specialist centre where they have facilities to provide a clean environment (free from pathogens). Live vaccines must not be given such as Bacillus Calmette-Guerin (BCG), as this is a weakened but live form of the bacteria that cause tuberculosis and can become disseminated in the absence of functioning T cells. Blood products should be irradiated, as immunocompetent cells in the blood may cause graft versus host disease (GVHD). Blood products should also be cytomegalovirus (CMV) negative as this could cause a fatal infection in an immunocompromised recipient. The prognosis in SCID is significantly worsened by any acquired infections.

There are many types of SCID (Table 11.3), and the phenotype reflects the type of defect. Many are inherited in an autosomal recessive manner (requiring an abnormal gene to be acquired from both parents) and consanguineous parents should increase the index of suspicion for SCID.

Most SCID is T cell negative; however leaky forms of SCID do occur where high T cell numbers can be seen. An example of this is Omenn's syndrome, which is described in Clinical correlation 11.2.

TABLE 11.3 SCID classifications.

Phenotype	Defect in	Mechanism	Inheritance
$T^{-}B^{-}NK^{-}$	ADA (adenosine deaminase)	Premature cell death due to purine metabolism defect	AR
	Reticular dysgenesis, also low monocytes and neutrophils. Platelets and red blood cells are normal	? Adenylate kinase 2—important for cell survival	AR
$T^{-}B^{+}NK^{-}$	Cytokine receptors are composed of 3 chains, α, β, and γ. In X-linked SCID the common γ chain (γc) of the receptors for the cytokines IL-2, 4, 7, 9, 15, and 21 is absent.	IL-7 is required for T cell development and survival, IL-15 is required for NK cell development	XL
	Janus kinase 3 (JAK3)	Kinase associated with γc	AR
$T^{-}B^{+}NK\downarrow$	CD45 (TCRγδ⁺)	CD45 important for TCR signalling	AR
	PNP (purine nucleoside phosphorylase)	Premature cell death due to purine metabolism defect	AR
$T^{-}B^{+}NK^{+}$	α Chain of the receptor for the cytokine IL-7	IL-7 required for T cell survival	AR
	The T cell receptor is held within the CD3 molecule which is made up of:		
$T^{-}B^{+}NK^{+}$	δ, ε chains	Pre-TCR and TCR signalling required for survival	AR
$T^{-}B^{+}NK^{+}$	ζ and γ (CD3 expression reduced, γδ T cells present)		
$T^{-}B^{-}NK^{+}$	RAG-1/2	Defective VDJ recombination required for both TCR and BCR (Ig)	AR
	Artemis (sensitive to ionizing radiation)	Artemis involved in VDJ recombination and DNA repair	

AR, autosomal recessive; XL, X-linked.

Another potential source of T cells in SCID is maternal foetal engraftment (MFE). In a normal foetus, T cells (which are absent in SCID) would destroy any maternal cells crossing the placenta. In SCID this does not occur and maternal T cells can survive and expand in the foetus. The presence of maternal T cells is considered to be one of the diagnostic criteria for SCID.

CLINICAL CORRELATION 11.2

Omenn's syndrome

Omenn's syndrome has been described in patients with mutations in RAG1/2, Artemis, and most other defects associated with SCID. Clinically it presents with often severe erythroderma (a general exfoliating dermatitis involving most of the patient's skin), and hepatosplenomegaly. Eosinophils can be increased, as can serum IgE levels. T cells can be greatly increased but are oligoclonal, highly activated, and do not proliferate in response to the mitogen phytohemagglutinin (PHA).

Key Point

The presence of T cells does not exclude a diagnosis of SCID.

The goal of treatment for SCID is for T and B cell function to be restored; this can be achieved by haematopoietic stem cell transplantation (HSCT). Success rates are good, especially if an HLA-matched sibling donor is available and the diagnosis was made prior to the acquisition of infections. For a limited number of SCID patients, such as those with defects in adenosine deaminase (ADA) or common gamma chain (γc), insertion of a corrected gene into the patient's own haematopoietic stem cells has been used to affect a cure. This is referred to as gene therapy but is only practicable if the genetic defect is well defined and discrete numbers of cells affected. Ideally cells expressing the transgene need to be long lived and have a selective advantage so that they can outgrow affected cells.

Patients with SCID caused by adenosine deaminase (ADA) deficiency are often profoundly lymphopenic but other cells are also affected. Skeletal, hepatic, renal, lung, and neurological abnormalities are also seen, in addition to the recurrent infections and failure to thrive caused by lack of lymphocytes. Lack of ADA causes a build-up of purine metabolites, which affects rapidly dividing cells such as lymphocytes. The defective enzyme (ADA) can be replaced conjugated to polyethylene glycol (PEG), which prolongs the half-life of the ADA by preventing it being excreted. This is often used only as a temporary measure to detoxify the metabolites but does not usually enable lymphocyte numbers to recover.

Di George and CHARGE syndromes

These are two other conditions that can present with absent T cells. Both, like most genetic diseases, have a large spectrum depending on multiple factors, including the specific mutation.

Di George is caused by a deletion in 22q11. This results in a number of defects including cardiac malformation, facial abnormalities, neonatal hypocalcaemia, and immunodeficiency. The immunodeficiency is caused by abnormalities in the thymus which can lead to low T cell numbers or, in

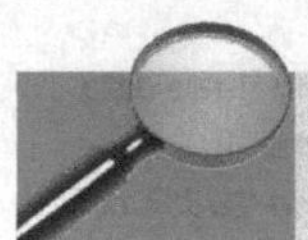

CASE STUDY 11.1 Omenn's syndrome

Patient history

Baby L was born at term to non-consanguineous parents. She presented at one week old with a facial rash, initially thought to be eczema, but that quickly developed into erythroderma. At 2 weeks she was admitted to hospital with rapid breathing that required oxygen. It was noted that she had a very high eosinophil count. The chest and skin improved with steroids and intravenous antibiotics. She was re-admitted at 6 weeks with worsening chest and skin and generalized lymphadenopathy.

Results

Her lymphocyte subsets were measured (see Figure 11.2).

Significance of results

T cell proliferation to PHA was absent.

A diagnosis of Omenn's syndrome was made and an appropriate underlying cause was then diagnosed.

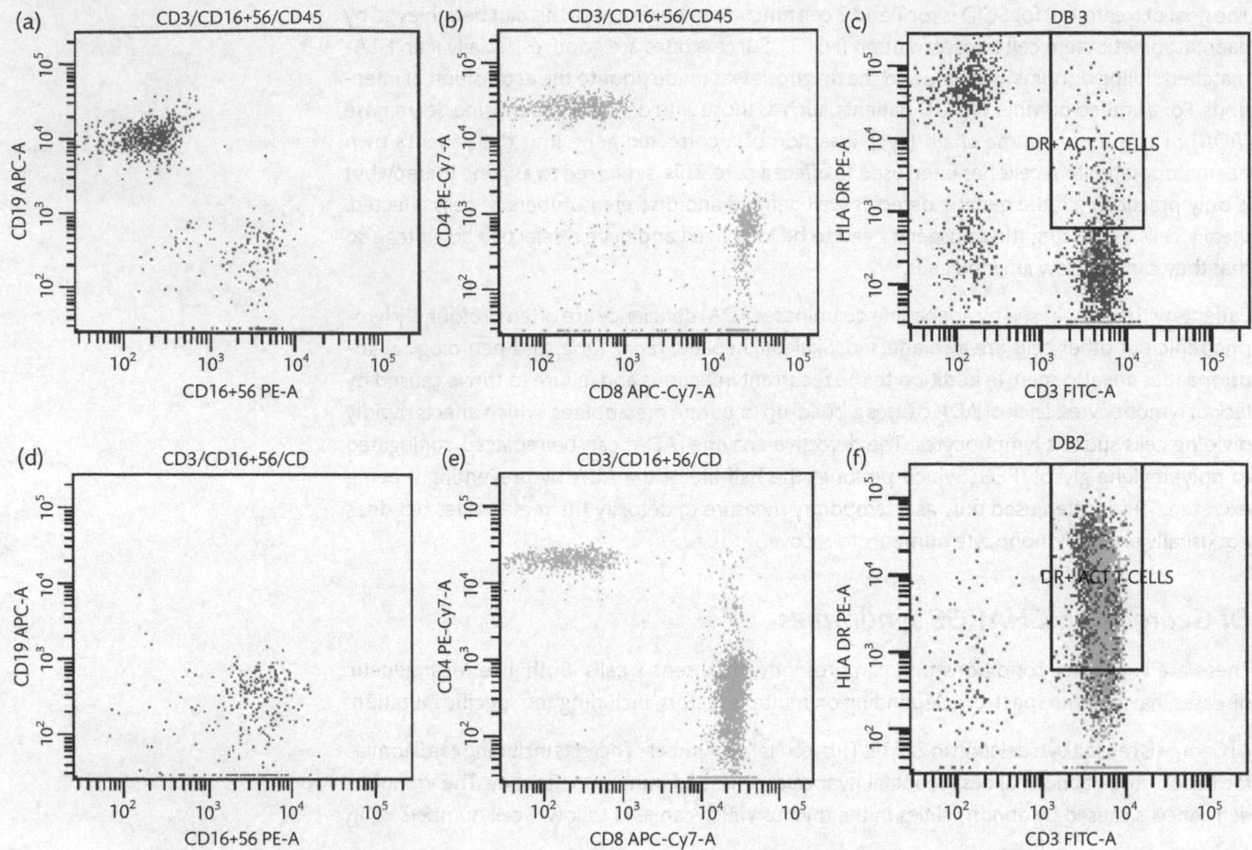

FIGURE 11.2

Omenn's syndrome. The top three plots show data from a normal child and the bottom three data from a patient with Omenn's. Plots (a) and (d) show data from CD3 positive lymphocytes. In (d) the B cell population is missing (CD19⁺). Plots (b) and (e) show CD3⁺ lymphocytes; CD4⁺ and CD8⁺ T cells are present in both. Plots (c) and (f) show all lymphocytes. The percentage of T cells expressing HLA-DR in (f) is increased compared to the normal, and the HLA-DR⁺, CD3– population (B cells) is missing.

the most severe form, the thymus can be absent. Unlike SCID there is no defect in the T cells, rather in the absence of a thymus in which to develop. HSCT has been used to treat T cell Di George, but with no thymus only peripheral expansion of the mature T cells given with the graft occurs. Recently thymic transplants have been successful and would now be the treatment of choice.

CHARGE syndromes consist of **c**oloboma (abnormal eye development), **h**eart defect, **a**tresia choanae (closure of one or both nasal cavities), **r**etarded growth and development, **g**enital hypoplasia, and characteristic **e**ar defects. CHARGE is due to mutations in CHD7 and can result in severely reduced or absent T cells. There is some overlap with Di George but the exact mechanism that causes complete absence of T cells is not yet known.

11.2.4 Low T cells

Low T cells can be seen in a number of immunodeficiencies. Updates on the classification of primary immunodeficiency are a good way to access the ever increasing list of disorders. Consider other factors, such as is it just T cells, or are other lymphocyte subsets decreased? For example DOCK8 patients have a generalized lymphopenia. In some conditions, such as

Wiskott–Aldrich syndrome, Nijmegen breakage syndrome, and ataxia telangiectasia, T cells will progressively decrease over time. Hypomorphic mutations (partial function) of the genes that generally cause SCID can present with low T cells. It is also important to take into consideration the ratio of $CD4^+$ T cells to $CD8^+$ T cells. A normal CD4:CD8 ratio is 1.5. Abnormal CD4:CD8 ratio may be an indication of maternal foetal engraftment (MFE), HIV infection, or leaky SCID. All of these will also have an increase in activation markers seen on the surface of the T cells.

Low $CD4^+$ T cells

When low $CD4^+$ T cells are seen, HIV should always be considered. In HIV the numbers of $CD8^+$ T cells are often increased, as are the percentages of T cells expressing activation markers such as HLA-DR.

Major histocompatibility complex (MHC) Class II deficiency also results in low $CD4^+$ T cells. Class II is constitutively expressed on antigen presenting cells such as B cells and monocytes. $CD4^+$ T cells only recognize antigen in the context of MHC class II and therefore cannot function normally. Measurements of T cell proliferation in response to stimulation by mitogens such as PHA are normal but responses to antigens are poor. Class II deficiency can be considered a form of SCID, and presentation, although slightly later, and treatment options are the same.

Defects in MAGT1 which causes impaired Mg^{2+} flux leads to reduced CD4 T cells.

Low $CD8^+$ T cells

Very low numbers of $CD8^+$ T cells (often < 50 cells/µl) are seen in zeta chain associated protein (ZAP) 70 deficiency. ZAP 70 is a kinase associated with the zeta chain of the CD3 molecule and is essential for T cell activation. Although T cell proliferation to PHA is absent, normal proliferation can be achieved by bypassing the TCR/CD3 complex using phorbol-myristate-acetate (PMA) and ionomycin. PMA acts directly to activate protein kinase C (PKC) which is a key kinase downstream in the T cell activation pathway of ZAP70. Ionomycin is a calcium ionophore, which works in synergy with PKC. ZAP 70 can be considered a form of SCID and the treatment is the same.

Patients with absent or reduced expression of MHC class I (sometimes also class II), also referred to as bare lymphocyte syndrome, have reduced $CD8^+$ T cells. There is a wide spectrum of severity of disease—some present with severe infections within the first few months of life and others are completely asymptomatic.

Key Points

- **Absent T cells can lead to a straightforward diagnosis of SCID.**
- **T cells, when present, should always be looked at closely, including CD4:CD8 ratio, numbers of cells, and the presence of activation markers. All these are present in the basic panel described. Any abnormalities will provide clues as to what further investigation are required.**

TCR gamma/delta T cells

TCRγδ T cells are $CD4^-/CD8^-$ or $CD8^+$. They represent about 5% of normal T cells. Their measurement can be useful as increases are seen in patients with DNA repair defects such as ataxia telangiectasia and cartilage hair hypoplasia.

They are absent in some defects of the NF-κB pathway.

11.3 B cells

11.3.1 Development

Like T cells, B cells are also derived from pluripotent haematopoietic stem cells. Unlike T cells, prior to birth B cells develop in the foetal liver and after birth in the bone marrow.

Pro-B cells are the earliest cells committed to the B cell lineage and express CD10 and CD19 on their surface. Surface immunoglobulin forms the receptor on a mature B cell, consisting of two light and two heavy chains associated with the Ig β and α subunits (these are responsible for intracellular signalling). The B cell receptor undergoes the same process of VDJ recombination as T cells to generate a diverse repertoire. The immunoglobulin heavy chain (IgH) undergoes rearrangement first. RAG and terminal deoxynucleotidyl transferase (TdT) (involved in the addition of new nucleotides during the joining of the VDJ gene rearrangement) are highly expressed at this pro-B cell stage. Successful synthesis of the μ protein enables progression to pre-B cell. At this stage no light chains have been rearranged and so Igμ protein associates with surrogate light chains λ5 and VpreB proteins. This plus Igα and β form the pre-B cell receptor. This receptor appears to send a survival message once assembled (no binding of the receptor with a ligand is required). Various proteins are important in this signalling pathway including B cell linker (BLNK) and Bruton's tyrosine kinase (Btk). This signal also inhibits IgH rearrangement of the other chromosome (allelic exclusion, when only one chromosome is used).

B cells have genes for two light chains, of which only one is required. The κ gene undergoes rearrangement first; if productive this will inhibit rearrangement of the λ light chain. This is why there are more B cells expressing kappa than lambda on their surface. The light chain will then combine with μ protein to form IgM; this is expressed on the surface of the cell now called an immature B cell. B cells now also undergo a process of negative selection similar to T cells. Any immature B cells that are auto-reactive have a chance of survival by undergoing a second gene rearrangement. If the receptor still reacts with self-antigens the B cell is deleted. This process occurs independently of T cells. Mature B cells now exit the bone marrow expressing IgM and IgD on their surface.

In the secondary lymphoid organs, B cells that recognize antigen, with appropriate help from a CD4$^+$ T cell, will undergo **class switch recombination** that leads to the production of antibody of various isotypes (i.e. IgG and IgA rather than just IgM). A further process called **somatic hypermutation**, in which mutations are introduced into the variable region at a very high frequency, will further increase the affinity of the antibody.

Class switch recombination
The process by which a B cell upon recognition of antigen will switch the production of immunoglobulin from IgM alone to other isotypes, e.g. IgG and IgA.

Somatic hypermutation
The introduction of mutations into the variable region of an antibody, to increase the antibody affinity.

11.3.2 Function

B cells recognize extra cellular pathogens and unlike T cells recognize antigen in its native or only partly denatured state. To respond effectively to protein antigens B cells require T cell help. Antigens with repeating segments such as polysaccharide and lipids can activate the B cells independently of T cells. Blood borne antigens will come into contact with B cells mainly in the spleen. Antigens entering through skin and other epithelial surfaces contact B cells in draining lymph nodes where mature B cells migrate. B cells found in mucosal lymphoid tissue will come into contact with inhaled or ingested antigens and tend to produce IgA.

The main function of a B cell is the production of antibody. The B cell receptor is the immunoglobulin molecule expressed on its surface. B cells express MHC class II and act as APCs presenting antigen to CD4$^+$ T cells from which they require signals to class switch.

11.3.3 Absent B cells

Key Point

SCID should always be considered in an infant with no B cells (MFE, Omenn's). The T cell subsets and activation markers should be looked at more closely to determine if the T cells appear normal.

X-linked Agammaglobulinaemia (XLA)

XLA occurs in 1/100 000–1/200 000 of the population. Affected boys present early from 4–6 months, after maternal antibodies start to decrease. They present with recurrent bacterial infections, small tonsils (absent germinal centres in the lymph nodes), and low immunoglobulins of all isotypes. Unlike T cell defects growth is usually normal. T cells will be normal in number and function and, although often completely absent, a small number of B cells may be present. XLA is caused by mutations in Btk (Bruton's tyrosine kinase). Btk is found downstream of the pre-B cell receptor, which is required for survival and maturation.

Treatment requires replacement of immunoglobulin with three-weekly intravenous or weekly subcutaneous injections. As with many immunodeficiencies recurrent infections can lead to irreversible long-term organ damage. Prompt and aggressive treatment of any breakthrough infections is required.

Mutations causing immunodeficiency carried on the X chromosome have some unique characteristics, which can be useful in diagnosis. Males only have one X chromosome and females randomly inactivate one of their two. In mutations resulting in failure of a cell type to develop, such as X-linked cyc SCID, all maternal T cells will have the normal X chromosome—this is referred to as non-random X-inactivation. In conditions where the mutation affects function and not development of a cell type, as in chronic granulomatous disease, the maternal cells will be about 50% normal and 50% will have the defect. In XLA Btk is found in monocytes, platelets, and B cells, but is only essential for B cell development.

Cross reference

Look at Section 11.9 for more information on chronic granulomatous disease. Figure 11.6 shows diagrammatically the maternal cells displaying 50% normal and 50% defected cells.

SELF-CHECK 11.2

When staining for Btk presence in a carrier, what would you expect to find?

Autosomal recessive forms of agammaglobulinaemia also occur due to mutations in the μ, Igα, BLNK, or λ5 genes.

GATA binding protein 2 (GATA2) deficiency, in which patients are susceptible to mycobacteria and papilloma viruses, and can progress to myelodysplasia/acute myeloid leukaemia, can present with no B cells, monocytes, or NK cells. This is one genetic cause of the clinical spectrum of disorders: MonoMAC, DCML deficiency, and Emberger syndrome.

11.3.4 Low B cells

Common variable immunodeficiency (CVID)

CVID occurs in 1/25 000–1/66 000 of the population. It is clinically heterogeneous and can occur at any age but often presents in the second or third decade with recurrent bacterial infections, hypogammaglobulinaemia (IgM can be normal), and impaired antibody responses. B cells are generally present but are often low in number. T cell function, as determined by proliferation responses to the mitogen PHA, can be poor. Patients can develop chronic lung disease and there is a strong association with inflammatory bowel disease. A sub-group develop granulomata and resemble sarcoidosis.

A diagnosis of CVID is made if:

(1) isotypes of antibodies are below two standard deviations of the mean

(2) there is an absence of antibody responses to specific pathogens

(3) there is a history of recurrent infection

(4) other causes have been excluded.

Cross reference

See Wehr (2008) for more detail about the EURO class trial.

The presence of autoimmunity is also included in some diagnostic criteria and profound T cell deficiency is an exclusion to the diagnosis.

Recently CVID patients have been further classified on the bases of their B cell phenotypes.

The diagnosis of CVID is only made when all other known causes have been eliminated. However, a number of genetic defects have now been identified in patients previously classified as having CVID or with decreased IgG and IgA and variable IgM deficiency.

Defects in the inducible co-stimulator (ICOS) and B cell activating factor (BAFF) can lead to reduced B cell numbers. BAFF is one of the family of tumour necrosis factor cytokines; it is secreted by mainly myeloid cells in the bone marrow and lymphoid follicles and provides maturation and survival signals to the B cells. ICOS expression on T cells is induced after stimulation by the T cell receptor and is essential for T–B cell interaction.

Defects in transmembrane activator, calcium-modulating, cyclophilin ligand interactor (TACI) and CD19, normally present with normal B cell numbers. CD19 forms part of a B cell co-receptor complex that includes a complement receptor that binds to C3d. When this complex is stimulated the signalling pathways of the B cell receptor are greatly enhanced. C3d is produced when complement is activated and can be found on microbes or antigen–antibody complexes. Although important in enhancing a B cell response, CD19 is not essential for its development. CD19 deficient patients have normal B cell numbers but low or undetectable CD19 on their surface.

Key Point

The percentages of T, B, and NK cells should account for 100% ± 5% of the lymphocytes. CD3 and CD19 expression can either be reduced or absent in some immunodeficiencies.

Treatment of CVID is very similar to that of XLA, with replacement of immunoglobulin with three-weekly intravenous or weekly subcutaneous injections.

11.4 Natural killer (NK) cells

11.4.1 Development and function

Natural killer cells are derived from pluripotent stem cells in the bone marrow. Unlike T and B cells they do not have unique receptors. As well as killing target cells NK cells also interact with other cells by secreting interferon γ (IFNγ) in response to IL-12 secreted by activated macrophages, enabling the macrophages to kill any ingested pathogens. NK cells kill by releasing granules containing perforin and granzyme B which kill the targeted cell.

NK cells have two mechanisms for recognizing a target. They express CD16 on their surface, which is a low affinity receptor for the Fc portion of IgG1 and IgG3. Pathogens coated in immunoglobulin will therefore be targeted. The second mechanism involves a balance between stimulatory and inhibitory signals. Cytotoxic T cells play an important role in killing virally infected cells, but rely on viral antigen being presented by MHC class I. However virally infected or malignant cells can downregulate MHC class I. NK cells express an activation receptor called NKG2D, the ligands for which are not expressed on normal cells but are upregulated by stress or DNA damage and are often expressed on virally infected or tumour cells.

Inhibitory receptors on NK cells such as the killer cell Ig-receptor (KIR) recognize different alleles of the HLA-A, B, and C molecules, ensuring that normal cells expressing HLA will not be killed. Only virally infected cells that have downregulated MHC class I would remove the NK cells' inhibition.

11.4.2 Absent NK cells

Key Point

T-B⁺ NK− SCID should always be considered in an infant with absent NK cells (MFE, Omenn's). The T cell subsets and activation markers should be looked at more closely to determine if the T cells appear normal.

There is a specific NK cell deficiency, but this is very rare with only a handful of cases reported. Clinical symptoms manifest in early childhood with increased susceptibility to viral infections, especially herpes virus (CMV, varicella zoster virus (VZV), herpes simplex virus (HSV)). Epstein-Barr virus (EBV) driven lymphoproliferative disease was reported in one of the cases.

The defect has not yet been identified but studies of affected families have mapped the defect to the centromeric region of chromosome 8.

NK cells can also be low or absent in GATA2 deficiency (see Section 11.3.3).

11.5 Additional antibodies

The next four sections (11.5–11.8) describe additional antibodies that can be used in the diagnosis of primary immunodeficiency. These include some that are absent in resting cells of peripheral blood and require stimulation before they can be detected. Antibodies can also be used to measure proteins found inside the cell, which require the cell membrane to be permeabilized (see Section 11.7).

There are a number of primary immunodeficiencies that would give normal results using the routine lymphocyte subset panel. Two examples are given of specific conditions which if suspected would require the setting up of additional antibodies. Also described is B cell phenotyping, useful for the classification of CVID and diagnosis of other primary immunodeficiencies.

11.5.1 Autoimmune lymphoproliferative syndrome (ALPS)

Clinically this condition presents with chronic, non-malignant lymphadenopathy with or without hepatosplenomegaly, severe autoimmune cytopenias (i.e. haemolytic anaemia, thrombocytopenia, and neutropenia), and susceptibility to malignancy. It can present early in the first few years of life.

ALPS is caused by a defect in apoptosis—there are a number described:

- **ALPS-FAS**

  Patients have a defect in Fas (tumour necrosis factor receptor superfamily member 6–TNFRSF6). They can have a germline and additional somatic mutation

  ALPS-sFAS- somatic mutations in Haematopoietic progenitor
- **ALPS-FASL**

  Patients have a defect in Fas Ligand.
- **ALPS-CASP10**

  Patients have a defect in Caspase 10.

  ALPS-U no mutations in known genes

  ALPS-phenotype increase in DNT but normal apoptosis

  ALPS -like diseases Caspase 8, FADD, Ras

A useful diagnostic finding is the presence of increased numbers of TCRαβ double negative T cells. Small numbers of double negative T cells can be detected in normal samples but these are generally TCRγδ. Increases in this population can be seen in viral infections. However DN TCRαβ T cells are usually < 1% of T cells. Antibodies against CD3, CD4, CD8, and TCRαβ would be required to detect this population. What is considered a significant level is variable but some quote figures as low as 1% of T cells. As with any low event group, when looking for these small populations, large numbers of events should be acquired.

Biomarkers, such as increased vitamin B12 and soluble FasL, can be very useful as part of an initial screen for defects in FAS.

HSCT has been used successfully to treat this condition. The patients have persistent benign lymphadenopathy, but with a high lifetime risk of lymphoma it is clinically very difficult to monitor and treat these rare patients.

11.5.2 Immune dysregulation, polyendocrinopathy, enteropathy, X-linked syndrome (IPEX)

Symptoms of IPEX often appear in early childhood as protracted diarrhoea, insulin dependent diabetes mellitus, thyroiditis, and hemolytic anaemia. There are often massive infiltration of T cells into the skin (resembles eczema) and gut. High levels of autoantibodies against thyroid and pancreatic cells can be seen.

Mutations in the Forkhead Box 3 (FOXP3) gene have been identified, leading to an absence of T regulatory cells (Tregs). Tregs are a small subset of $CD4^+$ T cells and classically have high $CD25^+$ expression and have been shown to be critical for the maintenance of peripheral tolerance. Although activated T cells express CD25, the absence of CD25 bright T cells can be a useful screen. An example of Tregs can be seen in Figure 11.3.

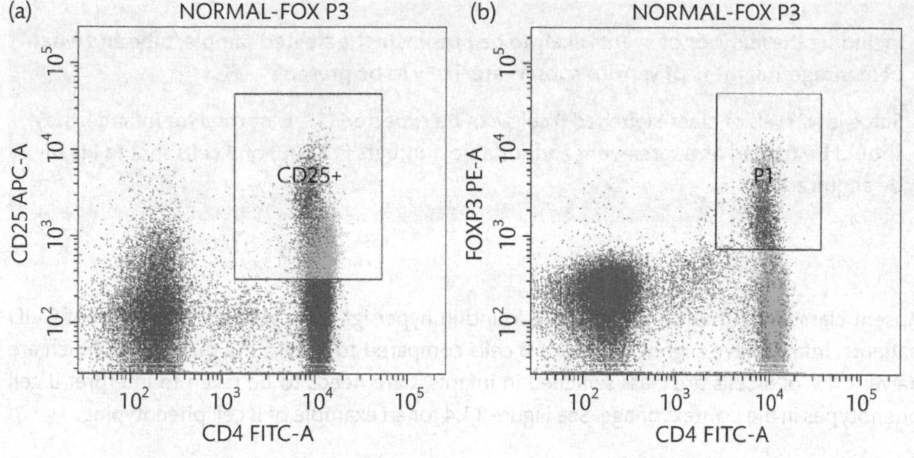

FIGURE 11.3

T regulatory cells. (a) and (b) show peripheral blood mononuclear cells first stained with anti-CD4 FITC and anti-CD25 APC antibodies, then permeabilized and stained with anti-FOXP3 PE. The FOXP3⁺ population denoted by the rectangle in (b) are seen as the purple population in the rectangle in (a). As shown, they are CD25 bright.

Early diagnosis is essential. Potent early immune suppression may control some features, but does not affect outcome and with an appropriate donor HSCT has been used to successfully to treat this condition.

Key Point

When diagnosing any immunodeficiency it is important to remember that there is usually a wide spectrum of presentations and laboratory findings. Absent protein expression may be diagnostic but the presence of protein does not exclude the diagnosis, as it may be non-functioning. The detection of mutations in a gene is an important addition to diagnosis but they are not always by themselves diagnostic.

11.5.3 B cell phenotype

Mature B cells on exiting the bone marrow are naïve in that they have not encountered antigen. IgM and IgD are expressed on their surface. They will preferentially home to the secondary lymphoid organs. Upon binding to antigen, CD27 is expressed. B cells process antigen and present to CD4⁺ T cells. Recognition of the antigen by the CD4⁺ T cell results in upregulation of CD40 ligand (CD154) on the T cells' surface which then binds to CD40 on the B cell, enabling the B cell to class switch from IgM to other isotypes. When this occurs IgM and IgD are no longer expressed. Antibodies against CD27, IgM, and/or IgD can be used to determine the presence of naïve, memory-activated, and class-switched B cells using flow cytometry.

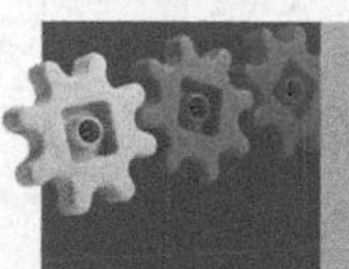

METHOD 11.3 Determination of naïve/memory-activated/class-switched B cells

If using whole blood, cells must be washed first to remove any IgM in the plasma. Antibodies will generally bind to free antigen first as opposed to bound antigen.

It is important to determine the number of events (usually cells) of a particular type to be acquired (i.e. data analysed) for each tube. A number of factors should be considered,

including the number of events likely to be present in the stained sample/tube and what percentage/numbers of various subsets are likely to be present.

Since low levels of class-switched B cells can be expected (1% is normal for infants), they should be treated as a rare event and suitable numbers (10 000) of B cells should ideally be acquired.

Absent class switch memory B cells are found in hyper IgM syndrome and a subset of CVID patients. Infants have high numbers of B cells compared to adults, the majority of which are naïve; < 1% of B cells are class switched in infants. Care needs to be taken to interpret B cell phenotypes in the context of age. See Figure 11.4 for an example of B cell phenotyping.

11.6 Inducible antigens

All of the antibodies described so far to identify lymphocyte subsets have been against structures present on the surface of resting peripheral blood lymphocytes. Some structures are only present for brief periods on the surface during activation, such as CD40 ligand. CD40 is constitutively expressed on B cells. Upon activation by antigen through the TCR/CD3 complex, $CD4^{+}$ T

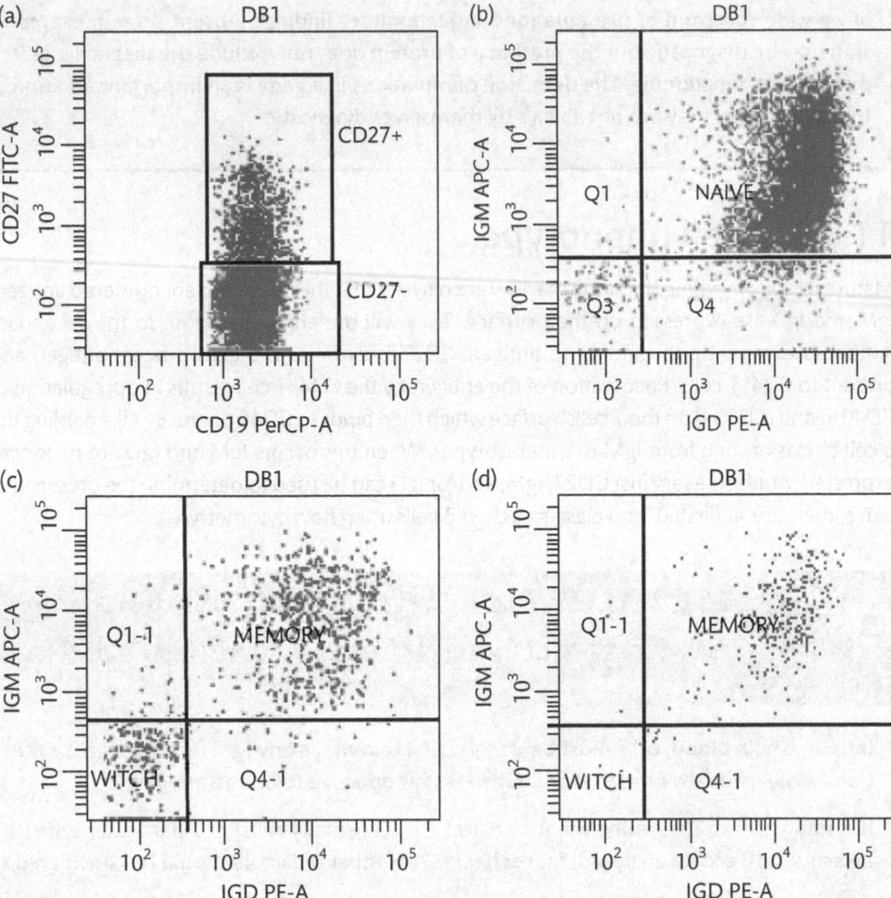

FIGURE 11.4

B cell phenotyping. These figures show lysed whole blood stained with anti-CD19 PerCP, anti-CD27 FITC, anti-IgD PE, and anti-IgM APC. (a)–(c) A normal child gated (a) on B cells; (b) on CD27– B cells; (c) on $CD27^{+}$ B cells. Pink represents CD27– and therefore naïve; the majority of these cells still express IgD and IgM on their surface. Blue represents activated B cells, some of which have class switched and no longer express IgD or IgM (bottom left-hand quadrant). (d) shows $CD27^{+}$ B cells from an infant with CD40-ligand deficiency; no class-switched B cells are present.

cells will upregulate CD40 ligand which binds to CD40 on B cells, resulting in the ability to class switch (i.e. make immunoglobulin classes other than IgM). CD40 ligand is expressed relatively briefly. An example can be seen in Figure 11.5.

Activation markers such as HLA-DR take a couple of days to upregulate and remain for a number of days, and are therefore readily detected on T cells in peripheral blood. HLA-DR expression on T cells is a useful marker since it will be increased in viral infections but also in oligoclonal T cell populations such as those found in Omenn's syndrome.

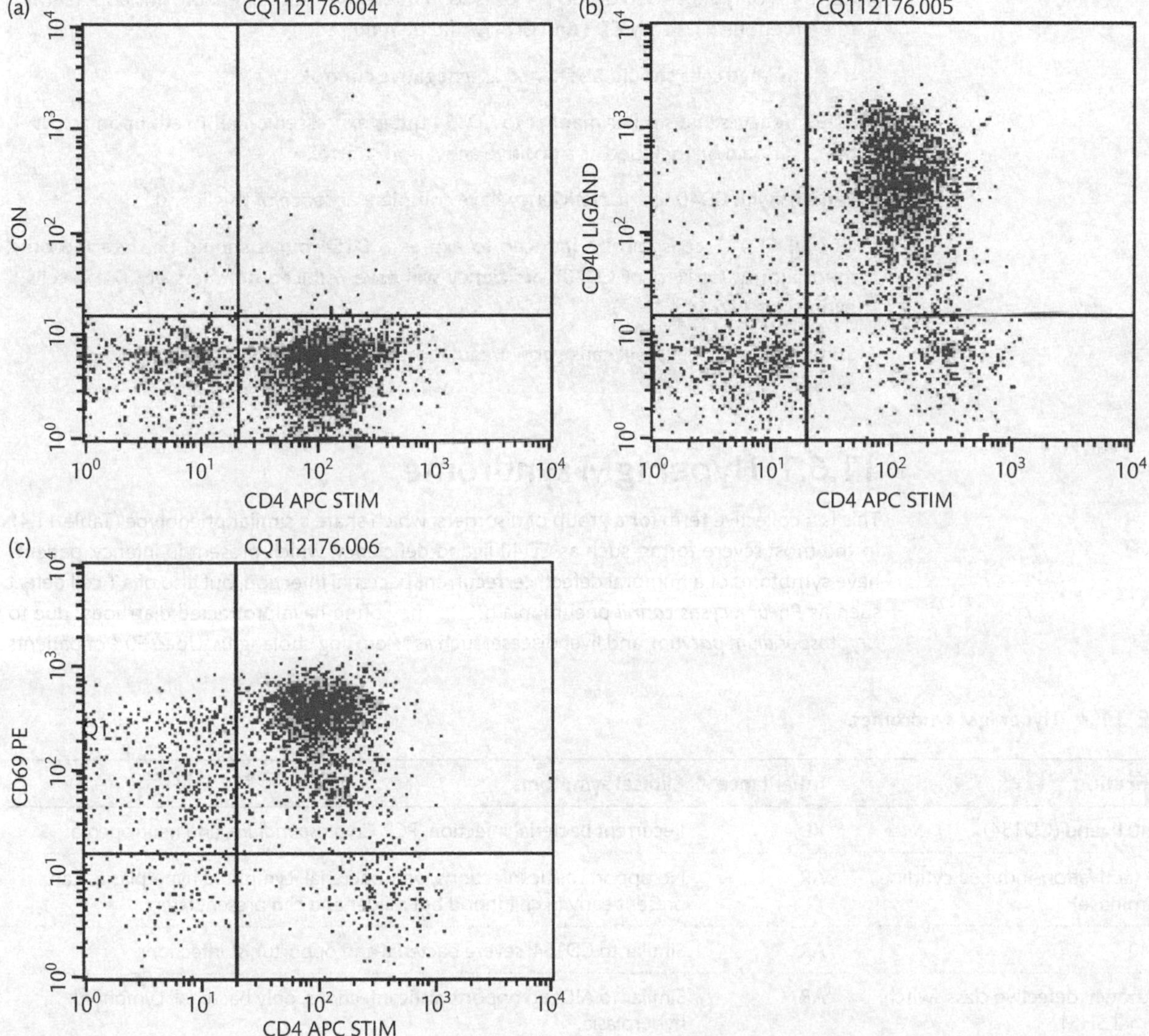

FIGURE 11.5

CD40 ligand assay. Peripheral blood mononuclear cells that have been stimulated with PMA and ionomycin for 4 hours at 37 °C and then stained with anti-CD3 and anti-CD4. All plots are gated on CD3⁺ expression. (a) Stained with the isotype control, which is negative; (b) stained with anti-CD40 ligand and shows the majority of CD4⁺ cells are positive; (c) stained with anti-CD69, which is positive for both CD4⁺ and CD4− cells.

METHOD 11.4 Detection of CD40 ligand (CD154)

Note: Not all defects in CD40 ligand will be detected by this assay.

This can be carried out on whole blood or PBMCs.

T cells will require stimulation, usually with PMA and ionomycin, for at least 4 hours. Antibodies against CD154 (CD40 ligand) can then be added, mixed, and incubated.

CD154 is only expressed on CD4$^+$ T cells so markers used should enable this population to be identified. Usually CD3 and CD4 would be required.

Unstimulated cells should be stained as a negative control.

CD69 behaves in a similar manner to CD154 but is expressed on all T cells upon activation. It should be included as a positive activation control.

Patients with CD40 ligand deficiency have complete absence of the ligand.

Not all CD4$^+$ T cells can be induced to express CD154 but it should be detected on the majority. Carriers of CD40L deficiency will have reduced numbers of CD4$^+$ T cells expressing CD154.

Stimulation of T cells will cause downregulation of CD3 and especially CD4.

11.6.1 Hyper IgM syndrome

This is a collective term for a group of disorders, which share a similar phenotype (Table 11.4). In the most severe forms, such as CD40 ligand deficiency, which present in infancy, patients have symptoms of a humoral defect, i.e. recurrent bacterial infection, but also of a T cell defect such as *Pneumocystis carinii* pneumonia (PCP). They often have protracted diarrhoea, due to *Cryptosporidium parvum*, and liver disease, such as sclerosing cholangitis. Up to 50% of patients

TABLE 11.4 **Hyper IgM syndromes.**

Classification	Inheritance	Clinical symptoms
1. CD40 ligand (CD154)	XL	Recurrent bacterial infection, PCP, *Cryptosporidium*, and neutropenia.
2. AID (activation-induced cytidine deaminase)	AR	No opportunistic infections, only bacterial. Lymphoid hyperplasia. Can present early in childhood but milder and can present later.
3. CD40	AR	Similar to CD154: severe bacterial and opportunist infections.
4. Unknown: defective class switch, normal SHM	AR	Similar to AID: no opportunistic infections, only bacterial. Lymphoid hyperplasia.
5. UNG	AR	Similar to AID: no opportunistic infections, only bacterial. Lymphoid hyperplasia.
6. NEMO (NFκB essential modulator)	AR	Ectodermal dysplasia (abnormal hair, teeth (pointed), and sweat glands). Severe bacterial and atypical mycobacteria infections.

AR, autosomal recessive; XL, X-linked.

will also have neutropenia. IgM levels are normal or increased whilst levels of all other isotypes are reduced.

Defects in the class switching of B cells are present and no class switch memory B cells are detected. CD40 is not only expressed on B cells but also on monocytes/dendritic cells and myeloid progenitors. This may explain the abnormal cellular T cell immune response, as monocytes and dendritic cell present antigen to CD4$^+$ T cells. This cannot be corrected for by immunoglobulin replacement therapy.

Haematopoietic stem cell transplantation has been used successfully to treat the more severe forms. Milder forms are generally treated with immunoglobulin replacement therapy, PCP and fungal prophylaxis, and careful surveillance for *Cryptosporidium*.

11.7 Intracellular staining

All staining described so far has been to structures on the cell surface. Intracellular proteins can also be detected by monoclonal antibodies if the cell is first fixed and the membrane is permeabilized. Many commercial reagents are now available. Many examples exist in the diagnosis of primary immunodeficiency where this technique is useful.

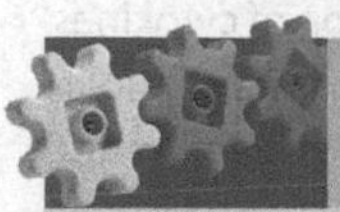

METHOD 11.5 Intracellular staining

To allow for the entry of an antibody inside a cell the membrane needs first to be fixed and then permeabilized.

It is not possible to determine if fluorescence detected by flow cytometry is intracellular or on the surface.

Some permeabilization procedures can alter the expression of certain structures both on the surface and inside the cell.

WASP and FOXP3 proteins absent in Wiskott-Aldrich syndrome and IPEX respectively can be determined by intracellular staining and flow cytometry.

Cytokines produced by cells after appropriate stimulation can be blocked from exiting the cell. This enables then to be detected intracellularly whilst simultaneously staining surface structures to identify the producing cell.

BrdU is a pyrimidine analogue and is incorporated in place of thymidine into the DNA of proliferating cells. Anti BrdU antibodies can be used to enumerate the proliferation of T cells in response to mitogens.

11.8 Functional assays

The presence of a cell type does not always mean it can function normally. B cell function can be determined in a number of ways, the simplest of which is to measure the immunoglobulins present. As described in Method 11.3, the presence of class switched B cells can also be detected. Specific antibody response to immunization antigens is a good method for assessing humoral immunity. T cell function is more diverse than B cells and therefore more difficult to measure.

Key Point

Live vaccines such as BCG should never be given to patients suspected of having a primary immunodeficiency.

11.8.1 Measuring T cell function

A basic function that can be measured is the T cell's ability to respond to stimulation, to become activated, and to proliferate. This is an essential requirement of T cells as part of the adaptive immune response.

In vivo T cells are stimulated by recognition of antigen in the context of MHC by the TCR with appropriate co-stimulatory signals. T cells can be activated *in vitro* by plant lectins such as phytohemagglutinin (PHA), antibodies such as anti-CD3, and antigens such as PPD (purified protein derivative -TB).

The most commonly used method is based on measuring tritiated thymidine incorporation into the DNA of proliferating cells. The major drawback of this method is the use of radioactive material. Other techniques that look at T cell activation involving the use of flow cytometry include the expression of various activation markers, such as CD69 and the secretion of cytokines. Methods that are equivalent to thymidine uptake, i.e. those that actually measure T cell proliferation, include the measurement of the number of T cells in S phase using DNA staining and antibodies to BrdU. Both these methods require permeabilization of the cells.

Another method uses carboxyfluorescein diacetate succinimidyl ester (CFSE), which labels intracellular molecules with fluorescence. With each cycle of cell division, the fluorescence is halved. This does not require a permeabilization step and allows for surface staining to identify specific cell populations.

11.8.2 Measuring NK cell function

The function of NK cells can be tested using a human leukaemia cell line K562 that does not express MHC class I. Killing assays using flow cytometry or chromium release can be used. Defects in cytotoxic cells such as NK cells and CD8⁺ T cells can result in a condition called familial haemophagocytic lymphohistiocytosis (FHL). This can be caused by a number of factors including deficiencies in perforin, Munc 13-4, 18-2, and syntaxin 11. Perforin expression can be measured by flow cytometry after first permeabilizing the cells. Other causes of FHL result in measurable defects in degranulation.

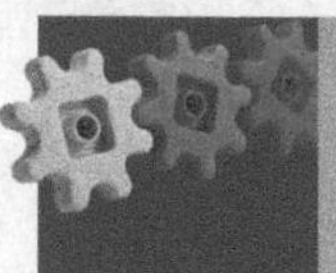

METHOD 11.6 NK cell degranulation assay

K562 cell line needs to be maintained.

PBMNCs are prepared from whole blood by density gradient. They are activated (stimulated with IL-2) or rested overnight in an incubator at 37 °C in 5% CO_2.

Rested and activated cells are then washed and incubated with and without K562 cells in the presence of conjugated anti CD107a for 2 hours. CD107a is expressed inside the

granules of NK cells and only detected on the surface once the granules have been released.

As with all functional assays a normal control is run alongside the patient samples.

Cells are then stained with CD3 and CD56 so that NK cells can be identified.

Cells are acquired by flow cytometry and the percentage of NK cells expressing CD107a determined. Activated cells will express a higher percentage than the resting cells.

Patients with some types of FHLH will have a reduced number.

Abnormal results would also be seen in patients with Chediak-Higashi or Griscelli syndromes.

11.9 Neutrophil defects

This section describes primary immunodeficiency due to neutrophil defects in which flow cytometry plays a role in diagnosis.

Neutrophils, like lymphocytes, are derived from haematopoietic pluripotent stem cells and develop in the bone marrow. They are short lived—10^{11} cells are generated daily—and are initially released into the peripheral blood circulation. To function effectively they need to be able to exit the circulation and migrate to the site of infection. They do this by responding to chemotactic signals such as one of the complement components C5a. To exit the blood vessels neutrophils need to adhere to the endothelium, which is facilitated by adhesion molecules present on both the neutrophils and endothelial cells. Neutrophils will then migrate to the site of infection. Neutrophils have various receptors on their surface involved in recognition of pathogens. These include toll-like receptors, sensing many common components of pathogens such as lipopolysaccharide found in bacterial cell walls, C-type lectins (dectin-1, dectin-2), and formyl-Met-Leu-Phe receptors (bacterial peptides). Patients with defects in dectin-1 or downstream in this pathway (CARD9) have problems with *Candida*. Pathogens coated in immunoglobulins and complement are termed **opsonized** and are readily phagocytosed by neutrophils as they have receptors for the Fc component of immunoglobulin and complement. Once the pathogen is in the phagosome, the activated neutrophil will undergo a respiratory burst during which highly toxic reactive oxygen species are produced and there is a significant ionic flux. Granule proteases are released as a result of this and these are primarily responsible for killing ingested bacteria.

Opsonization
The binding of complement and antibodies to the surface of a pathogen or foreign substance to aid phagocytosis.

There are many congenital neutrophil defects, but only two will be discussed here as flow cytometry plays a useful role in their diagnosis.

11.9.1 Leukocyte adhesion deficiency (LAD)

LAD is a very rare condition. In the severe form patients present very early with recurrent severe bacterial infections, especially on mucosal surfaces (perianal abscess). Those that survive into early childhood have severe periodontitis and gingivitis. They have poor wound healing with lack of pus and one of the earliest signs is delayed separation of the umbilical cord. A leukocytosis is also present as neutrophils are unable to leave the circulation. The defect in LAD1 is in the synthesis of the common beta chain (CD18) shared by three leukocyte integrins: LFA-1, Mac-1 (CR3), and p150.95 (CR4). These can be readily detected on the surface of neutrophils with appropriate antibodies. The severity of the disease relates to the degree of CD18 that is detectable, < 1% of normal CD18 in severely affected children. LAD1 can be treated by HSCT.

LAD2 presents in a very similar fashion to LAD1 but with no delayed cord separation and also includes mental retardation and the Bombay or hh blood group. CD15 (Sialy–Lewis X) is absent. It is a much less severe condition and infections are generally not life threatening.

11.9.2 Chronic granulomatous disease (CGD)

This is one of the more severe neutrophil defects and affected children do not usually survive beyond early adulthood. There is a failure in intracellular killing especially of catalase positive organisms, such as staphylococci, as well as fungi such as aspergillus. There is formation of granulomas especially in the liver, lungs, and gut.

The defect is in one of five components of NADPH oxidase that produces reactive oxygen intermediates (ROIs) important for the killing of phagocytosed pathogens. One of these components is coded for on the X chromosome, gp91phox. The other four components are inherited in an autosomal recessive fashion: p22phox, p67phox, p40phox, and p47phox.

Dihydrorhodamine is a dye that when oxidized by H_2O_2 in the presence of a peroxidase will change to a fluorescent form, rhodamine. This can be used to detect the respiratory burst by flow cytometry (Figure 11.7).

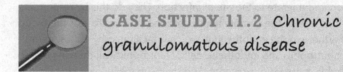

CASE STUDY 11.2 Chronic granulomatous disease

Patient history

A 4-year-old boy presented with cervical lymphadenopathy. He had a biopsy taken of his right cervical lymph node, which showed caseous granuloma. He was started on IV antibiotics for high inflammatory markers and spiking temperature. He was also started on anti-tubercular medication, but was still continuing to spike temperatures. On transfer to a paediatric infectious disease unit it was noted that he had had a mild failure to thrive and previously had a perianal abscess, which needed to be incised and drained.

Results

Following abnormalities noticed on a chest X-ray, a CT scan was performed which showed a lung abscess. A biopsy from this grew Burkholderia cepacia.

A neutrophil oxidative burst assay was performed on both his neutrophils and his mother's. Results are shown in Figure 11.6.

Significance of results

A diagnosis of chronic granulomatous disease (CGD) was made. Appropriate treatment planned. An X-linked defect in gp91Phox was confirmed and family testing/counselling arranged.

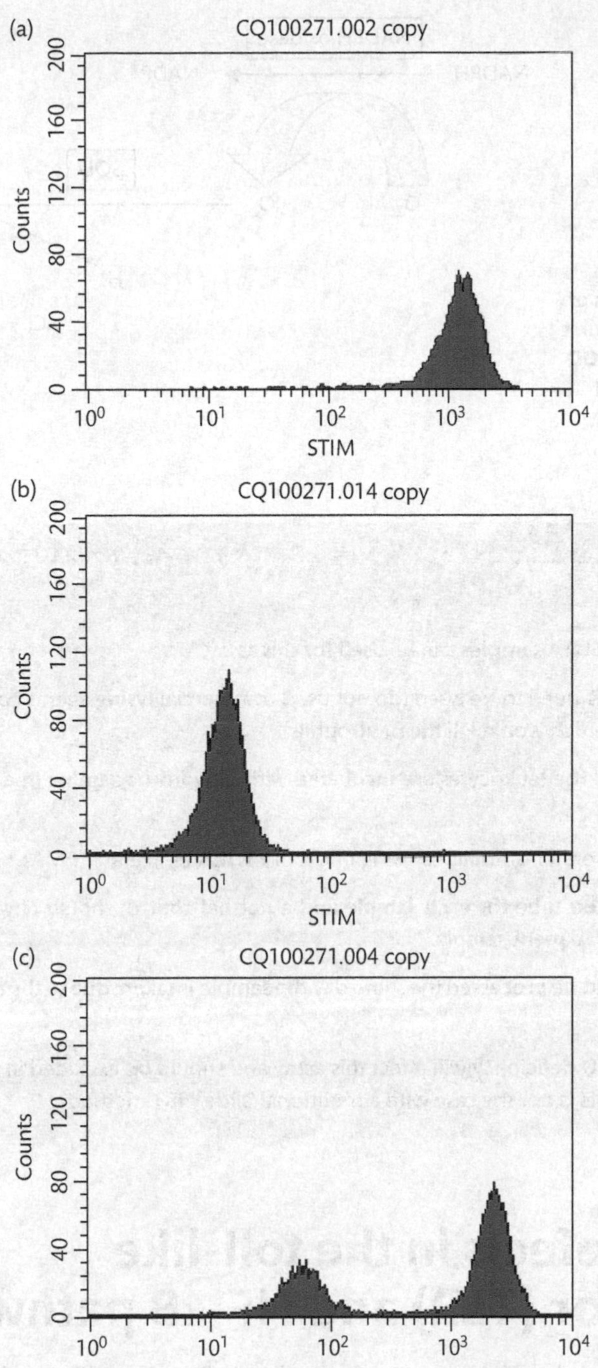

FIGURE 11.6

Dihydrorhodamine assay in chronic granulomatous disease. (a) A normal DHR shift after stimulation of neutrophils with PMA. The histogram shows data gated on neutrophils on the basis of forward and side scatter; (b) a CGD patient with no shift in DHR; (c) the mother of the CGD patient in (b)—she has two populations demonstrating that she is a carrier.

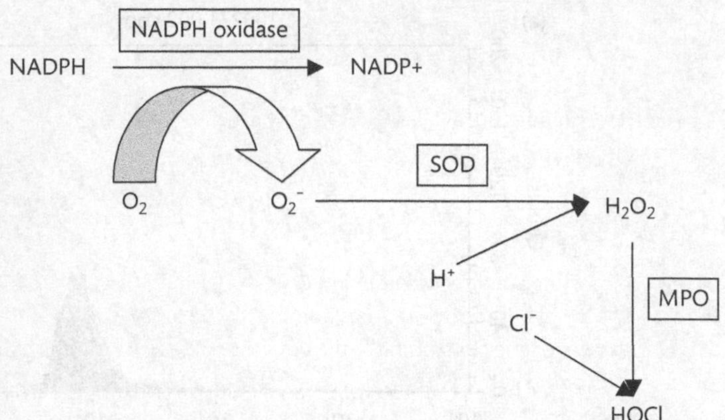

FIGURE 11.7
Neutrophil oxidative mechanisms for the production of reactive oxygen species (ROS) during the oxidative burst process. O2⁻ Superoxide, H_2O_2 Hydrogen peroxide, SOD Superoxide dismutase, MPO Myeloperoxidase, HOCl Hypochlorous acid.

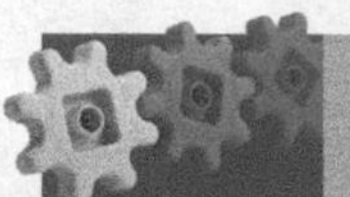

METHOD 11.7 *Neutrophil oxidative burst*

Whole blood EDTA samples can be used for this assay.

Red blood cells need to be lysed (do not used commercial lysing agents containing formaldehydes which would kill the neutrophils).

After washing, the leukocytes are incubated with dihydrorhodamine in a 37 °C waterbath.

Neutrophils are then stimulated using phorbol-myristate-acetate (PMA).

An unstimulated tube for each sample and a normal control should always be tested alongside each patient sample.

Samples should be processed the same day the sample is taken, due to the short half-life of neutrophils.

MPO and G6PD deficiency will affect this assay and should be excluded in an abnormal result. Note this is not the case with a traditional 'slide' NBT method.

11.10 Defects in the toll-like receptor (TLR) and NF-κB pathways

There are 10 TLRs in humans found on various cells including neutrophils, dendritic cells, T cells, and B cells, as well as vascular endothelial cells. They recognize foreign products found on pathogens such as lipopolysaccharide (LPS) from bacterial cell walls, and various nucleic acids produced in the course of viral infections. Some are found on the cell surface and others are intracellular; see Figure 11.8.

Stimulation of these TLRs leads to activation of a number of pathways, most important of which involves the nuclear factor of kappa light polypeptide gene enhancer in B cells (NF-κB); see Figure 11.8. The activation of this pathway leads to production of proinflammatory cytokines and type 1 interferons. These play a critical role in the initial inflammatory response.

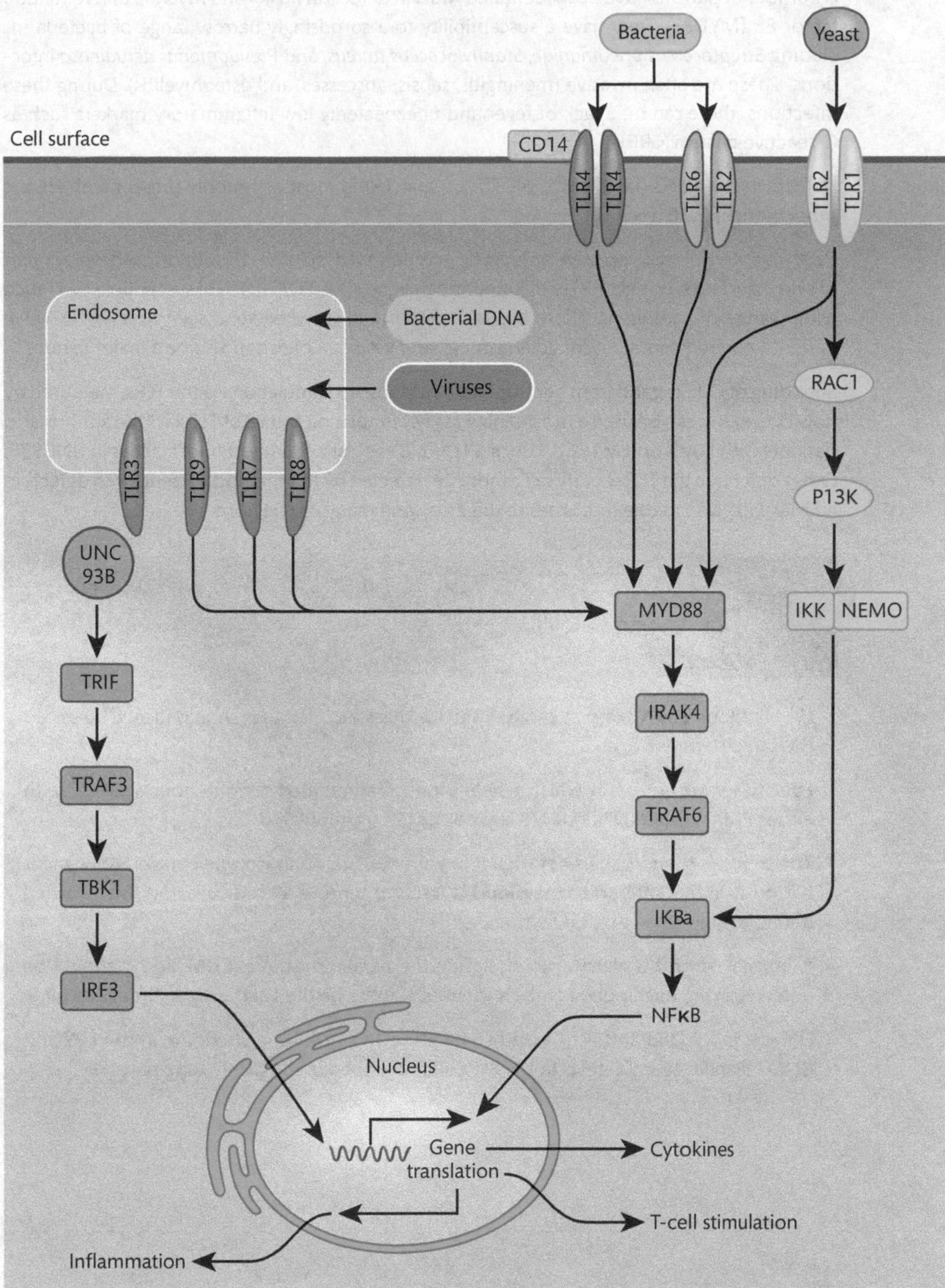

FIGURE 11.8

TLR signalling pathway and known defects. IKBα, inhibitory kappa B proteins; IKK, IκB kinase; IRF3, IFN regulatory factors; MYD88, myeloid differentiation factor 88; NEMO, NF-κB essential modulator; NF-κB, nuclear factor of kappa light chain gene enhancer in B cells; TBK1, TANK-binding kinase 1; TCR, T cell receptor; TLR, toll-like receptors; TRAF, TNF receptor associated factor; TRIF, toll/IL-1 domain; UNC93B, UNC 93 homologue B1.

A number of patients have been identified with AR defects in IRAK4 and myeloid differentiation factor 88 (MYD88). They have a susceptibility to a surprisingly narrow range of bacteria including *Streptococcus pneumoniae*, *Staphylococcus aureus*, and *Pseudomonas aeruginosa* infections. These are often invasive (meningitis, sepsis, abscesses, and osteomyelitis). During these infections, there can be a lack of fever and unexpectedly low inflammatory markers such as C-reactive protein (CRP).

Defects in the TLR-3 (UNC93B, TRIF, TB1K1, and TRAF) most commonly present with *Herpes simplex* encephalitis (HSE).

Patients with X-linked recessive anhidrotic ectodermal dysplasia—ED (abnormal development of skin, hair, and sweat glands) with immunodeficiency (XR-EDA-ID)—are susceptible to a much wider range of pathogens. These include the same invasive bacteria seen in IRAK4/MYD88 patients, environmental mycobacteria, fungi, and viruses. Colitis can also be a major feature.

Shedding of CD62 ligand from neutrophils in response to stimulation via the TLRs, measured by flow cytometry, can be used as a screening assay. Stimulation by LPS of TLR4 will be abnormal in patients with IRAK4 and MYD88. Use of a TLR-7/8 agonist will detect abnormalities in UNC93B. Other defects in the TLR-3 pathway cannot be detected by this method. Patients with defects in NEMO will give variable responses to this assay and many will be normal.

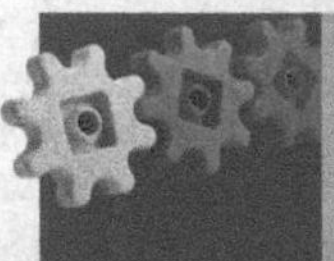

METHOD 11.8 CD62 ligand shedding assay

Whole blood EDTA samples can be used for this assay. Samples should ideally be tested the same day.

Four tubes are set up in which whole blood is stimulated for one hour at 37 °C with either PMA, LPS, CL097 (TLR 7/8 Ligand), or left unstimulated.

The blood is then washed before adding anti-CD62L or an isotype control. After incubation with the antibodies the blood is lysed to remove all red cells and then washed before acquiring on the flow cytometer.

A normal control is always run alongside the patient's sample. CD62 ligand should be detected in the unstimulated tube and should always be shed in the PMA stimulated tube.

Defects in MYD88 and IRAK4 and some NEMO will result in shedding in the LPS and CL097. Patients with defects in UN93B will fail to shed in the CL097 tube only.

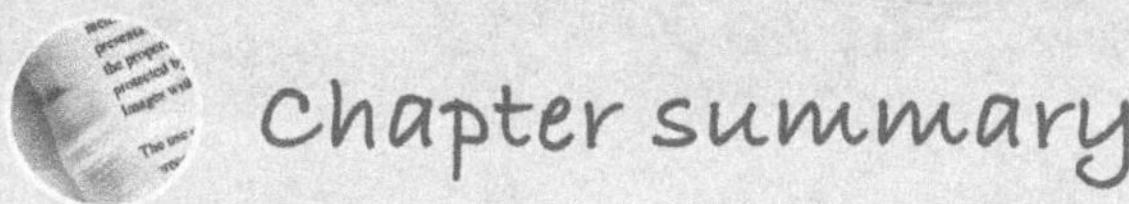

Chapter summary

- Flow cytometry plays a role in the diagnosis of a number of primary immunodeficiencies.
- A basic panel of antibodies can be used to screen for certain diseases such as SCID.
- The presence of a cell type or protein does not exclude a functional defect.

- For many primary immunodeficiencies a more directed approach is required to ensure the correct test is carried out.
- A number of techniques are available enabling intracellular proteins and cell function to be assessed.

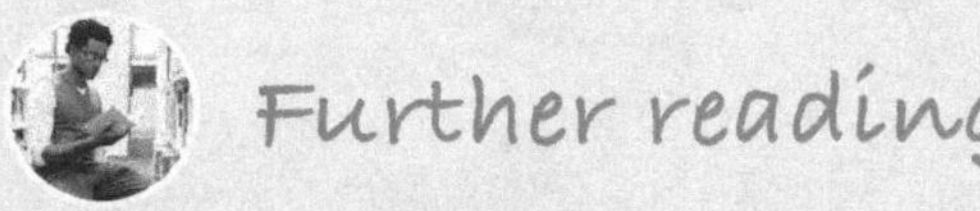

- **Male D, Brostoff J, Roth D, Roitt I (2012). *Immunology*, 8th edition. Mosby, St Louis.**
- **Murphy K (2011) *Janeway's Immunobiology*, 8th edition. Garland Science, New York.**
- **Ochs HD, Smith CIE, Puck JM (2013) *Primary Immunodeficiency Diseases: A Molecular and Cellular Approach*, 3rd edition. Oxford University Press, New York.**
- **Owen J, Punt J, Stranford S (2013) *Kuby Immunology*, 7th edition. W.H. Freeman, New York.**
- **Wehr C, Kivioja T, Schmitt C, *et al.* (2008). The EUROclass trial: defining subgroups in common variable immunodeficiency. *Blood*, 111, 77–85.**

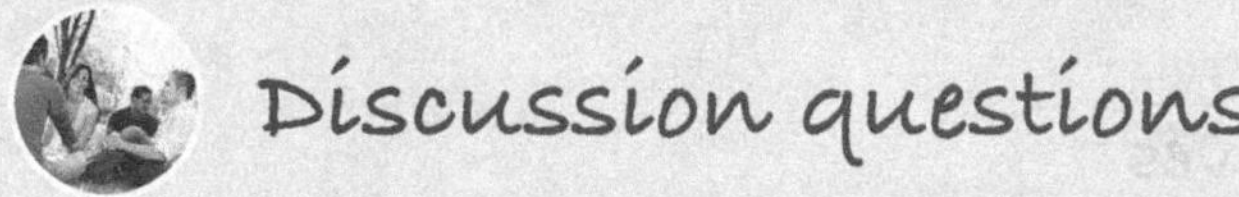

11.1 Describe the functions of T cells.

11.2 Which primary immunodeficiency would have absent B cells? How would you differentiate between them?

11.3 What are the clinical symptoms of autoimmune lymphoproliferative syndrome (ALPS)? What is the defect? What test could you do to help with diagnosis?

11.4 What would you expect to see in the mother carriers of the following conditions: X-linxed SCID, XLA, and CGD?

Answers to self-check questions are provided in the book's Online Resource Centre.

 Visit www.oxfordtextbooks.co.uk/orc/hall2e

12

Human immunodeficiency virus (HIV)

Learning Objectives

After studying this chapter you should be able to:

- describe how HIV transmission occurs
- understand how HIV infects cells and replicates
- describe the clinical features of HIV disease
- outline the assays and techniques used to test for HIV infection
- describe how the disease is monitored
- outline the treatment regimens for HIV disease
- discuss how drug resistance may occur
- understand how HIV transmission and infection may be prevented.

Introduction

The human immunodeficiency virus (HIV) affects over 35 million people worldwide and it is the most widespread cause of immunodeficiency. It is estimated that in the time since the first case of HIV was identified over 36 million people have died as a result of HIV infection (World Health Organization 2012) and over 1.6 million died in 2012 alone of HIV infection/AIDS.

12.1 The human immunodeficiency virus

HIV is a member of the retrovirus family and sub-classified within the lentivirus family. HIV can be subdivided into two main families, HIV-1 and HIV-2. At a molecular level HIV-2 is more homologous with simian immunodeficiency virus (SIV), a virus which when introduced into macaque monkeys causes an AIDS-like disease.

HIV-1 has three main classes; M (Major), O (Outlying), and N (New). HIV-1 class M accounts for around 90% of HIV-1 infections and can be further subdivided into nine different clades (or sub-types), A, B, C, D, F, G, H, J, and H. Due to continuous transmission, mutation, and recombination, the distinction between different clades has become blurred.

The HIV virus is shown in Figure 12.1; it is around 20 nm in diameter and almost spherical. The plasma membrane is derived from the host plasma membrane which encloses a capsid. The capsid contains two copies of single-stranded RNA which is tightly bound to the nucleocapsid proteins. Also enclosed within are the regulatory proteins Vif (Virus infectivity factor), Vpr (Viral protein U), Nef (Negative regulatory factor), p7, and viral protease.

12.2 The life cycle of HIV

Knowledge of the HIV life cycle is necessary for the design of strategies to help prevent infection and disease progression. You can see the stages of the life cycle in Figure 12.2.

HIV-1 uses the CD4 receptor and a chemokine co-receptor, either CXCR4 or CCR5, to bind to and infect CD4 positive cells. CXCR4 was the first HIV co-receptor to be discovered. CCR5-utilizing viruses are macrophage-trophic and more important in the infection of macrophages and early HIV disease: there are now selective CCR5 antiviral therapies. Viral HIV-1 strains differ in their ability to infect different cell populations and in their ability to utilize the different co-receptors. Mutations or deletions in the CCR5 co-receptor have been shown to render some individuals less susceptible to HIV-1 infection (Quillent *et al.* 1998, Libert *et al.* 1998).

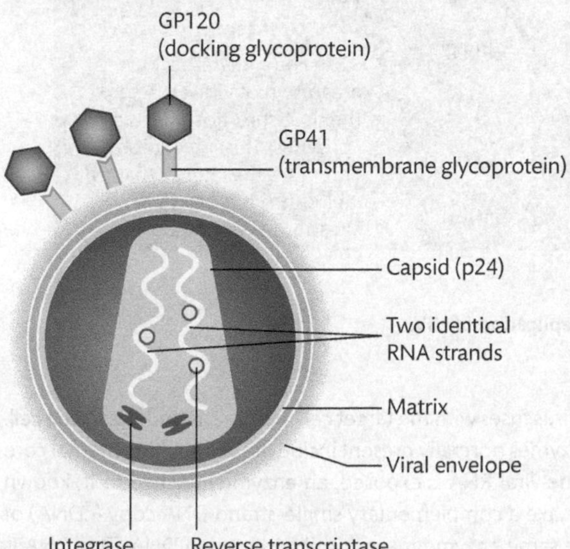

FIGURE 12.1
Diagrammatic representation of HIV virus.

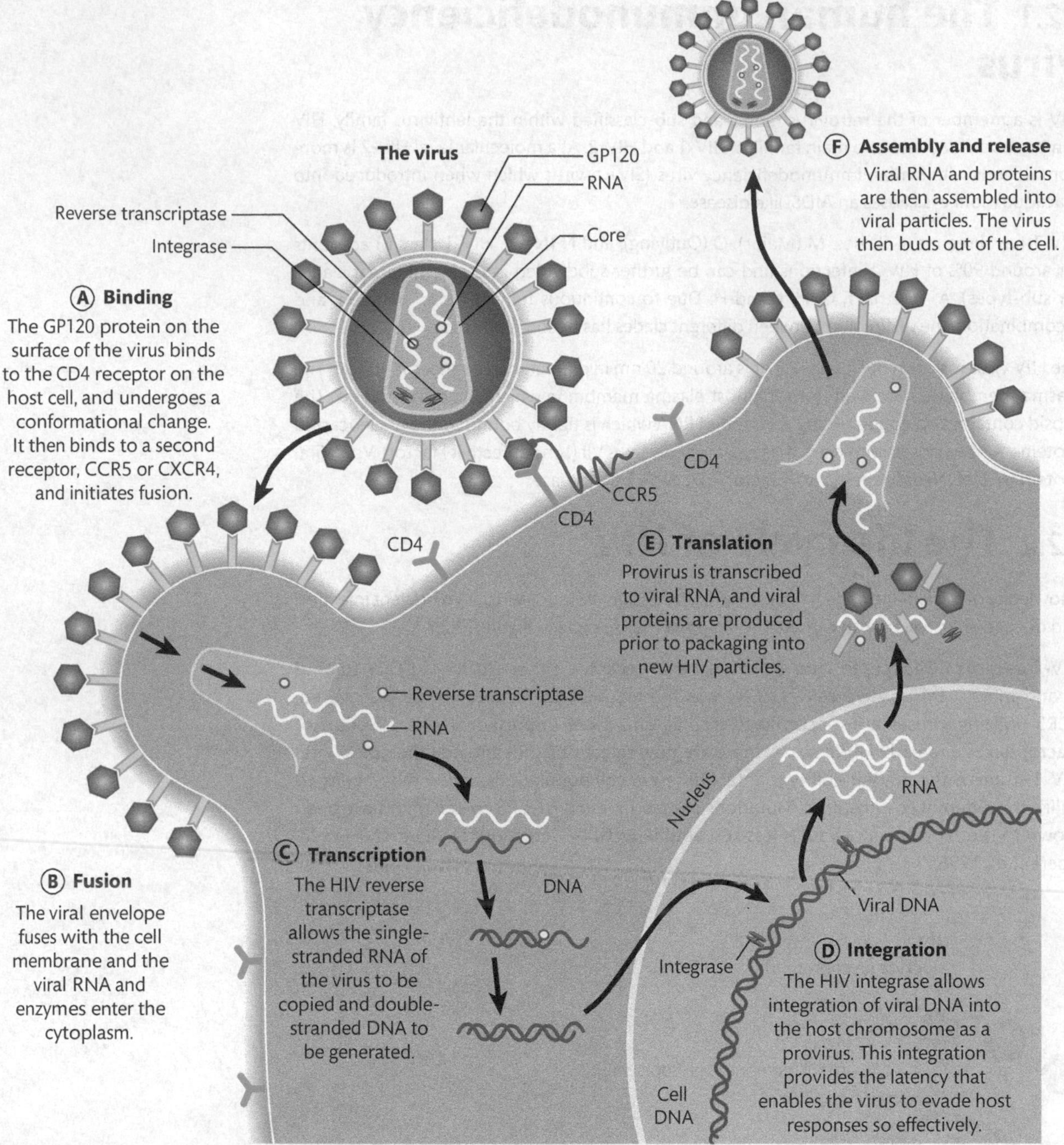

The virus
GP120
RNA
Reverse transcriptase
Integrase
Core
(A) Binding
The GP120 protein on the surface of the virus binds to the CD4 receptor on the host cell, and undergoes a conformational change. It then binds to a second receptor, CCR5 or CXCR4, and initiates fusion.
(F) Assembly and release
Viral RNA and proteins are then assembled into viral particles. The virus then buds out of the cell.
CD4
CCR5
CD4
CD4
(E) Translation
Provirus is transcribed to viral RNA, and viral proteins are produced prior to packaging into new HIV particles.
Reverse transcriptase
RNA
Nucleus
RNA
(B) Fusion
The viral envelope fuses with the cell membrane and the viral RNA and enzymes enter the cytoplasm.
(C) Transcription
The HIV reverse transcriptase allows the single-stranded RNA of the virus to be copied and double-stranded DNA to be generated.
DNA
Viral DNA
Integrase
(D) Integration
The HIV integrase allows integration of viral DNA into the host chromosome as a provirus. This integration provides the latency that enables the virus to evade host responses so effectively.
Cell DNA

FIGURE 12.2
Schematic representation showing replication of HIV.

Following cellular attachment, the virus fuses with the target cell membrane and enters the cell. The viral envelope is removed by enzymes normally present inside the cell and the internal core exposed and broken down. Once the viral RNA is exposed, an enzyme attached to it, known as reverse transcriptase, begins to make a complementary single-strand DNA copy (cDNA) of the viral RNA and subsequently the same enzyme makes double-stranded DNA. This DNA is then integrated into the host T cell DNA where it may remain quiescent ('latent infection') or be used as a template to make new viral particles. Multiple copies of mRNA are transcribed and the subsequent translation of mRNA results in the synthesis of viral polypeptides and proteases. RNA and structural proteins then gather at the host cell surface where they are cleaved by polypeptides into functional HIV-1 proteins. The virus then buds from the cell's surface and infects further CD4 cells.

Viral RNA copies are integrated into the host genome in the form of proviral DNA. The detection of such integrated, replication-competent proviral DNA is an important diagnostic marker in the evaluation of HIV-1 infection of newborns born to HIV-1 seropositive women. It is clear that viral integration and viral reservoirs established early in infection serve as a major obstacle in eradication of HIV-1 infection. Several anatomical reservoirs may exist, including the lymphatic system, the male urino-genital tract and the central nervous system. However, it is the presence of latently infected CD4 cells that provide a long-term reservoir of HIV-1 replication-competent cells. Proviral DNA can be used to evaluate viral infection in the absence of measurable amounts of the viral RNA in the plasma.

12.3 Transmission of HIV

Infection with HIV may occur following sexual contact with an HIV positive individual, sharing of contaminated needles and/or syringes amongst drug users, or very rarely through transfusion of contaminated blood or blood products. The latter cause is now extremely rare in countries compliant with the WHO standards for blood products for transfusion, due to improved screening of donations and pre-donation questionnaires—individuals with high risk behaviours such as drug addicts and/or those with a history of unsafe sexual practices are discouraged from giving blood. Maternal–foetal transmission may affect up to 25% of pregnancies to HIV positive women, though this has been reduced dramatically to less than 1% by successful antiretroviral therapy (ART) or delivery by caesarean section. A further 5–20% of babies born to HIV positive women may be infected through breastfeeding and consequently this is discouraged.

Maternal–foetal transmission is still a serious problem in the developing world, due to poor education about disease transmission and prevention, poor or non-existent access to antiretroviral drugs, and taboos surrounding bottle-feeding. The advice is further confused by the observation that transmission occurs more readily in babies receiving mixed feeding (breast and bottle) and mothers are now advised to choose only one type of feeding.

While healthcare workers have been infected with HIV after needlestick injury and through blood entering an open wound or mucous membrane, this is extremely rare. Transmission by a healthcare worker to a patient is also extremely rare—a case has been described whereby six patients were infected by a dentist following dental treatment. There is no evidence to suggest transmission through mosquito bites or other insect or animal bites.

12.4 Effects of HIV on the immune system

CD4 is a specific receptor for HIV-1. By infecting the very cell required to mediate B cells and coordinate cytotoxic cell responses, the body's ability to raise antibodies or kill virally infected cells is compromised. In response to HIV-1 infection, more T cells are produced which mature to become T helper cells, but then also become targets for viral infection themselves, thus helping to provide a fresh reservoir of susceptible cells.

With time, infection with HIV results in a progressive decline in the number of CD4 T cells and reversal in the normal CD4:CD8 ratio, causing a severe, progressive immunodeficiency. In particular, HIV-1 infects CCR5$^+$ CD4$^+$ T cells. Effector memory T cells (T_{EM}), which express CCR5 (CD4$^+$ CD45RA$^-$, CD27$^-$, CCR5$^+$), are prime targets for HIV infection, comprising around 15% of the peripheral blood T cells and regenerated from naïve and central memory T cells, and it is this population which is initially depleted in early HIV infection. The loss in the CD4 T cell count may be a result of a number of different mechanisms. These include killing of infected cells by the virus itself by the development of pores in the cell membrane of infected cells as a result of viral budding, fusion of uninfected cells with infected cells, and apoptosis or programmed cell death of HIV infected and uninfected 'bystander' cells.

Cells other than CD4$^+$ T cells also expressing the CD4 antigen are susceptible to HIV infection; these include monocytes/macrophages, follicular dendritic cells, microglial cells, and Langerhans cells, and may serve as a further reservoir for HIV infection and exacerbate the pathogenesis of the disease due to abnormal function. CD4 cells are necessary for the proper functioning of the immune system, through their interaction with antigen presenting cells, B cells, cytotoxic T cells, and natural killer cells. Lack of T cell help may lead to a number of disorders as described below.

The gut also serves as a large reservoir for HIV-infected CD4 T cells. In acute infection, there is an enormous depletion in the number of GALT-associated CD4 cells. Since the majority of intestinal lymphocytes express CCR5, it is not surprising that lymphocyte depletion is most significant within this subset of T cells.

There is strong evidence that HIV infection is associated with severe damage to the B cell compartment. **Hypergammaglobulinaemia**, exhausted tissue-like CD21 low B cells, and polyclonal B cell activation are hallmarks of the extensive B cell dysregulation in HIV infection and may be reversed by antiretroviral therapy. Memory B cells expressing CD27 may consist of around 40% of the peripheral blood B cells; these cells can be further sub-classified into IgM and class switched memory B cells—a pool of antigen-specific B cells which can rapidly differentiate into antibody-secreting **plasmoblasts** on restimulation. The IgM memory subset is extensively lost during acute HIV infection and this effect is not reversed by anti-retroviral therapy. HIV infection results in progressive damage to the memory B cells population (CD19$^+$ CD27$^+$) and impaired vaccination responses to common antigens like tetanus toxoid, and is associated with increased susceptibility to invasive bacterial disease.

Hypergammaglobulinaemia

An increase of gammaglobulins in serum.

Plasmoblast

A precursor cell of the plasmocyte, which constitutes 1% of the nucleated white blood cells. Not commonly seen in the peripheral blood of normal people, but can be seen in chronic infections, granulomatous and allergic diseases, and plasma cell myeloma.

Seroconversion

The detection of antibodies in response to an antigen (infectious organism). In HIV infection, the conversion from an antibody-negative to an antibody-positive state can take from one week to several months.

Infectious mononucleosis

Also known as glandular fever. An acute disease characterized by fever and swollen lymph nodes and an abnormal increase of mononuclear leukocytes or monocytes.

CLINICAL CORRELATIONS 12.1

Effects of depletion in CD4 cells

- **Hypergammaglobulinaemia through lack of CD4 cell control of B cell function.**
- **Autoimmune disease such as rheumatological disorders, SLE, Graves' disease, idiopathic thrombocytopenic purpura (ITP) and anti-phospholipid syndrome.**
- **Increased infections—viral, fungal and bacterial.**
- **Dementia.**
- **Inflammation and symptomatic bowel disease is common. The gut has been proposed as a major site of HIV replication.**

12.5 Clinical features of HIV infection

Following infection with HIV-1, around 10% of individuals develop an acute illness, called **seroconversion** illness. Seroconversion illness usually occurs 2–6 weeks after infection but may occur up to 3 months post infection and resembles **infectious mononucleosis**. The

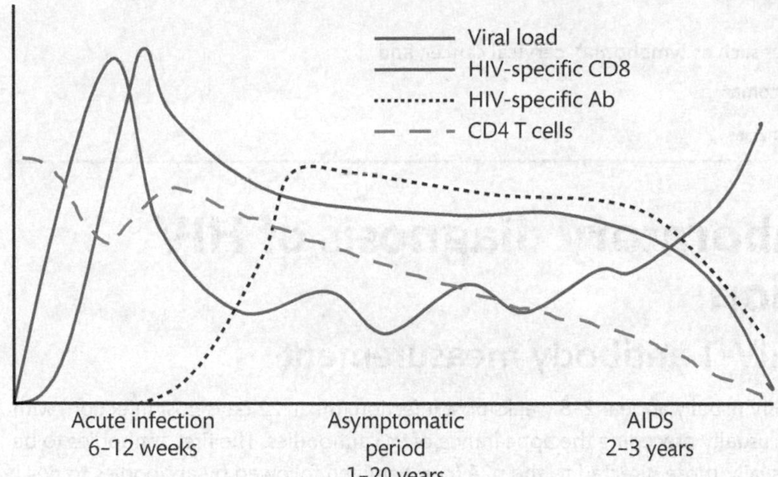

FIGURE 12.3

Effect of HIV disease progression on CD4 counts and viral load with time. Seroconversion illness is associated with a sharp increase in HIV-1 viral load and decrease in CD4 count. Following this, there is some regeneration of the immune system as seen by an increase in CD4 count to slightly subnormal levels and controlled viraemia. Over time, without treatment, the regenerative capacity of the immune system is lost, as seen by increase in viral load and steady decline in CD4 cell count.

symptoms may include fever, headache, sore throat, enlarged or swollen lymph nodes, malaise, and rash. Following infection, most individuals will remain asymptomatic for periods of between 2 and 15 years. The course of the disease varies considerably from individual to individual; in the absence of treatment, some individuals may rapidly progress to Acquired Immunodeficiency Syndrome (AIDS) while others are termed long-term non-progressors or 'elite controllers' and even after many years of infection remain asymptomatic with normal levels of CD4 cells, undetectable plasma HIV-1 viral load, and an absence of opportunistic infections. In the absence of antiretroviral treatment, progressive damage to the immune system eventually leads to the development of symptoms and recurrent infections with other viruses, such as herpes zoster and bacterial or fungal infections. These infections often involve the skin or mucous membranes, frequently in the buccal cavity. Skin disorders such as eczema or psoriasis may also be present and the virus may affect the gastrointestinal tract, causing weight loss, diarrhoea, and appetite loss. Figure 12.3 shows the laboratory observations at different stages in the disease.

12.6 Progression to AIDS

Continued damage to the immune system eventually leads to the development of AIDS—this is the most advanced stage of HIV infection. The Centre for Disease Control and Prevention's definition of AIDS includes all HIV-1 positive individuals with a CD4 count of less than 200 cells per microlitre or a percentage of less than 14. This late stage of the disease is characterized by a collection of opportunistic infections which would not normally occur in individuals with a healthy immune system. The UK definition of AIDS is based on specific clinical criteria such as opportunistic infections, e.g. pneumocystis pneumonia, rather than a laboratory surrogate.

CLINICAL CORRELATIONS 12.2

Opportunistic infections frequently found in AIDS

- **Pneumocystis jirovecii pneumonia (PCP)***
- **Toxoplasmosis***
- **Tuberculosis***
- **Extreme weight loss and wasting*; exacerbated by diarrhoea which can be experienced in up to 90% of HIV patients worldwide**
- **Meningitis and other brain infections**
- **Fungal infections**

- **Syphilis**
- **Malignancies such as lymphoma*, cervical cancer, and**
- **Kaposi's sarcoma***

*** AIDS defining illnesses**

12.7 Laboratory diagnosis of HIV infection

12.7.1 HIV-1 antibody measurement

Antibodies to HIV usually appear 2–8 weeks post infection (mean 22 days post infection) with IgM antibodies usually preceding the appearance of IgG antibodies. The first antibodies to be detected are usually those directed to the p24 (core) antigen followed by antibodies to gp41 (transmembrane) proteins.

Antibody screening alone may not identify HIV infected individuals in the 'window period' prior to seroconversion, and hence diagnosis in the acute phase of infection can be improved by the measurement of p24 antigen, which usually precedes that of the antibody (mean 16 days post exposure). However, p24 antigen levels in serum decline shortly after seroconversion so this antigen alone may only be present in approximately 70% of patients. The formation of p24 antigen–antibody complexes may account for the apparent decline in level of p24.

Immunoassays such as ELISAs and chemiluminescent assays are commonly used to determine the presence of HIV-1 p24 antigen, antibodies to HIV-1 (group M and group O), and antibodies to HIV-2 in human serum or plasma. Immunoassays are the most common way of identifying HIV infection and many commercial HIV screening tests combine the testing of p24 antigen and anti-HIV antibodies to enhance assay sensitivity. ELISA plates may be coated with anti-p24 antibodies to identify the presence of p24 antigen, together with HIV-1 antigens such as gp160, gp41, and/or peptides from HIV-2 envelope proteins, to identify antibodies with reactivity to both HIV-1 and HIV-2. The presence of HIV antigen or HIV-reactive antibody is determined by reactivity with an enzyme-conjugated anti-human antibody which, following the addition of a suitable substrate, will catalyse a colour reaction.

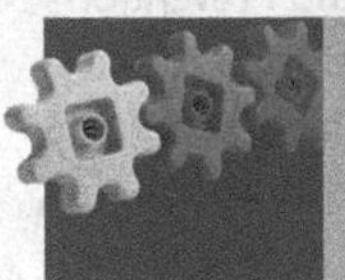

METHOD 12.1 Analytical sensitivity and specificity of HIV antibody tests

HIV ELISA tests have a high sensitivity and specificity of 98.4–99.9% and 99.3–100% respectively.

It is important to remember that false negatives may occur in the window period before seroconversion.

Depending on laboratory practice, negative results may be retested with another assay or automatically released. If recent exposure is suggested, then repeat testing may be recommended after a suitable time interval. Positive HIV tests are confirmed using one or more assays using a different test principle to the first so that it is unlikely to give a second false positive result. In addition, confirmation testing should be with a test of higher specificity to the screening test. Specialized confirmatory tests may include western blot or a line immunoassay or immunofluorescence antibody tests—these confirmatory tests can be costly and labour intensive but helpful when indeterminate results obtained. In line immunoassays, different HIV-1 and HIV-2 antigens are coated at discrete locations on a test strip and the reactivity of the antibody to particular antigens determined. For example, an HIV-1 positive sample may bind to gp120 and gp41 but not gp105 and gp36, while a sample positive for HIV-2 may react with gp105 and gp36 but not with gp120 and gp41.

Rapid screening tests or point-of-care testing using whole blood have a major role in the developing world where access to laboratory equipment is limited. The three main rapid methods available are described below:

- Particle agglutination: HIV-1 positive whole blood is mixed with latex particles coated with specific HIV antigens; the antibody cross-links the latex particles, resulting in the visual agglutination of the particles.
- Immunoconcentration: HIV antigens are immobilized on a solid-phase column and blood samples applied to the column. These assays require sequential additions of washing buffers and detection substrate and are thus slightly more complex to perform. A positive sample is identified by antibody binding to the specific antigens and visualization is colorimetric. Some immunoconcentration assays allow for differentiation of HIV-1 from HIV-2.
- Immunochromatography: In this rapid assay, antigen and signal reagents are combined on a nitrocellulose strip. Samples applied to an absorbent pad move by capillary action along the strip and if antibody is present it will combine with the HIV antigen and signal reagents to produce a visual band at a defined position.

A number of laboratories will attempt to determine the duration of infection by the use of 'detuned' assays under the Serological Testing Algorithm for Recent HIV Seroconversion (STARHS). Detuned assays take positive sera and then retest at sequential dilution and with reduced incubation times, thus reducing assay sensitivity. More recent infection is indicated by negativity in the detuned (less sensitive) assay. There are alternative methods, but with the common goal of assisting public health agencies in providing accurate incidence statistics by identifying recent and established infection.

12.7.2 HIV-1 viral load measurement

HIV-1 infected patients are monitored through measurement of plasma HIV-1 viral load, which measures the degree of **viraemia** (the concentration of viral RNA in the plasma). The prognosis for patients is worse for those with a high HIV viral load. Although the HIV-1 viral load test is not usually recommended as a diagnostic test, it may well be positive before seroconversion and hence when the HIV test such as those described above is negative.

Antiretroviral therapy may reduce the plasma viral load to levels below that of detection—routinely to a lower limit of detection of less than 20 or 40 copies HIV-1 RNA per ml.

The main method for detecting viral RNA is reverse transcription-PCR (RT-PCR). The RT-PCR based methods involve three main processes:

1) Isolation of RNA from the viral particle.
2) Reverse transcription of the target RNA to generate complementary DNA (cDNA) using HIV-1 specific primers.
3) PCR amplification of the target cDNA and detection by fluorescent probe.

It is essential that the design of the primer and detection probes are such that they bind to highly conserved regions in the genome and thus are not affected by the mutations which occur frequently during viral replication.

Quantification is made possible by the addition of an internal standard of known copy number, with identical primer binding region but reconfigured probe binding region. The internal standard generates a DNA product of the same length as the target RNA, but, by using two different detection probes with different emission spectra, the HIV DNA product can be discriminated from the internal standard—put simply, quantification is possible by comparing the fluorescent output from the DNA amplification product and that of the internal standard.

Real-time PCR enables the scientist to view the increase in DNA with sequential PCR cycles. Essentially, there are three main types of Real-time PCR methods, differing in the way the increase in PCR product is visualized; these utilize TaqMan Probes, Molecular Beacons, and SYBR green respectively.

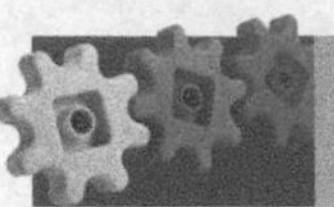

METHOD 12.2 Real-time PCR probes

- TaqMan Probes consist of oligonucleotide probes labelled with two different types of fluorophore, a green reporter protein and quencher fluorophore which bind to specific regions in the target DNA. When the probe is intact, the fluorescence of the reporter probe is suppressed by the proximity of the quencher. With sequential cycles of PCR, the reporter and quencher dyes are separated and fluorescence from the reporter protein is released and can be quantified. Each cycle of PCR is represented by an increase in fluorescence intensity.
- Molecular beacons also consist of reporter and quencher dyes, but with this system the reporter dye is wrapped around into a hairpin-like configuration, bringing the reporter and quencher dye into close proximity, eliminating the reporter's ability to fluoresce. In contrast to the TaqMan probe, the quencher and reporter dyes remain intact with each round of PCR. On binding to a complementary strand of DNA, however, the probe elongates, removing the reporter dye from the quenchers' influence, enabling a fluorescent signal to be released.
- SYBR Green is a dye which binds to all double-stranded DNA and can be used in Real-time PCR methods. SYBR Green, however, has no sequence specification and therefore may lack specificity.

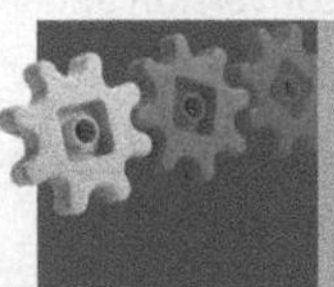

METHOD 12.3 Analytical sensitivity of real-time or kinetic PCR

The concentration of HIV RNA within EDTA plasma can be detected to a lower limit of 20 copies/ml with a positivity rate exceeding 95%.

The dynamic range is 20–10 × 10^7 copies/ml

Some laboratories have developed in-house HIV-1 viral load assays, which are used routinely to determine HIV-1 viral load.

Sometimes viral loads may become positive after a series of previously undetectable results; this is referred to as a 'blip'. Blips may be due to the sensitivity of the assay at the lower detection limit or may suggest adherence problems, developing drug resistance, illness, or vaccination. Following a blip, it is usually recommended to repeat the viral load to establish if this is a true one off, or a trend to a rising viral load. Repeated blips can be a sign of imminent antiretroviral failure, but may be a prominent feature of some newer generation assays and without overt clinical sequelae.

In addition to plasma, HIV-1 viral load can also be measured in other tissues such as the cerebral spinal fluid (CSF), seminal fluid, and breast milk.

The detection of HIV-1 in the CSF may be linked with dementia and CSF may serve as an important reservoir for HIV-1.

HIV-1 can also be detected in the seminal fluid of HIV-1 positive men. Many HIV discordant couples, (HIV +ve male and HIV –ve female) may wish to conceive their own biological child; however, unprotected sex will necessarily put mother and child at risk of infection. To reduce this risk, some couples chose artificial insemination using 'washed sperm'; this process can reduce the viral load to levels below the detection limit, commonly around 100 copies/ml, and significantly reduce the risk of infection.

Only a handful of laboratories also measure HIV-2 viral load and there is currently no commercially available HIV-2 viral load assay.

12.7.3 CD4 count measurement

HIV infection is characterized by a progressive depletion in $CD4^+$ T cells and a decrease in the CD4:CD8 ratio. The CD4 count is a good prognostic marker for the clinical progression of HIV disease. The likelihood of an individual progressing to an AIDS defining diagnosis in the absence of treatment increases with decreasing CD4 count. CD4 (and CD8) count can be measured by flow cytometry.

Cross reference

More information on measurement of $CD4^+$ and $CD8^+$ T cells by flow cytometry can be found in Chapter 11.

Lymphocytes may be gated by forward and side scatter characteristics, or a pan leukocyte marker, such as CD45, and side scatter characteristics, to distinguish them from other leukocytes such as granulocytes and monocytes. Then $CD4^+$ and $CD8^+$ T lymphocytes may then be stained with fluorescently labelled specific monoclonal antibodies. By using antibodies labelled with different fluorescent dyes and specific filters to detect each dye, multiple sub-populations of lymphocytes can then be analysed in a single tube and identified by their differing fluorescence emission profiles. While the percentage of CD4 and CD8 cells and the CD4:CD8 ratio is important, absolute counts are important prognostic indicators of disease progression. An absolute CD4 count can be obtained by adding to each tube a preparation containing a known number of fluorescent beads and comparing the number of cellular flow cytometric events with that in the bead preparation or by analysing only those cells within a predefined volume. A CD4 count of between 200 and 500 indicates that some damage has already occurred to the immune system and the current BHIVA guidelines advocate therapy at CD4 counts less than 350 and higher if there is clinical evidence of immune compromise. At less than 200 cells/microlitre there is a high risk of opportunistic infection and an AIDS defining diagnosis. Therefore, most laboratories now measure the absolute CD4 count as standard. Future flow cytometric tests to monitor HIV infection and disease progression may address the expression of CD45RA (a marker of naïve T and B cells) and CD27 to differentiate between naïve, memory, and effector memory T cells and the effect of HIV infection on these cell populations.

The effects of HIV infection on B cells may also be examined by flow cytometry although presently measurement of B cells dysregulation is more likely to be carried out in a research setting rather than a routine diagnostic laboratory. Deficiencies in B cell memory can be determined by the expression of $CD19^+$ $CD27^+$ IgD^+/IgD^- cells while exhausted B cell populations by the expression of $CD19^+$ $CD10^-CD27^-CD21^{low}$ cells. HIV-induced B cell immune activation may be evidenced by the increased expression of B cell activation markers CD70, CD71 (Transferin receptor; TFRC), CD80, and CD86.

12.7.4 Proviral DNA measurement

HIV-1 proviral DNA is integrated into the host genome. The identification of proviral DNA is a useful tool in the early diagnosis of infection in neonates. Neonates born to HIV+ mothers may have maternal antibodies in the circulation in the absence of HIV-1 infection and therefore a positive HIV-1 antibody test may be misleading. Demonstration of proviral DNA in neonates provides direct evidence of HIV-1 infection and active viral replication. It is a useful tool in the diagnosis of these infants enabling prompt initiation of antiretroviral therapy as needed.

Antiretroviral therapy may reduce the plasma HIV viral load to below the limit of detection, but does not completely eliminate infection or replication as evidenced by positive proviral DNA. Proviral DNA can be measured in isolated peripheral blood mononuclear cells/cell lines (PBMCs) using RT-PCR.

12.8 Treatment regimens for HIV-1 infections

Presently there are now multiple therapies available for treatment and/or suppression of HIV infection, each targeting different aspects of the viral lifecycle. The mainstay of therapy is induction and maintenance with three active agents; however, trials are currently looking at single agent maintenance to reduce therapeutic toxicity to patients in the long term.

- **Nucleoside reverse transcriptase inhibitors (NRTIs)** are analogues of DNA building blocks which must be phosphorylated by the body before they become active. During replication, the reverse transcription enzyme may insert NRTIs instead of natural DNA bases and terminate transcription; in this way NRTIs prevent HIV from copying its genetic information and replicating. NRTIs include AZT (Retrovir), which was the first ever anti-HIV drug. When first used on its own, AZT had serious side-effects. Now it is used in much lower doses in combination with other drugs. Other NRTIs include lamivudine, abacavir, zidovu dine, stavudine, etc.
- **Non-nucleoside reverse transcriptase inhibitors (NNRTIs)** bind to an adjacent area to the enzymatically active pocket of RT and inhibit its activity. They include efavirenz, nevirapine, delaviridine, etravirine, etc.
- **Protease inhibitors (PIs)** prevent the virus from assembling correctly before leaving CD4 cells. They include Darunavir, Atazanavir, Tipranavir, saquinavir, nelfinavir, and ritonavir. These drugs differ in their lipid solubility and their necessity for pharmacologic boosting to achieve therapeutic levels in the patient.

CLINICAL CORRELATIONS 12.3

HLA-B*5701 and HIV

Abacavir is associated with a severe hypersensitivity reaction in some HLA-B*5701 individuals. Screening is now becoming increasingly common before deciding on a particular course of antiretroviral therapy.

HLA-B*5701 is much more common in Caucasians–the incidence is 5–8% as compared with Asian or sub-Saharan African individuals (<1%).

12.8.1 New classes of antiretroviral drug

The new classes of antiretroviral drugs include HIV fusion-inhibitors, integrase inhibitors, and entry inhibitors.

Fusion inhibitors work by attaching themselves to proteins on the surface of T cells or proteins on the surface of HIV and prevent HIV binding to T cells and consequently from entering the cell. Currently there is only one FDA approved fusion inhibitor, Fuzeon (T-20). This drug targets the gp41 protein on HIV's surface. Some experimental drugs target proteins on T cells: TNX-355 targets the CD4 protein, and Vicriviroc and Celsentri target the CCR5 protein. These drugs are designed to prevent HIV infection of CD4 cells by blocking the receptors recognized by the virus.

Integrase inhibitors on the other hand work by inhibiting integration of the viral DNA (after the action of the viral reverse transcriptase to convert RNA to DNA). There is apparently no functional equivalent of this enzyme in human cells.

Maraviroc from Pfizer was the first drug of its class to be licensed for use as an entry inhibitor. Maraviroc binds allosterically to CCR5 causing a conformational change in the CCR5 receptor, thereby inhibiting viral binding and entry.

Cross reference

A list of currently licensed therapies can be found at: http://www.aidsmap.com/v635494203890000000/file/1187469/drug_chart_october_2014_web.pdf

12.8.2 Immune based therapies

Other treatment options may include immune based therapies using interleukin-2. This naturally occurring cytokine boosts CD4 production and hence strengthens the immune response. To date clinical trials have been disappointing in this area.

12.8.3 Drug resistance

The HIV-1 virus shows great heterogeneity both phenotypically and genotypically. During HIV-1 replication, reverse transcriptase encoded by the virus makes a RNA:DNA hybrid from which a double-stranded DNA copy is generated. However, as the HIV-1 RT enzyme lacks 3′ exonuclease activity, errors made during transcription cannot be repaired, and as the virus replicates variants may appear which can survive and replicate despite antiretroviral therapy, i.e. the virus becomes 'resistant'. In patients taking antiretroviral therapy, pre-existing drug resistant strains of the virus confer a selective advantage and, assuming replicative fitness, they may rapidly predominate and become resistant to antiretroviral therapy.

Two main techniques are available to identify drug resistant strains of HIV-1: phenotypic resistance and genotypic resistance.

12.8.4 Phenotypic resistance

Phenotypic testing is a direct measure of drug resistance, whereby the patient's virus is cultured in the presence of antiretroviral drugs and the ability of the virus to replicate is measured. This procedure can be time consuming as the virus must be cultured *in vitro*. However, by amplifying key portions of the genes within the patient's virus and inserting them into a laboratory strain of HIV deficient in those genes, this allows the production of a laboratory strain of HIV which is genetically identical to the patient's virus. The ability of the virus to grow in the presence of antiretroviral drugs is compared to that of a completely susceptible strain of the virus. One particular benefit of phenotypic testing is that combinations of drugs may be tested in combination or in parallel and it mimics the situation *in vivo*.

12.8.5 Genotypic resistance

Genotypic resistance testing involves analysing the viral genotype to determine the arrangement of nucleotides in the genome of the virus. When a mutation occurs in the virus which alters the coding for a particular amino acid, this may affect the viral susceptibility to antiretroviral therapy.

There are two main types of resistance testing: sequencing assays and point mutation assays or LiPAs. Both methods look for mutations at specific locations within the protease and reverse transcriptase enzymes of the viral RNA. Sequencing involves determining the nucleotide order of the amplified RT-PCR product and hence the amino acids encoded for, while LiPAs identify only a limited selection of mutation-associated changes in the genome.

Differences detected in the viral genome are compared with those known to be associated with drug resistance. If a particular mutation is found, for example, in the reverse transcription enzyme, this could mean that the virus is not susceptible to the antiretroviral drug targeting this part of the genome. This enables the clinician to prescribe only drugs to which the patient is susceptible. Mixed viral populations may also be detected suggesting emerging resistance.

The commercial sequencing assays generally have integral software packages with which the patient's HIV viral sequence can be compared, which highlights the currently known resistance-associated mutations and the viral susceptibility or resistance to particular antiretrovirals. Databases are also available on the internet, such as the Stanford University database, with which viral sequences can be compared to determine whether a certain mutation confers resistance to a particular antiretroviral. These databases are continually developing to keep up with novel observations regarding resistance.

Future genotyping tests will need to remain up to date with the newly developed antiretrovirals and look for resistance to integrase inhibitors, etc.

Sequencing assays can also be used to determine the clade (or subtype) of infecting virus and this can be useful in determining the likely origin of that strain of virus.

CLINICAL CORRELATIONS 12.4

Testing guidelines for HIV

The Current European Resistance Testing Guidelines, published in AIDS(2001; 15: 309-320) suggest testing for:

- **Treatment naïve patients, especially if transmission is suspected from an antiretroviral 'experienced' individual.**
- **Chronic infection, especially where transmission rates are high as evidenced by high viral loads.**
- **Post exposure–if a sample from the index case is available, this may be tested, although antiretroviral treatment may be initiated prior to an HIV genotype.**
- **Virologic failure, i.e. where the viral load is increasing despite antiretroviral therapy.**
- **Pregnancy–if the mother has a detectable viral load.**
- **Paediatrics–in infants with detectable viraemia.**

SELF-CHECK 12.1

Why is it so important to ensure that antiretroviral drugs are taken at regular intervals/consistently and that missed doses are avoided?

12.8.6 HIV tropism measurement

As discussed above, HIV-1 gains entry to CD4 positive cells by binding to the CD4 receptor and the co-receptors, or CCR5. Some patients are infected with a strain of HIV-1 which preferentially uses either the CCR5 or CXCR4 receptor or a combination of both, and this is referred to as the virus's 'tropism'. In the majority of patients CCR5 viruses are found early on in infection, but with disease progression CXCR4 viruses become more predominant. CXCR4 viruses are significantly more virulent. Since CCR5 blockers are only effective in those patients in whom the virus is predominantly CCR5, a knowledge of the predominant virus is important to determine which patients may benefit from treatment with CCR5 antagonists.

Assays are available to determine viral tropism; HIV particles constructed from the patient envelope protein are cultured in the presence of cells expressing CXCR4 or CCR5. These viral constructs or vectors are also encoded with the gene for luciferase. On infecting a cell and replicating, luciferase is released, oxidizing luciferin, a bioluminescent molecule, which can be quantified. Genetic tropism testing is a cheaper and quicker alternative to phenotypic testing.

12.9 Prevention of HIV transmission and infection

Given the latest epidemiological data, it is clear that new diagnoses are not falling, and indeed new diagnoses in Europe now outnumber deaths from AIDS, meaning that the number of people living with HIV is increasing, with major implications for health care, economic growth, cost, and suffering.

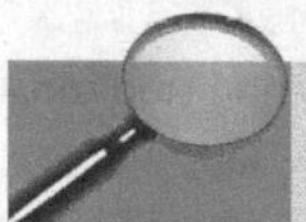

CASE STUDY 12.1 Grievous bodily harm

A couple (A & B) in a long-term relationship attend two separate sexual health clinics for HIV tests in June of the given year—both state that the test results are negative for HIV.

Several months later, one of them (A) attends the local hospital A&E complaining of severe flu-like symptoms, night sweats, and an unusual skin rash. The symptoms are consistent with HIV seroconversion illness and A is tested again for HIV and found to be HIV positive. A insisted has had no sexual relationships with anyone other than partner B. However, when B had a second HIV test, it was also found to be positive.

On reviewing the couple's HIV test results from June, it was found that B had in fact tested HIV+ on initial screening. It was suggested that B had lied to A about HIV status and was the source of A's seroconversion illness. B denied this.

Questions:

What blood tests would you perform to confirm HIV infection?

What other tests could you perform to confirm HIV infection?

Why might A's HIV antibody test be negative at the time of seroconversion?

What tests could you perform to determine the origin of A's HIV infection?

Novel methods of preventing both infection and disease progression are therefore necessary—behavioural changes including circumcision, microbicides, and prophylactic drugs and vaccines have all been considered. In the US a fixed dose combination of Tenofovir and Emtricitabine is licensed for pre-exposure prophylaxis.

12.9.1 Vaccines

Special challenges for a successful HIV vaccine are due to HIV integration, HIV variation, and its early harm to the immune system. These factors make the challenge of an HIV vaccine uniquely difficult compared to past successful vaccines.

Potential vaccines are being considered, developed and put into trial which:

1. Reduce susceptibility to infection (prophylactic vaccines).
2. Slow disease progression (therapeutic vaccines).
3. Reduce infectivity and therefore make transmission less likely.

A prophylactic vaccine should offer sterilizing cross-protective immunity to all the different clades of virus which are circulating. It should be safe, effective, and cheap. Current vaccines in trials include some designed to induce humoral immunity (antibodies) only, some designed to induce HIV-specific cell-mediated responses alone, and some designed to produce both. Many small phase 1 trials have been performed or are being undertaken, only two large trials have been performed, and neither has shown the vaccine to be effective.

Few therapeutic vaccine trials (with or without other immunomodulatory therapy) have been carried out. Some hopeful, although relatively short-lived, responses have been observed and it seems certain that such novel therapy will be most appropriate in individuals already receiving successful ART.

The possibility of modifying disease with a vaccine which, although not offering sterilizing immunity, may allow extra years of disease-free, ART-free life for the patient, and may also have an impact on the infectivity of the HIV+ individual, is exciting. It has been predicted that the numbers of new infections averted in 15 years could range from 5.5 million to 28 million from the most modest scenario (30% efficacy and 20% coverage) to the most optimistic (70% efficacy and 40% coverage).

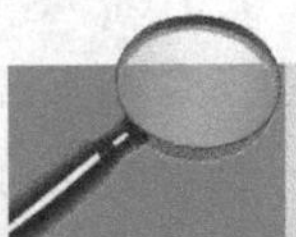

CASE STUDY 12.2 *Atypical pneumonia*

Patient history

A 23-year-old man is admitted via the emergency department with a three-day history of dry cough and increasing shortness of breath with a fever on and off for 2 weeks. He has no history of recent foreign travel, works in an office job, and on direct questioning had not previously been tested for HIV. He is a man who has sex with men and does not use condoms with multiple partners.

Results 1

Full Blood Count–Hb 110, MCV 89, WCC 5 (Lymphs 0.5, Neuts 4.5)

U&E–normal

LFT–normal

CXR–bilateral interstitial shadowing bilaterally

PO_2 8 kPa, PCO_2 7 kPa, PH 7.35 Room air

Significance of results

The patient is hypoxic on room air with Type 1 respiratory failure. His chest X-ray is consistent with but not diagnostic of PCP and he is mildly lymphopenic.

The patient was started on empirical treatment for PCP and an urgent bronchoscopy was arranged.

Results 2

Bronchoalveolar lavage (BAL):

Routine smear negative

WCC++

CRAG Negative

CMV Negative

PCP DIF = Positive

HIV1/2 Ab and P24 ag screen–Positive

CD4–34 × 10^6/L

Significance of results

The BAL confirms the presence of PCP and absence of concomitant pathogens such as cryptococcus (CRAG or Cryptococcal Antigen Test) and CMV (cytomegalovirus). HIV ab and P24 antigen testing confirm the underlying diagnosis. The CD4 count is consistent with an opportunistic infection, but may rise out of the acute illness and should be repeated once.

Patient outcome

When the patient had received 3 days of PCP treatment and had clinically stabilized a viral load and resistance test was sent. Wild type virus (HIV-1) was identified with no resistance mutations. Prior to discharge after 10 days of PCP treatment the patient was commenced on antiretroviral therapy, with a confirmed CD4 count of <50 ×10^6/L. He was virologically suppressed within 8 weeks and had a good immune reconstitution with no further specific HIV related problems.

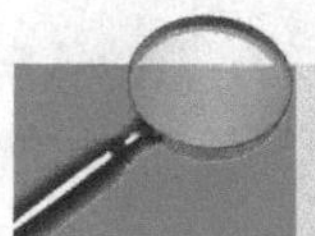

CASE STUDY 12.3 Kaposi's sarcoma

Patient history

A 23-year-old female presented to her GP with a rash on her legs. It had been present for some weeks and was painless. On examination the GP noticed a purplish rash which was nodular and non-blanching. The patient also had generalized lymphadenopathy and oral candidiasis. A biopsy of the lesion was arranged and taken.

Results

Histology: Non-communicating vascular sinusoids with immunostaining positive for HHV8/KSHV, consistent with Kaposi's sarcoma.

Significance of results

The patient was given a diagnosis of KS (Kaposi's sarcoma) and a careful sexual history taken prior to consenting for an HIV test. The HIV test was positive and her CD4 count was 10 ×10^6/L. A CT scan confirmed that there was no visceral involvement with the KS and the patient was started on antiretroviral therapy. The KS flared with immune reconstitution and then regressed, with a good long-term outcome.

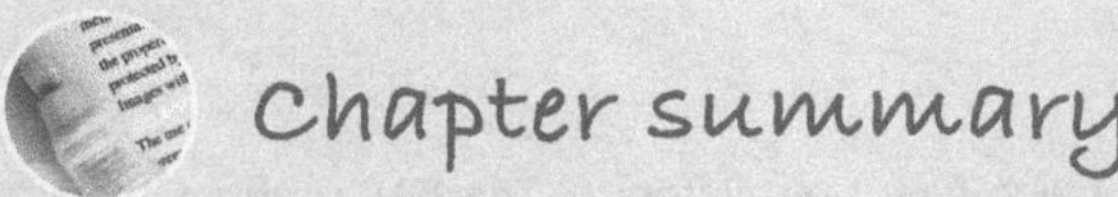

Chapter summary

- HIV-1 infection is the most common cause of immunodeficiency, and continues to be a major problem throughout the world.
- As yet there is no cure, though disease progression can be slowed significantly by the use of antiretroviral therapy.
- The ultimate goal is to eradicate the disease by production of a vaccine which protects against all the clades of virus and is realistic/practical for use in the developing world.
- Diagnosis relies on the detection of antibodies and/or viral proteins, usually by ELISA, although some rapid tests are available which can prove particularly useful in the developing world.
- Prognosis is generally worse for those individuals with high viral loads and low CD4 counts.
- Response to treatment is determined by monitoring CD4 count and viral load.
- Failure to control the adverse effects on the immune system, as seen by decreasing CD4 count and increasing viral load, may suggest treatment failure (developing resistance) or poor patient compliance–the former can be determined by genotypic and phenotypic resistance testing.

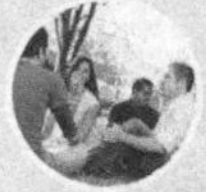

Discussion questions

12.1 How can you test for HIV?

12.2 Do the current methods for HIV also detect HIV-2?

12.3 What do you understand by the term seroconversion?

12.4 What symptoms might you expect to see during seroconversion?

12.5 What do you understand by the term long-term non-progressor?

12.6 How can you monitor disease progression and/or therapy efficacy?

12.7 How can you determine why a treatment regimen is failing?

12.8 If no resistance mutations are detected, why else might the antiretroviral therapy be failing?

12.9 Why do you think there is no effective HIV-1 vaccine?

Answers to self-check questions are provided in the book's Online Resource Centre.

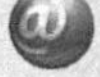

Visit www.oxfordtextbooks.co.uk/orc/hall2e

13

Histocompatibility and immunogenetics

Learning Objectives

After studying this chapter you should be able to:

- outline the immunological basis of histocompatibility and immunogenetics
- describe the major features of the HLA system
- describe the clinical and laboratory techniques used to HLA type, identify HLA antibodies, and crossmatch for transplants
- discuss the advantages and limitations of these techniques
- outline the role of HLA in transplantation and disease
- discuss the use of HLA in the allocation of organs and tissue
- explain how HLA is associated with autoimmune disease and drug hypersensitivity.

Introduction

In this chapter we will look at the human leukocyte antigen (HLA) system and describe the evolution of techniques for determining HLA antigen presentation and gives an insight into the role of HLA in clinical transplantation and disease association. The chapter describes in detail the methods used in the clinical Histocompatibility and Immunogenetics (H&I) laboratory to determine these antigens, details the genes involved, and explains the nomenclature system currently in use. Furthermore, we will look at laboratory techniques for determining the specificity of antibodies to the HLA system, the laboratory techniques employed to ensure there are no antibodies present at the time of transplant, and the implication of HLA antibodies detected post transplantation.

The chapter describes the role of the HLA system in disease, and demonstrates how, via several different mechanisms, HLA genes/molecules are associated or involved in the pathogenesis of autoimmune diseases and drug hypersensitivity.

13.1 The major histocompatibility complex (MHC)

Major histocompatibility complex (MHC)
A group of genes that code for cell-surface histocompatibility antigens and are the principal determinants of tissue type and transplant compatibility.

Human leukocyte antigen (HLA)
A genetically determined series of markers (antigens) present on human white blood cells (leukocytes) and on tissues that are important in histocompatibility.

Cross reference
You can read more about complement in Chapter 4.

The **major histocompatibility complex (MHC)** is a gene-dense region, which in humans is located on the short arm of chromosome 6. The MHC in humans is located at 6p21.3 and spans four megabases, encapsulating the greatest number of genes involved in immune responsiveness. The MHC is split into three major regions—class I, class II, and class III—each encoding different proteins/molecules, including the polymorphic class I and class II **human leukocyte antigens (HLA)**. The class III region may arguably be regarded as misnamed as it does not contain genes that produce the classical HLA molecules. The class III region consists of a collection of immunologically functional genes such as complement, tumour necrosis factor, and heat shock protein genes.

HLA class I is involved in the presentation of antigens of intracellular origin and HLA class II is involved in the presentation of extracellular antigens. Both of these molecules present peptides to T cells via the T cell receptors (TCR). HLA class I presents peptides to $CD8^+$ cytotoxic T cells and HLA class II presents peptides to $CD4^+$ helper T cells.

13.1.1 HLA Class I

A HLA class I molecule consists of an alpha chain consisting of three extracellular domains, a transmembrane region, and a cytoplasmic tail, closely associated with and stabilized by a non-polymorphic β chain beta-2-microglobulin, a protein encoded on chromosome 15. Most of the polymorphism of HLA class I is seen in the membrane distal α1 and α2 domains, the area of the molecule where peptides are bound; the α3 domain of the HLA class I molecule also contains a ligand for the CD8 molecule. HLA class I is expressed on the surface of most nucleated cells. HLA class I molecules have a 'closed' peptide binding groove and preferentially bind peptides of eight to ten amino acids in length. They have six side-chain pockets to accommodate side chains of amino acids, although all of the pockets are not always occupied. These two features determine which amino acids readily bind to the HLA class I molecule. Look at Figure 13.1 to see the structure of the HLA class I molecule.

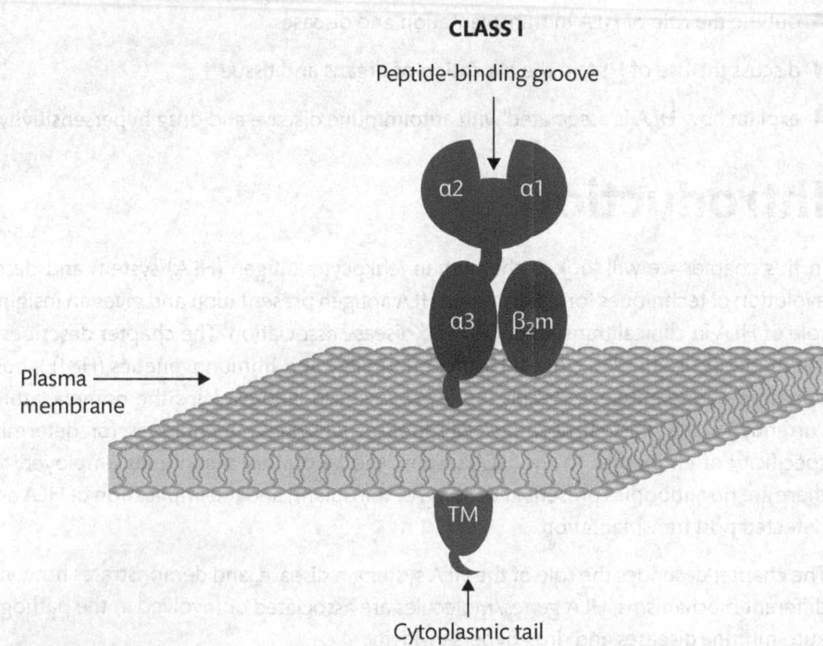

FIGURE 13.1
HLA class I molecule showing the peptide binding grove between the alpha 1 and alpha 2 domains, beta-2-microglobulin, and cytoplasmic tail.

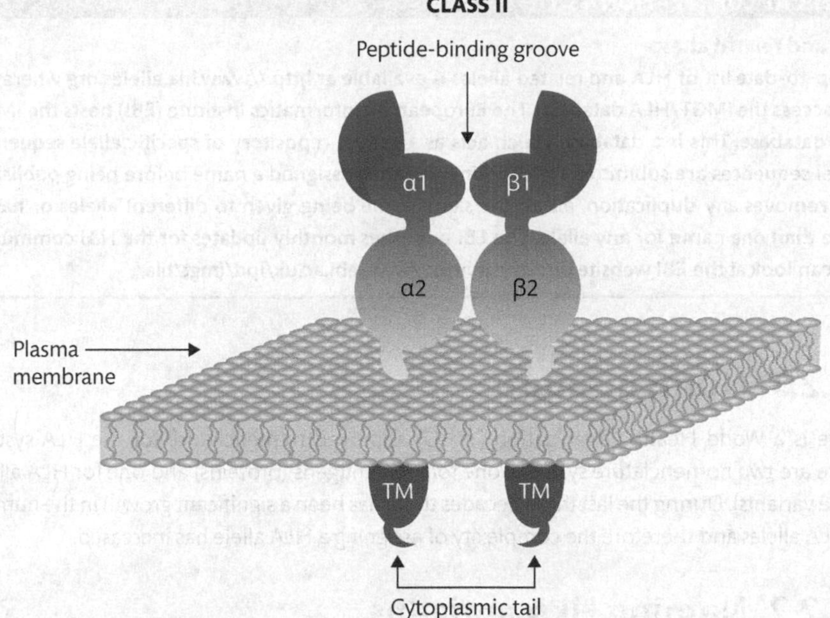

FIGURE 13.2
HLA class II molecule showing separate alpha and beta chains, the peptide-binding groove between the alpha 1 and beta 1 domains, and cytoplasmic tails.

13.1.2 HLA Class II

The HLA class II molecule consists of an alpha chain and a beta chain, both consisting of two extracellular domains a transmembrane region and a cytoplasmic tail. HLA class II is expressed on the surface of macrophages, monocytes, dendritic cells, B cells, and activated T cells, and is also gamma-interferon inducible on many other cell types. HLA class II molecules bind longer peptides than HLA class I, these generally being between 12 and 24 amino acids in length. However, as the peptide-binding groove of HLA class II molecules is open these can be any length. The β2 domain of the HLA class II molecule also contains a ligand for the CD4 molecule expressed on T helper cells. HLA class II molecules have five amino acid side-chain pockets in the peptide-binding groove, made up from both the alpha and beta chains. Similarly to HLA class I, these features determine the repertoire of amino acids that can stably bind to HLA class II molecules. Look at Figure 13.2 to see the structure of the HLA class II molecule.

SELF-CHECK 13.1

What is the difference between HLA class I and HLA class II? How does this affect their function?

13.2 HLA system

The HLA genes are the most polymorphic part of the MHC, and, although there are several other genes, these tend to have different functions in antigen processing and presentation and immunity. HLA is not only polymorphic, it is also polygenic, and these two factors make HLA matching very difficult. This system is highly complex with 12,672 HLA and related alleles described (correct as of February 2015).

CLINICAL CORRELATION 13.1

HLA and related alleles

An up-to-date list of HLA and related alleles is available at http://www.hla.alleles.org where you can access the IMGT/HLA database. The European Bioinformatics Institute (EBI) hosts the IMGT/HLA database. This is a database which acts as a central repository of specific allele sequences. Novel sequences are submitted for checking and then assigned a name before being published. This removes any duplication, either the same name being given to different alleles or having more than one name for any allele. The EBI publishes monthly updates for the H&I community. You can look at the EBI website directly at http://www.ebi.ac.uk/ipd/imgt/hla/.

13.2.1 Nomenclature

There is a World Health Organization (WHO) approved nomenclature for the HLA system. There are two nomenclature systems, one for HLA antigens (proteins) and one for HLA alleles (gene variants). During the last three decades there has been a significant growth in the number of HLA alleles and therefore the complexity of assigning a HLA allele has increased.

13.2.2 Naming HLA antigens

The naming of HLA antigens is determined by the WHO Committee for Factors of the HLA System who met following the International Histocompatibility Workshops. This committee named antigens once there was significant evidence to support the antigen's existence, historically assigning a 'w' to demonstrate it had been 'workshop' assigned. Antigens were named on the basis of their protein structure and epitopes presented, i.e. their serological similarity and differences with other HLA antigens.

13.2.3 Naming HLA alleles

HLA alleles are named in a systematic way (see Figure 13.3). The position and syntax of the naming indicates information about the HLA allele and is dependent on the DNA and protein sequence of the allele and its similarity to other HLA alleles. All HLA alleles have a minimum of four digits following the prefix HLA, the name of the gene (or the locus identifier), and a

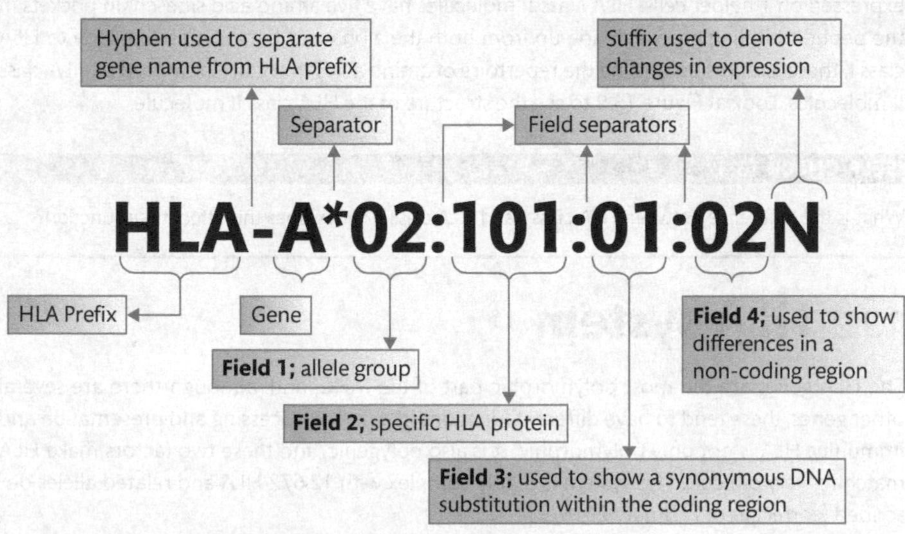

FIGURE 13.3
HLA allele nomenclature system showing the structure using '*' and ':' as separators. Figure kindly provided by Professor Steven GE Marsh, Anthony Nolan Research Institute, London, UK and is from the website hla.alleles.org.

separator '*'. The first two digits, the ones before a colon (used to separate different characteristics of the allele), describe the type of HLA allele. Very often this will correspond to the HLA antigen found in serological typing. For example, the majority of HLA alleles beginning HLA-A*02 will HLA type as HLA-A2 by serological typing. The next set of digits following the colon refer to the amino acid sequence of the allele, (*HLA-A*02:01*). This is followed by a second colon. Changes in these digits indicate a change in DNA sequence within the coding region that does not change the amino acid sequence–for example, GCT, GCC, GCA, and GCG all code for alanine, (*HLA-A*02:01:01*). This is followed by a final colon and digits which show changes in the DNA sequence of the non-coding regions of the gene or changes in the leader sequence, (*HLA-A*02:01:01:01*). Finally, there is an optional suffix. This can be any of the following:

N	Null allele
L	Low cell surface expression
S	Secreted
C	Cytoplasmic (not on cell surface)
A	Aberrant (we are not sure it is expressed)
Q	Questionable (this mutation has been shown to affect expression).

SELF-CHECK 13.2

What is the structure of the HLA allele naming system?

13.3 HLA typing

HLA typing is now normally performed using molecular methods based on polymerase chain reaction (PCR). Serological HLA typing is included within this chapter for historical reasons, to demonstrate all of the techniques available for HLA typing.

13.3.1 Serological HLA typing

The main serological typing technique is the complement dependent cytotoxicity test (CDC) which was described by Terasaki et al. (1965). This technique involves addition of a preparation of lymphocytes to multiple wells containing HLA antibodies specific for differing HLA antigens. Following incubation, rabbit complement is added to cause cell lysis in the presence of an antigen–antibody reaction. This is followed by a further incubation before adding staining reagents such as propidium iodide or acridine orange and ethidium bromide to all the wells. The activity of complement is arrested by adding ink to quench background fluorescence. Each of the wells is read microscopically on a fluorescent microscope and scored for the percentage of cells that are dead. Live cells stain green while dead cells stain red (see Figure 13.4).

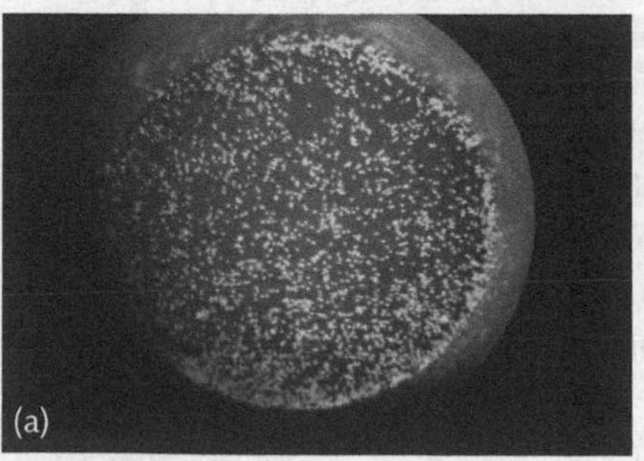

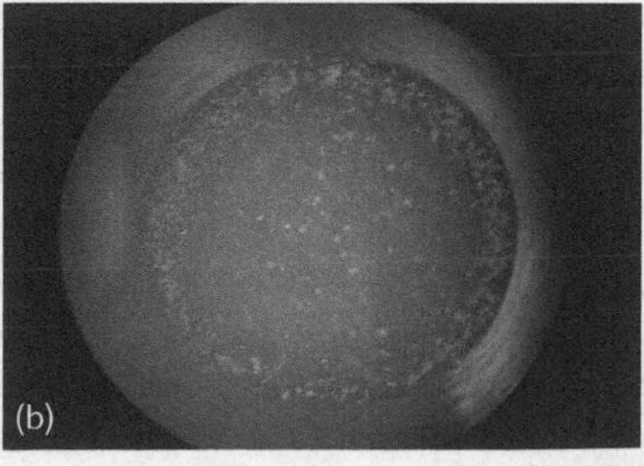

FIGURE 13.4
CDC tests: negative (a) and positive (b).

While the CDC test remains in use today for HLA typing, it has been mainly replaced by molecular methods which offer significant advantages in terms of accuracy and resolution for HLA typing, but serology still has a role in demonstrating surface antigen expression.

Key Points

- **Serological HLA typing has now been replaced in the clinical laboratory by molecular HLA typing.**
- **Live lymphocytes must be prepared for serological typing.**
- **Serological typing is dependent on complement mediated cell lysis.**

Cross reference

You may find it helpful to read more about molecular biology techniques to support your learning in this chapter. You can read more in the *Biomedical Science Practice* textbook of this series.

13.3.2 Molecular HLA typing

Molecular HLA typing can be used to give a higher resolution type than can be derived by serological HLA typing, and is the technique of choice for HLA typing. Molecular HLA typing can also provide a variety of different levels of resolution; from low resolution serological equivalent to high resolution gene sequencing.

13.3.3 Polymerase chain reaction with sequence-specific primers (PCR-SSP)

Polymerase Chain Reaction with Sequence Specific Primers (PCR-SSP) is a technique where multiple PCR reactions are used to identify the HLA alleles present. This technique uses pairs of primers to detect the sequence of interest, but only identifies known HLA genes, as primers are developed around a known sequence. An internal control consisting of primers to a non-polymorphic gene sequence is used to assure that the conditions are suitable for PCR. Once PCR is complete the PCR reactions are electrophoresed on an agarose gel containing ethidium bromide. The gel is visualized by UV light, photographed, and the presence of HLA alleles determined from the absence and presence of PCR products.

13.3.4 Polymerase chain reaction using sequence-specific oligonucleotide probes (PCR-SSOP)

Polymerase Chain Reaction using Sequence-Specific Oligonucleotide Probes (PCR-SSOP) is a technique where the exon(s) of the HLA gene to be examined are amplified by PCR then the PCR product is hybridized with a series of probes which are bound to a solid matrix such as nylon membrane. One of the PCR primers will have a reporter molecule conjugated to it so that a positive hybridization can be identified by a colour change at the position of the probe on the solid matrix. As with PCR-SSP, probes are designed around known sequences and therefore only known alleles can be identified.

A variant of this technique is Luminex PCR-SSOP typing where the probes are bound to a fluorescent colour-coded bead and one of the PCR primers has been conjugated to a fluorescent protein. This allows up to one hundred of these beads with differing probes to be analysed quickly and simultaneously on a dedicated flow cytometer.

13.3.5 PCR-sequence based typing (PCR-SBT)

Sequenced Based Typing (SBT) is a system where the exon(s) of interest are amplified by PCR similarly to PCR-SSOP. With SBT the amplicons are directly analysed on a DNA sequencer and compared to a database of known DNA sequences to determine which alleles are present. As DNA is directly sequenced new alleles can be identified and characterized using DNA sequencing.

Key Points

- **Molecular HLA typing can be used for low- to high-resolution typing.**
- **There are a variety of techniques that can be used for molecular typing.**

SELF-CHECK 13.3

What are the advantages and disadvantages to each of the HLA typing methods?

13.4 HLA antibody testing

Laboratory techniques for the detection of HLA antibodies have been revolutionized in the last decade with new technologies increasing both the sensitivity and the specificity of detection. Particular benefits include the reproducibility, accuracy, and timeliness of tests, making them ideal for antibody screening of patients presenting in acute clinical situations and for monitoring of patients post-transplant. Once detected, HLA antibodies can now be defined for the majority of HLA-A, -B, -Cw, -DR, -DQ, and -DP specificities. Further guidance on the application of HLA antibody testing is available from the 'Guidelines for the detection and characterization of clinically relevant antibodies in allotransplantation', British Society for Histocompatibility & Immunogenetics and British Transplantation Society.

13.4.1 Complement-dependent cytotoxicity test

The same test used for HLA typing can be used for detection and identification of HLA antibodies. However, in this case the patient's serum is added to cells of known HLA type. The specificity of the antibody can be determined through analysis of the pattern of positive and negative reactions.

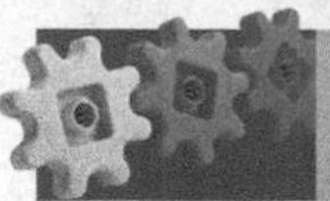

METHOD 13.1 ELISA

- **ELISA can detect antibodies against HLA Class I and Class II.**
- **ELISA can either utilize a pool of antigens used to screen for the presence of antibodies or can be the antigens from a single donor in each well of a multi-well plate.**
- **ELISA is more sensitive and more specific than CDC in that it separates class I and class II antigens and doesn't rely on the antibody being complement fixing (see Table 13.1).**
- **HLA ELISA tests are similar to most ELISA techniques:**
  - **Add patient serum to the well and incubate.**
  - **Wash the wells with buffered saline.**

- Add an enzyme-conjugated anti-IgG and incubate.
- Wash again with buffered saline.
- Add enzyme substrate and incubate.
- Measure optical density of the colour developed on a reader at the specified wavelength.

TABLE 13.1 The different sensitivity and specificity for the different HLA antibody detection and identification methods.

	Sensitivity	Specificity
CDC	+	+
ELISA	++	++
Luminex	+++	+++
Luminex single antigen beads	+++	++++

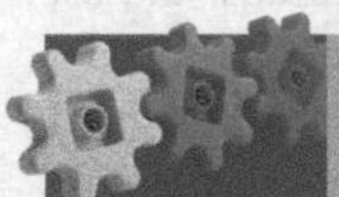

METHOD 13.2 Luminex

Luminex is a hybrid of the ELISA and flow cytometric techniques. The features of Luminex are:

- Antigens are coated onto colour coded polymer beads.
- There can be up to one hundred beads read simultaneously.
- Each population of beads can be coated with the antigens from a single individual or a single recombinant HLA antigen.
- Fluorescently conjugated anti-IgG is used for detection of the presence of an antibody.
- A dedicated flow cytometer is used to read the test results.
- Luminex is a much more sensitive technique than CDC and ELISA but there are some questions raised about the clinical relevance of antibodies detected by this method.

Online Resource Centre

To see an online video demonstrating Luminex, log on to www.oxfordtextbooks.co.uk/orc/fbs

SELF-CHECK 13.4

What are the advantages and disadvantages of the different techniques used for HLA antibody detection and identification?

13.5 Solid organ transplantation

In recent years there have been many developments, such as improved immunosuppression and reduction in organ ischaemic time, which have significantly improved transplant graft survival. Even with these significant improvements, matching for HLA antigens plays a significant role in graft survival and patient survival. Süsal and Opelz (2013) showed that, even with

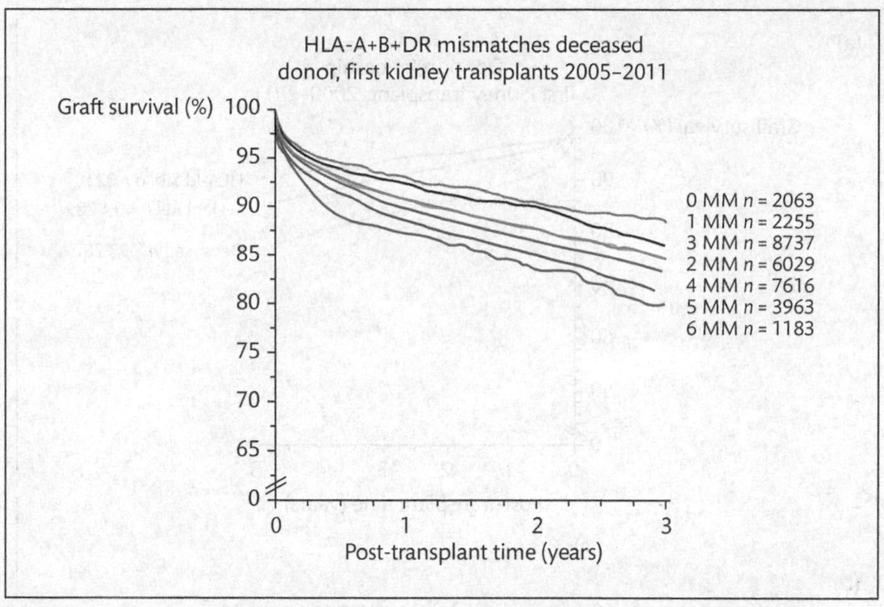

FIGURE 13.5
HLA matching in deceased donor transplants showing the decreasing graft survival when HLA antigens are mismatched (Süsal and Opelz 2013). Reprinted with permission from Süsal and Opelz (2013). Copyright © 2013 Wolters Kluwer Health/Lippincott Williams.

improved surgical techniques and improved immunosuppression (see Figure 13.5), transplantation of well-matched kidneys showed a greater than ten percent graft survival advantage compared to poorly matched kidneys at 3 years post-transplant. In living donor transplants, where the ischaemic times are usually very short, we continue to see an HLA matching effect. This can be seen in Figure 13.6.

13.5.1 HLA matching and organ allocation

The benefits of HLA matching in solid organ transplantation have been well described. However, there are several factors which can reduce the benefits of HLA matching in solid organ transplantation. Look at Table 13.2 to see these factors.

Although clearly of benefit in most forms of solid organ transplantation, generally HLA matching is limited to kidney transplantation where the benefits have been recognized for a long time. In the UK these benefits were formalized in the 1998 National Kidney Allocation Scheme (NKAS). This scheme had a significant component based on HLA matching, and segregated nationally allocated kidneys into three tiers, depending on the number of HLA mismatches. Allocating fully matched tier 1 (referred to as a 000 mismatch, i.e. no mismatches at HLA-A, B, or DR) and tier 2 (100, 010, and 110 mismatched) kidneys nationally, preferentially trying to match patients at HLA-DR.

The scheme was redefined in 2006 to address observed inequities in access to transplantation, but still gave absolute priority to 000 HLA-A, B, and DR mismatched grafts and gave points for age and HLA mismatch to ensure well matched grafts for young patients. The scheme also continued to recognize the problems of highly sensitized patients with patients divided into five tiers (A–E) as described in Table 13.3. Patients in tiers A and B are prioritized on waiting time and

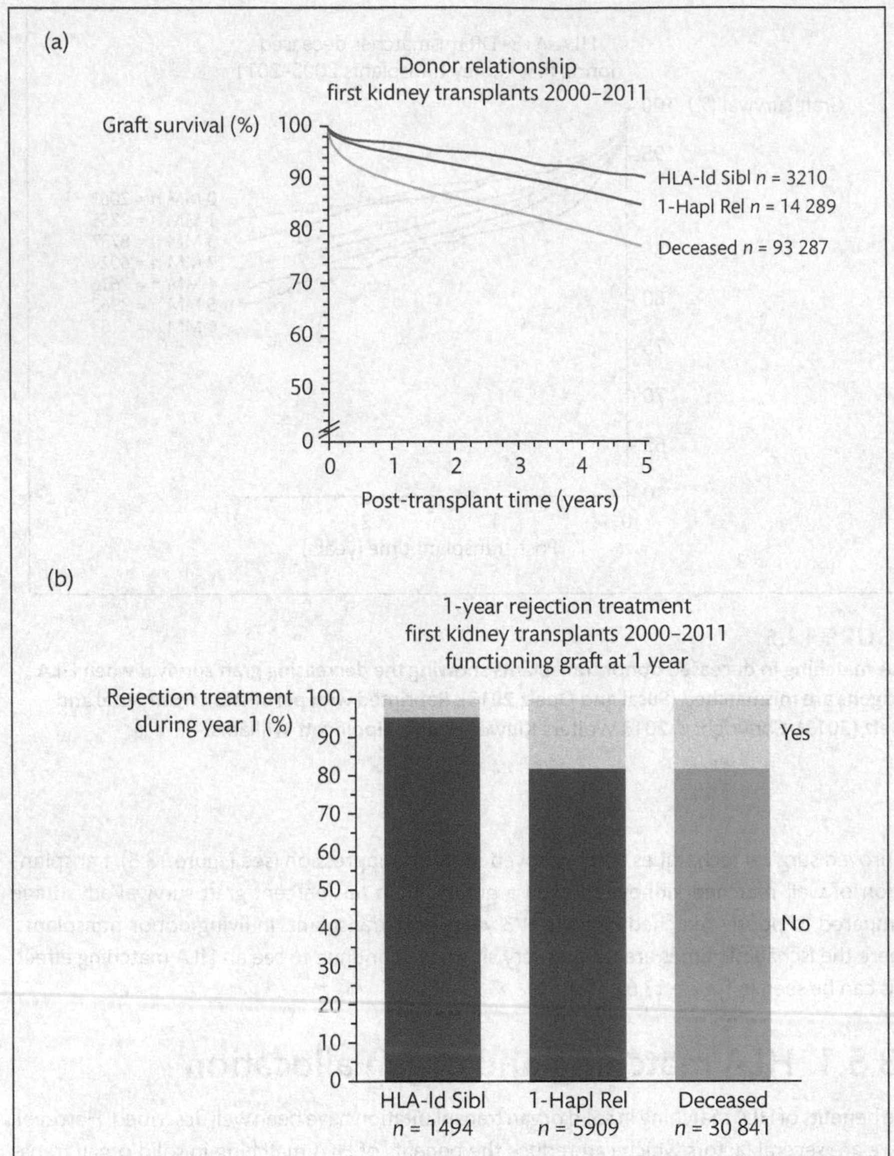

FIGURE 13.6

HLA matching in related live donor transplants shows HLA matching effect (Süsal and Opelz 2013). Reprinted with permission from Süsal and Opelz (2013). Copyright © 2013 Wolters Kluwer Health/Lippincott Williams.

patients in tiers C, D, and E according to a points-based system as described by NHS Blood and Transplant (NHSBT)/Organ Donation and Transplant (ODT).

In 2010 NHSBT/ODT also introduced a national pancreas allocation scheme covering rules for allocation of simultaneous pancreas and kidney transplants, pancreas transplant alone, and pancreas after kidney along with pancreatic islets, which included HLA match grade between recipient and donor and sensitization points for HLA sensitization as part of the allocation process.

Cross reference

You can read more at the NHSBT/Organ Donation and Transplantation (ODT) website at http://www.odt.nhs.uk/

TABLE 13.2 Factors which can reduce the benefits of HLA matching in solid organ transplantation.

Patient clinical condition–some patients cannot wait for a matched donor.
Lack of replacement therapy–for example lungs and livers.
Patient waiting list–if the waiting list is small there is little chance of finding a match.
Donor pool–if there are a limited number of donors it may be difficult to find a patient that matches.
Physical barriers–such as patient size and weight.

SELF-CHECK 13.5

Why do we need to HLA match for kidney transplants? What are the advantages for patients and for organ transplant programs?

13.5.2 Crossmatching

Crossmatching of donor organs with recipients is a prerequisite in kidney, pancreas, heart, lung, intestinal and multi-visceral transplantation and pancreatic islet transplantation. Crossmatching protocols are driven via the clinical parameters required for each organ being transplanted. The role of the crossmatch test in transplantation is to determine whether there are patient antibodies that will react with donor antigens and, therefore, the crossmatch allows an immunological risk assessment of patient/donor combinations. The techniques currently in use include complement-dependent cytotoxicity crossmatching, flow cytometric crossmatching, solid phase assay crossmatching, and virtual (or electronic) crossmatching. The requirements of the crossmatch tests are described in the current European Federation of Immunogenetics standards.

Cross reference

You can read more about the European Federation of Immunogenetics and the associated standards at http://www.efiweb.eu/

13.5.3 Complement-dependent cytotoxic (CDC) crossmatching

Complement-dependent cytotoxicity (CDC) is a relatively insensitive crossmatching technique, which has been clinically validated. Patients transplanted against a positive IgG CDC crossmatch are at high risk of hyperacute rejection. The crossmatching technique is similar to the CDC described in Section 13.3.1, with separated donor T and B cells added to patient sera to

TABLE 13.3 The additional factors NHSBT/ODT use for highly sensitized patients.

A. 000 mismatched paediatric patients highly sensitized or HLA-DR homozygous.
B. 000 mismatched paediatric patients–others.
C. 000 mismatched adult patients highly sensitized or HLA-DR homozygous.
D. 000 mismatched adult patients–others. Favourably matched paediatric patients.
E. All other eligible patients.

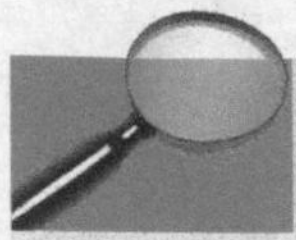

CASE STUDY 13.1 *Living donor kidney transplant*

Patient history

A 38-year-old male was diagnosed with IgA nephropathy. The disease is caused by a genetic defect which results in the formation of an abnormal galactose-deficient O-glycan hinge region of IgA1 antibody. As a result, anti-IgA1 IgG antibodies are formed, followed by the formation of immune complexes, activation of the alternative complement system, and deposition in the glomeruli. Glomeruli in turn produce different inflammatory cytokines and proliferative mediators inducing kidney injury and fibrosis. The patient was given haemodialysis and was referred to the transplant unit for listing on a deceased donor waiting list. The clinician also discussed the option of living donation with the patient and an older brother offered to donate. Samples from the donor and the patient were sent to the H&I laboratory for testing.

Results

The HLA genotyping was performed by PCR-SSOP for HLA-A, B, C, DRB1, and DQB1 were at medium resolution. The patient's HLA antibody profile was determined by Luminex for registration on the waiting list and to assess the donor compatibility. The screening test for HLA antibodies gave equivocal results so further testing was required using a HLA antibody identification test. This further test was negative for HLA antibodes. Crossmatching was performed both by CDC and flow cytometry.

Results:

HLA type	A*	B*	C*	DRB1*	DQB1*	ABO/ Rh
Patient	03	13	06	07	02	O+
		47		04	03:01	
Donor	03	13	06	07	02	O-
		55	03:03	01:01	05	

Note: The patient and the donor were haploidentical—they shared one haplotype which is A*03, B*13, C*06, DRB1*07, and DQB1*02.

HLA antibody tests were negative in all four samples tested pre-transplant.

Crossmatching was performed on two occasions, the second of which was immediately prior to transplant, using both current and historic serum samples.

First crossmatch

CDC T cell	CDC B cell	Flow T cell	Flow B cell
Neg	Neg	Neg	Neg

Pre-transplant crossmatch

CDC T cell	CDC B cell	Flow T cell	Flow B cell
Neg	Neg	Neg	Neg

Significance of results

The patient was subsequently transplanted. There was immediate graft function and a CT scan after the transplantation showed normal perfusion. The patient was discharged from the hospital on triple immunosuppressive therapy: tacrolimus, mycophenolate mofetil (MMF), and prednisolone. First week assessment showed a normal creatinine blood level (139 μM/L) with no haematuria or proteinuria. HLA antibody screening was performed and there were no HLA class I or class II donor specific antibodies; however a non-donor specific HLA-DR18 antibody was detected, which is assumed to be from a previous sensitizing event such as a blood transfusion.

BOX 13.1 Quality assurance in the H&I laboratory: EFI and UKAS

H&I laboratories are accredited by several authoritative bodies, with laboratory accreditation being dependent of the repertoire of the laboratory and the transplant programs supported. The main accrediting bodies for H&I labs in the UK are UKAS/CPA, who accredit laboratories to ISO15189 and CPA standards, and the European Federation of Immunogenetics (EFI). Although accreditation of H&I laboratories is not mandatory, certain transplant service providers require services to be provided by an accredited laboratory. For example, a stem cell transplant unit requiring accreditation from the Joint Accreditation Committee of the ISCT and EBMT (JACIE) must procure services from a laboratory with EFI accreditation for its stem cell procedures. With regard to HLA typing of deceased donors, NHS Blood and Transplant Organ Donation and Transplant requires a laboratory to have either EFI or CPA accreditation. Samples for H&I testing, particularly those referred for disease association testing, are often referred on from CPA accredited laboratories which requires the testing laboratory to have CPA accreditation.

assess compatibility by identifying any complement fixing donor-specific antibodies. The test detects both HLA specific and non-HLA complement fixing IgG and IgM antibodies. IgG and IgM antibody differential is demonstrated by addition of a disulphide reducing agent, dithiothreitol (DTT).

13.5.4 Flow cytometric crossmatch (FCXM)

The flow cytometric crossmatching (FCXM) is a reliable and highly sensitive method for the detection of donor specific antibodies. Like the CDC test, this technique detects both HLA-specific and non-HLA antibodies; however, unlike CDC this test detects both complement fixing and non-complement fixing antibodies. This test can be adapted to detect different immunoglobulin classes and also gives a semi-quantitative value of antibody binding. Therefore the FCXM can be used to detect some antibody classes that are not identified by the standard CDC test. Although a positive flow crossmatch is linked to episodes of early rejection and shorter graft survival, in many cases its significance is still under debate.

As with CDC, lymphocytes isolated from the donor blood are used for this crossmatch, but with flow cytometry cell populations are sorted by fluorescently labelled markers. Patient serum is mixed with the donor lymphocytes to allow antibody binding. Labelled anti-IgG antibody is then added, incubated, washed, and detected by flow cytometry. Anti-CD3 and either CD19 or CD20 conjugated antibodies are often used to separate T and B cells, respectively.

13.5.5 Solid phase assay crossmatching

To make the crossmatch HLA specific, solid phase assay crossmatching has been developed. This test relies on the removal of donor HLA antigens from donor cells and subsequently binding these to synthetic beads coated with capture antigens. The take-up of solid phase crossmatch tests has been very low, and there are only a few publications describing their use, and therefore little evidence available presently to support their use. The advantage of these tests is that any reactivity observed can be attributed to HLA antibody. They can also be used to give a result in the presence of cytotoxic drugs and antibody based therapies such as anti-thymocyte globulin and rituximab.

13.5.6 Virtual crossmatching

Virtual crossmatching was developed out of necessity firstly in cardiothoracic transplantation, due to the limited organ ischaemia time available. At first this relied on results generated out of the aforementioned insensitive CDC assays for antibody screening and HLA typing, but the recent introduction of specific and sensitive tests described in Section 13.4 and DNA typing techniques described in Section 13.3 has allowed the use of virtual crossmatching in all forms of transplantation. This test relies on accurate HLA antibody screening and definitive donor HLA typing to perform a paper-based crossmatch prior to transplant.

Virtual crossmatching is possible where HLA antibodies are fully defined and donor HLA typing information is available to assess suitability. Unfortunately this approach is not available for all patients as some may still have undefined HLA specificities while others may have specificities for which donors are not routinely typed, such as HLA-DPA and -DQA. In this situation it may still be necessary to perform a CDC and/or FCXM, although this may limit the donors available for such patients.

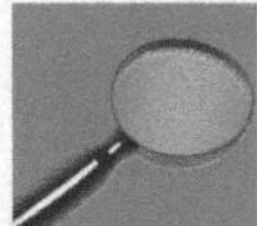

CASE STUDY 13.2 Passive transfer of HLA antibodies has serious implications for cardiothoracic patients requiring virtual crossmatching

Patient history

A 6-year-old, 20 kg female, previously well with no history of prior surgery or transfusions, presented with dilated cardiomyopathy following a short two-week history of increasing breathlessness. 12 hours later she was transferred to the intensive care unit for mechanical support and was listed for urgent transplantation. She received a blood transfusion as part of the process of introducing mechanical support and was subsequently transplanted 3 weeks later. Pre-transplant testing for HLA antibodies was positive, revealing defined HLA specificities, even though there were no reported sensitizing events, except for the transfusion of red cells one day before testing. Testing of the donor and longitudinal testing of patient samples demonstrated that one of the antibody specificities detected in the patient was of donor origin, and this allowed an insight into the dynamics of such passively transferred antibodies.

Results

Patient HLA genotyping was performed by PCR-SSOP for HLA-A, B, C, DRB1, and DQB1 at low/medium resolution and the patient's and blood donor HLA antibody profile was determined by Luminex.

Results:

	HLA -A*	HLA-B*	HLA-C*	HLA-DRB1*	HLA-DQB1*	HLA antibodies detected
Patient HLA	02, 24	07, 55	07, 03:03	04, 14	05, 03:01	A33, A10, A68, A69, Cw5
Donor HLA	NT	NT	NT	NT	NT	Cw5, Cw6, Cw15, Cw17, Cw18

IgG has a half-life of approximately 21-3 days and the level of the passively transferred Cw5 antibody decreased over the next 3 weeks, as can be seen in Figure 13.7, showing that there was no primary synthesis of the antibody, whereas the other HLA antibodies remained at the same level.

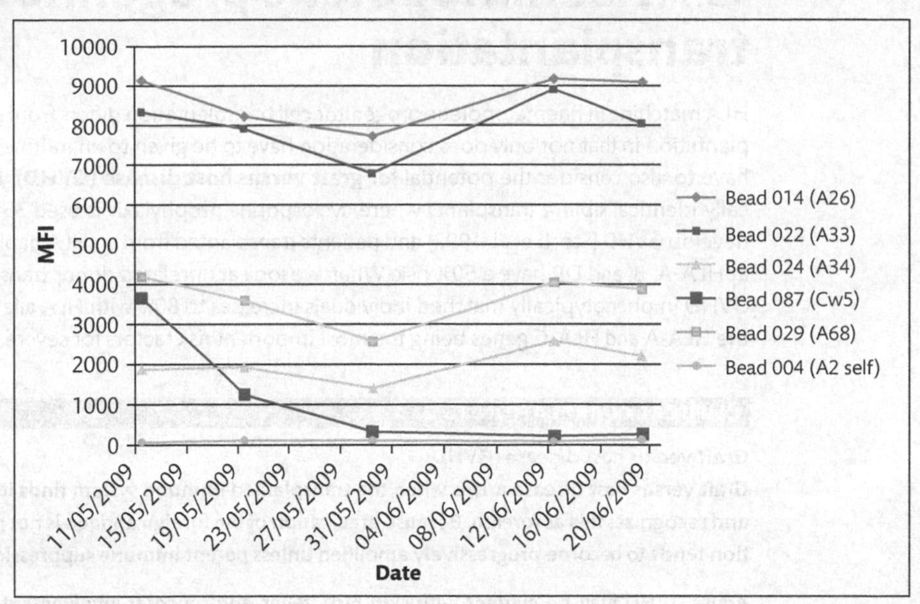

FIGURE 13.7

Longitudinal titres of donor-specific antibodies.

Significance of results

Transfer of HLA antibodies via blood transfusion is reasonably well documented, and can be the cause of transfusion associated acute lung injury (TRALI), a rare but potentially life-threatening condition. The incidence and severity of TRALI has led to the predominant use of male-only plasma components in the UK (www.shotuk.org). In this case the detection of the antibody in the patient serum meant that certain potential donors would be precluded for donation if there was thought to be a immune response, or the patient may have been at risk of TRALI had the transfusion contained patient-specific antibodies. The frequency of HLA antibodies and their implications for transplanted allografts need to be considered when patients receive blood products.

13.6 Post-transplant monitoring

The need for post-transplant monitoring for HLA antibodies is debatable, and requirements are different for different cases. However, testing should always be performed if there is graft dysfunction or a biopsy for graft impairment to assist with categorization of the rejection process.

If high risk transplants such as antibody incompatible transplants are performed, patients are at high risk of antibody mediated rejection and require regular monitoring of donor-specific antibody (DSA) levels post-transplant. Patients who have a low risk transplant, for example those with no evidence of DSA at the time of transplant, should be tested in the first year post-transplant and should always be tested if rejection is suspected. It is important that samples are collected post-transplant to identify any donor-specific response. Failure to collect samples may decrease the patient's chance of receiving a subsequent transplant as regular testing can define antigens that should not be crossed on a future graft. Local policies should define the frequency of testing post-transplant.

13.7 Haematopoietic progenitor cell transplantation

HLA matching in haematopoietic progenitor cell transplantation differs from solid organ transplantation in that not only does consideration have to be given to engraftment of the cells, we have to also consider the potential for **graft versus host disease (GVHD)**. In HLA genotypically identical sibling transplants where cyclosporine prophylaxis is used 35% of patients will develop GVHD (Storb et al. 1992) and patients transplanted from an HLA haploidentical sibling at HLA-A, B, and DR have a 50% risk. When we look at unrelated donor transplants, the risk of GVHD in phenotypically matched individuals increases to 80% with HLA allelic mismatches at the HLA-A and HLA-C genes being the most important risk factors for severe GVHD.

CLINICAL CORRELATION 13.2

Graft versus host disease (GVHD)

Graft versus host disease arises when the transplanted immune system finds itself in a new host and recognizes this as foreign. Because eradication of the foreign antigen is not possible, the reaction tends to become progressively amplified unless potent immune suppression is employed.

Acute GVHD may be evident with skin rash, fever, and mucosal involvement–mouth and gut, which can bleed, even fatally.

The treatment of acute GVHD is high dose steroids and then increasing amounts of oral immunosuppression like cyclosporine.

Chronic GVHD can be manifest in much the same way as acute GVHD, but the symptoms are usually more subtle, with progressive rash if skin is involved, scarring of the liver, diarrhoea if the GI tract is involved, or shortness of breath if it is the lungs.

Chronic GVHD is treated in the same way as the acute form.

There is some evidence that GVHD may be driven as well by certain infections that activate the immune system as it develops in the new host (such as CMV). For patients who have had a transplant for leukaemia, GVHD may have a beneficial anti-tumour effect, but the goal is always to control this process.

However, the true measure of transplant outcome is the overall patient survival. Patients with chronic myeloid leukaemia (CML) who have been given a haploidentical transplant that mismatched for only one HLA antigen have been shown to have comparable survival to those who received an HLA identical transplant, but those with a greater mismatch do not.

13.8 HLA and disease

Polymorphisms in HLA molecules determine the repertoire of peptides bound and presented to T cells. Subsequently many HLA associations have been described with disease. Most of the diseases with HLA associations are autoimmune diseases, in some of which we are now starting to understand the underlying mechanisms.

13.8.1 Ankylosing spondylitis

Ankylosing spondylitis (AS) is a debilitating spinal arthropathy where the spinal joints, ligaments, and sacroiliac joints become inflamed and painful. Peripheral joints and uvea and

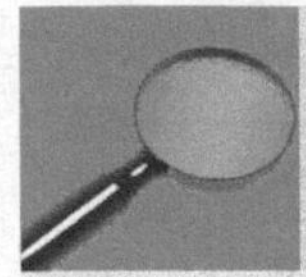

CASE STUDY 13.3 Marrow unrelated donor haematopoietic progenitor cell transplant

Patient history

A 7-year-old child presented with a history of bloody diarrhoea due to colitis, weight loss, and a chesty cough with an adenovirus infection. The neutrophil oxidative burst test was abnormally low and immunogenetic analysis revealed an autosomal recessive P22-phox mutation. He was diagnosed with chronic granulomatous disease (CGD) and was referred for transplant assessment. Patient samples were sent to a Histocompatibility and Immunogenetics laboratory (H&I) for HLA typing to identify a donor. Samples from the parents, siblings, and a maternal uncle were sent for HLA typing.

Results

HLA genotyping was performed by polymerase chain reaction-sequence-specific oligonucleotide probes (PCR-SSOP). The method provides an intermediate resolution typing. The patient, parents, and unrelated donors were typed for HLA-A, B, C, DRB, and DQB (±DPB), while the relatives were first typed for DRB1 to identify any matches.

HLA type	A*	B*	C*	DRB1*	DQB1*	DPB1*	ABO/gender	CMV
Patient	01:01	51:01	15:01	15:02	06:01	17:01	A+/M	Neg
	03:02	13:01	06:02	07:01	02:02	26:01		
Mother	01	51	15	15	06	NT	A+/F	NT
	02	52	12	01	05			
Father	11	35	04	15	05	NT	A+/M	NT
	03	13	06	07	02			

HLA-DRB1* types of other relatives were:

Sibling 1: 01:01, 15:01; Sibling 2: 01:01,15:01; Sibling 3: 15:01,15:02; Uncle: 01:01, 15:02.

None of the family matched the patient, therefore an unrelated donor search was initiated by sending the patient HLA and ABO types to the Anthony Nolan Trust. The search of the UK registries showed no potential donors (only allele/antigen mismatches at one or two HLA loci were found). A search of the international registries Bone Marrow Donors Worldwide (BMDW) revealed five potential donors: one each in Italy, Lithuania, and Israel, and two in the USA. As the full HLA type of the majority of the donors was not provided (only HLA ABDR type at low resolution antigen level), three donors mismatched at one HLA-A antigen were also selected as a backup. Samples were requested from all donors and confirmatory/extended HLA typing was performed using PCR-SSOP.

International donors selected for confirmatory typing:

HLA type	A*	B*	C*	DRB1*	DQB1*	DPB1*	ABO & Rh/gender	CMV
Donor 1	01:01	51:01	15:01	15:02	06:01	04:02	B-/F	Neg
	03:01	13:01	06:02	07:01	02:02	14:01		
Donor 2*	01:01	51:01	15:01	15:02	06:01	02:01	A+/M	Neg
	03:01	13:01	06:02	07:01	02:02	04:01		

HLA type	A*	B*	C*	DRB1*	DQB1*	DPB1*	ABO & Rh/gender	CMV
Donor 3	01	51	15	15:02	06:01	04:01	O+/M	Pos
*	31	13	06	07:01	02:02	04:02		
Donor 4	01	13	06	15:02	06:01	13:01	O+/M	Pos
	30	51	07	07:01	02:02	17:01		
Donor 5	01	13	15	15:01	06:01	NT	O-/M	Pos
	03	51	06	07:01	02:02			
Donor 6	01	13	12	15:02	06:01	NT	O+/M	Neg
	30	52	06	07:01	02:02			

* The final donor selected. Male donor matched for ABO blood and CMV status. The transplant was performed in April 2014 after reduced intensity conditioning with campath, treosulfan, and fludarabine.

Significance of results

This case shows several issues which should be considered when selecting a donor for stem cell transplantation. A matched related donor for this patient was not available. Although two of the siblings matched each other (1:4 chance of being identical siblings), they did not match the patient. Only the international registry search identified potential donors; there were none in the UK.

Patient follow-up

There were no adverse reactions after infusion of donor cells and no incidence of GVHD was reported 4 weeks post-transplant. Immunosuppression consists of cyclosporine and mycophenolate mofetil (MMF) as GVHD prophylaxis. To prevent infection, prophylactic anti-fungal (amphotericin), anti-CMV (aciclovir), and anti-bacterials were given. Neutrophils recovered to > 0.7×10^9/L, demonstrating early engraftment.

tendon insertions can also be affected. Unlike most autoimmune diseases, AS is predominantly found in males and onset is usually in early adulthood.

The genetic predictability of AS is extremely high, as is the disease severity and age of onset. The association of AS with HLA-B27 was one of the earliest described HLA associations and remains one of the strongest associations identified by Brewerton et al. (1973). The pathogenic mechanism was described by Fussell et al. (2008) and describes that this HLA association is due to the particular folding of the HLA-B27 molecule and its subsequent binding of auto-antigen peptides.

CLINICAL CORRELATION 13.3

Ankylosing spondylitis

The main symptoms are:

- Back pain and stiffness:
  - the pain lessens and is better with exercise
  - the pain and stiffness is worse in the morning and at night
  - the pain may be around the buttocks.
- Arthritis:
  - pain on moving the affected joint

- tenderness when the affected joint is examined
- swelling and warmth in the affected area.

- **Enthesitis and fatigue.**

Enthesitis is a painful inflammation where a bone is joined to a tendon. Common sites for enthesitis are:

- **top of the shin bone**
- **Achilles tendon**
- **under the heel**
- **where the ribs join to the sternum.**

90–95% of AS patients have HLA-B27 in comparison to approximately 10% of the general population.

13.8.2 Coeliac disease

Ninety percent of patients with Coeliac disease (CD) have the HLA-DQ2 beta chain, encoded by the *HLA-DQA1*05:01; HLA-DQB*02:01* haplotye, and to a much lesser extent the *DQA1*02:01; DQB1*02:02* haplotype; the majority of the remaining patients have HLA-DQ8 beta chain encoded by *HLA-DQA1*03; HLA-DQB1*03:02*. $CD4^+$ T cells which carry the HLA antigens have been shown to be reactive to transglutaminase 2 and subsequently it has been demonstrated that the reactivity of T cells to transglutaminase 2 peptides is restricted by these HLA molecules. The strong HLA association with CD plays a pivotal role in the disease pathogenesis, and the association is so strong that 2012 guidelines from the European Society of Paediatric Gastroenterology, Hepatology, and Nutrition suggest that not all children with symptoms of CD and high levels of IgA antibodies to transglutaminase 2 require a diagnostic biopsy. If the patient is positive for tTg and EMA IgA antibodies, testing for HLA-DQ2 and DQ8 is recommended, and, if positive, the guidelines say there is no need to perform a diagnostic biopsy.

Cross reference

You can read more about coeliac disease in Chapter 7.

13.8.3 HLA and rheumatoid arthritis

HLA polymorphisms have been shown to be associated with the production of rheumatoid arthritis associated auto-antibodies and have been shown to correlate with the severity and aggressiveness of articular and extra-articular disease. HLA-DRB1 alleles, particularly *DRB1*04:01, 04:04, 04:05*, and, to a lesser extent, *01:01* and *14:02*, confer the risk of severe synovitis with accelerated joint damage. Several studies have shown a correlation between homozygosity for *HLA-DRB1*04* and increased levels of anti-CCP.

Cross reference

You can read more about rheumatoid arthritis, rheumatoid factor, and anti-CCP in Chapter 5.

13.8.4 HLA and drug hypersensitivity

There are several examples of HLA associations with drug hypersensitivity in different populations, with the majority of associations being with HLA class I molecules. Look at Cheng et al. (2014) for a review of these.

The most well-characterized hypersensitivity reaction is seen in HIV positive individuals who are given the antiretroviral drug abacavir. *HLA-B*57:01* individuals were shown to be the only group who had reactions to abacavir. The reactions to abacavir are caused by the patients' own cytotoxic T cells recognizing altered 'self' peptides presented in the HLA molecules of the *B*57:01* molecule. Abacavir binds non-covalently to the *HLA-B*57:01* molecule, changing the structure of the antigen-binding groove and therefore causing the HLA molecule to bind different peptides

Cross reference

You can read more about HIV in Chapter 12.

to those normally presented. In such cases, the peptides presented are aberrant and recognized as foreign by the recipient's T cells. The peptides have not been identified as self-peptides during the thymic selection processes, therefore this generates a severe immune response.

13.8.5 HLA and other diseases

Due to the nature of the HLA molecule and its role in immunity, there have been associations made with several diseases and conditions, too many to list all here, and the majority for which the pathogenic mechanisms still remain unknown.

There are HLA linked associations with Behçet's disease (HLA-B51), birdshot retinochoroidopathy (HLA-A29), narcolepsy (*DQB1*06:02*), type 1 diabetes (predominately *DQB1*03:02*), and actinic prurigo (*DRB1* 04:07*), as well as rapid disease progression from HIV to AIDS (HLA-B35), or slow progression (HLA-B27 and B57). Several other studies have described linkages with systemic lupus erythmatosus (SLE) and psoriatic arthritis, as well as HLA associated carbamazepine and allopurinol hypersensitivity, leading to Stevens–Johnson syndrome, in certain populations.

An interesting association was made in the 1970s linking HLA-A3 to haemochromatosis. In 1996 the candidate gene for haemochromatosis was identified as the HFE gene (a mutation of which severely affects iron absorption). This was found on chromosome 6 approximately 4.6Mb telomeric of the HLA-A locus, likely meaning the association was not due to the function of the HLA molecule, only its proximity to the candidate gene.

SELF-CHECK 13.6

Reflecting on the different HLA associated diseases, what are the different mechanisms in place and what are the HLA associations?

SELF-CHECK 13.7

Can you list the different HLA disease associations and explain the mechanisms of four of these?

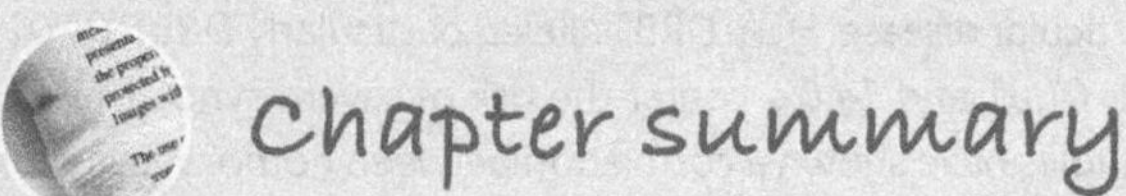

Chapter summary

- HLA molecules come in two main forms, class I and class II.
- There is a structured nomenclature for HLA allele names.
- HLA typing is mainly performed using molecular, PCR based methods.
- HLA antibodies can be detected by CDC, ELISA, or Luminex.
- HLA matching is important in transplant organ survival.
- There are HLA matching schemes, which are used to assist in organs being transplanted into patients who will benefit from the transplant.
- HLA alleles are associated with many autoimmune diseases.
- HLA alleles are associated with some drug hypersensitivity.

Acknowledgements

The authors would like to thank Dr Fatmah Naemi for the initial work on Case Studies 13.1 and 13.2.

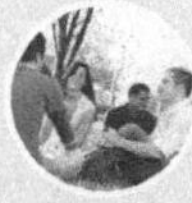

Discussion questions

13.1 Draw the structure of the HLA class I and class II molecules.

13.2 How do HLA class I and II molecules interact differently with T cells?

13.3 Describe the nomenclature for HLA alleles.

13.4 Describe the techniques used for HLA molecular typing and discuss their advantages and disadvantages.

13.5 Describe the methods for detection and identification of HLA antibodies.

13.6 On what basis are kidneys allocated in the UK?

13.7 Briefly discuss the different approaches that can be used for crossmatching.

13.8 Discuss the HLA association with autoimmune disease, using examples.

Answers to self-check questions are provided in the book's Online Resource Centre.

 Visit www.oxfordtextbooks.co.uk/orc/hall2e

References

Chapter 2

Beetham R (1979) Power functions for statistical control rules. *Clin Chem*, **25**(6), 863–9.

Brouet JC, et al. (1974) Biologic and clinical significance of cryoglobulins. A report of 86 cases. *Am J Med*, **57**(5), 775–88.

Dierlamm T, et al. (2002) IgM myeloma: a report of four cases. *Ann Hematol*, **81**(3), 136–9.

Ferri C, Zignego AL, Pileri SA (2002) Cryoglobulins. *J Clin Pathol*, **55**(1), 4–13.

Graziani M, Merlini G, Petrini C (2003) Guidelines for the analysis of Bence Jones protein. *Clin Chem Lab Med*, **41**(3), 338–46.

Maharaja VS, *et al.* (2014) IgG4 related disease. *Annul Rev Pathol*, **9**, 315–47.

Milford Ward A, Shelton J, Rowbottom A, Wild GD (2007) *Protein Reference Unit Handbook of Clinical Immunochemistry*. 9th Edition, PR Publications, Sheffield.

Miller D, *et al.* (2008) Differential diagnosis of suspected multiple sclerosis: a consensus approach. *Mult Scler*, **14**(9), 1157–74.

Owen RG (2014) Guidelines in the diagnosis and management of Waldenström's macroglobulinaemia. *Br J Haematol*, **165**(3), 316–33.

Pieringer H, *et al.* (2014) IgG4-related disease: an orphan disease with many faces. *Orphanet J Rare*, **9**, 110.

UK Myeloma Forum (2004) Guidelines on the diagnosis and management of AL amyloidosis. *Br J Haematol*, **125**, 681–700.

Vermeersch V, Gijbels K, Marien G, *et al.* (2008) A critical appraisal of current practice in the detection, analysis and reporting of cryoglobulins. *Clin Chemistry*, **54**(1), 39–44.

Vladutiu AO (2000) Immunoglobulin D: properties, measurement, and clinical relevance. *Clin Diagn Lab Immunol*, **7**(2), 131–40.

Westgard JO, Groth T (2000) Detection of Bence-Jones protein in practice. *Ann Clin Biochem*, **37**(5), 563–70.

Chapter 3

Ahlstedt S, Murray CS (2006) In vitro diagnosis of allergy: how to interpret IgE antibody results in clinical practice. *Primary Care Resp J*, **15**, 228–36.

Crameri R (2006) Allergy diagnosis, allergen repertoires and their implications for allergen specific immunotherapy. *Immunology Allergy Clin North Am*, **26**, 179–89.

Ebo DG, Sainte-Laudy J, Bridts CH, *et al.* (2006) Flow-assisted allergy diagnosis: current applications and future perspectives. *Allergy*, **61**, 1028–39.

Gell PGH, Coombs RRA (eds) (1963) *Clinical Aspects of Immunology*. 1st Edition, Blackwell, Oxford.

GINA (2015) *From the Global Strategy for Asthma Management and Prevention*, Global Initiative for Asthma. Available from: http://www.ginasthma.org/

Hamilton RG, Adkinson NF (2004) In vitro assays for the diagnosis of IgE-mediated disorders. *J Allergy Clin Immunol*, **114**, 213–25.

Milford Ward A, Shelton J, Rowbottom A, Wild GD (2007) *Protein Reference Unit Handbook of Clinical Immunochemistry*. 9th Edition, PR Publications, Sheffield.

Murphy K (2014) *Janeway's Immunobiology*. 8th Edition, Garland Science, New York.

Royal College of Physicians Working Party (2003) *Allergy—the unmet need: a blueprint for better patient care*. Report of a working party. RCP, London.

Sanz ML, Ganboa PM, De Weck AL (2007) In vitro tests: Basophil activation tests. In Pichler WJ, *Drug Hypersensitivity*, pp. 391–402. Karger, Basel.

Schwartz LB (2006) Diagnostic value of tryptase in anaphylaxis and mastocytosis. *Immunology Allergy Clin North Am*, **26**, 451–63.

Simons FER., *et al.* (2007) Risk assessment in anaphylaxis: current and future approaches. *J Allergy Clin Immunol*, **120**, S2–24.

Vrtala S (2008) From allergen genes to new forms of allergy diagnosis and treatment. *Allergy*, **63**, 299–309.

Way MG, Baxendine CL (2004) The significance of post mortem tryptase levels in supporting a diagnosis of anaphylaxis. *Anaesthesia*, **57**, 310–1.

Wohrl S, *et al.* (2006) The performance of a component based allergen microarray in clinical practice. *Allergy*, **61**, 633–9.

Chapter 4

Agostoni A, Cicardi M (1992) Hereditary and acquired C1-inhibitor deficiency: Biological and clinical characteristics in 235 patients. *Medicine*, **71**, 206.

Bork K, Barnstedt SE, Koch P, Traupe H (2000) Hereditary angioedema with normal C1-inhibitor activity in women. *Lancet*, **356**(9225), 213–7.

Bork K, Hardt J, Witzke G (2012) Fatal laryngeal attacks and mortality in hereditary angioedema due to C1-INH deficiency. *J Allergy Clin Immunol*, **130**(3), 692–7.

Bowden DW, Rising M, Akots G, *et al.* (1986) Homogeneous, liposome-based assay for total complement activity in serum. *Clin Chem*, **32**, 275.

Canova-Davis E, Redemann CT, Vollmer YP, Kung VT (1986) Use of a reversed-phase evaporation vesicle formulation for a homogeneous liposome immunoassay. *Clin Chem*, **32**, 1687.

Cicardi M, Beretta A, Colombo M, *et al.* (1996) Relevance of lymphoproliferative disorders and of anti-C1 inhibitor autoantibodies in acquired angio-oedema. *Clin Exp Immunol*, **106**, 475.

Colten HR, Rosen FS (1992) Complement deficiencies. *Annu Rev Immunol*, **10**, 809.

Daha MR, Fearon DT, Austen KF (1976) C3 nephritic factor (C3NeF): Stabilization of fluid phase and cell-bound alternative pathway convertase. *J Immunol*, **116**, 1.

Davis AE, (1988) 3rd C1 inhibitor and hereditary angioneurotic edema. *Annu Rev Immunol*, **6**, 595.

Davis AE, (1989) Hereditary and acquired deficiencies of C1 inhibitor. *Immunodeficiency Rev*, **1**, 207.

Davis AE, Aulak KS, Zahedi K, Bissler JJ, Harrison RA (1993a) C1 inhibitor. *Meth Enzymol*, 223, 97.

Davis AE, Bissler JJ, Cicardi M (1993b) Mutations in the C1 inhibitor gene that result in hereditary angioneurotic edema. *Behring Inst Mitt*, **93**, 313.

Ebanks RO, Jaikaran AS, Carroll MC, *et al.* (1992) A single arginine to tryptophan interchange at beta-chain residue 458 of human complement component C4 accounts for the defect in classical pathway C5 convertase activity of allotype C4 A6. Implications for the location of a C5 binding site in C4. *J Immunol*, **148**, 2803.

Egan LJ, Orren A, Doherty J, Wurzner R, McCarthy CF (1994) Hereditary deficiency of the seventh component of complement and recurrent meningococcal infection: Investigations in an Irish family using a novel haemolytic screening assay for complement activity and C7 M/N allotyping. *Epidemiol Infect*, **113**, 275.

Figueroa J, Andreoni J, Densen P (1993) Complement deficiency states and meningococcal disease. *Immunol Res*, **12**, 295.

Fijen CA, van den Bogaard R, Schipper M, *et al.* (1999) Properdin deficiency: molecular basis and disease association. *Mol Immunol*, **36**(13–14), 863–7.

Frank MM, Gelfand JA, Atkinson JP (1976) Hereditary angioedema: The clinical syndrome and its management. *Ann Intern Med*, **84**, 580.

Goldberg B, Lad P, Ghekierre L, Wolde-Tsadik G (1997) Comparison between assays for complement fragments and total hemolytic complement in the routine assessment of complement activation. *J Clin Ligand Assay*, **20**, 212.

Gotze O (1986) Components and Reactivity. In Rother K, Till GO (eds) *The Complement System* p 154. Springer, Heidelberg.

Holmskov U, Malhotra R, Sim RB, Jensenius JC (1994) Collectins: Collagenous C-type lectins of the innate immune defense system. *Immunol Today*, **15**, 67.

Janatova J, Tack BF (1981) Fourth component of human complement: Studies of an amine-sensitive site comprised of a thiol component. *Biochemistry*, **20**, 2394.

Jolles S, Williams P, Carne E, *et al.* (2014) A UK national audit of hereditary and acquired angioedema. *Clin Exp Immunol*, **175**(1), 59–67.

Kozono H, Kinoshita T, Kim YU, *et al.* (1990) Localization of the covalent C3b-binding site on C4b within the complement classical pathway C5 convertase, C4b2a3b. *J Biol Chem*, **265**, 14444.

Lachmann PJ (1991) The control of homologous lysis. *Immunol Today*, **12**, 312.

Lachmann PJ, Hughes-Jones NC (1984) Initiation of complement activation. *Semin Immunopathol*, **7**, 143.

Lambris JD (1988) The multifunctional role of C-3, the third component of complement. *Immunol Today*, **9**, 387.

Law SK, Dodds AW (1990) C3, C4 and C5: The thioester site. *Biochem Soc Trans*, **18**, 1155.

Mandle R, Baron C, Roux E, *et al.* (1994) Acquired Cl inhibitor deficiency as a result of an autoantibody to the reactive center region of Cl inhibitor. *J Immunol*, **152**, 4680.

Morgan BP, Harris CL (1999) *Complement regulatory proteins.* Academic Press, London.

Morgan BP, Orren A (1998) Vaccination against meningococcus in complement-deficient individuals. *Clin Exp Immunol*, **114**, 327.

Morgan BP, Walport MJ (1991) Complement deficiency and disease. *Immunol Today*, **12**, 301.

Reid KB (1986) Activation and control of the complement system. *Essays Biochem*, **22**, 27.

Reid KB, Day AJ (1989) Structure-function relationships of the complement components. *Immunol Today*, **10**, 177.

Reid KB, Turner MW (1994) Mammalian lectins in activation and clearance mechanisms involving the complement system. *Semin Immunopathol*, **15**, 307.

Schreiber RD, Muller-Eberhard HJ (1974) Fourth component of human complement: Description of a three polypeptide chain structure. *J Exp Med*, **140**, 1324.

Strife CF, Leahy AE, West CD (1989) Antibody to a cryptic solid phase C1q antigen in membranoproliferative nephritis. *Kidney Int*, **35**, 836.

Turner MW (1991) Deficiency of mannan binding protein—a new complement deficiency syndrome. *Clin Exp Immunol* **86** (Suppl 1), 53.

Waytes AT, Rosen FS, Frank MM (1996) Treatment of hereditary angioedema with a vapor-heated C1 inhibitor concentrate. *N Engl J Med*, **334**, 1630.

Wener MH, Uwatoko S, Mannik M (1989) Antibodies to the collagen-like region of C1q in sera of patients with autoimmune rheumatic diseases. *Arth Rheum*, **32**, 544.

Wisnieski JJ, Naff GB (1989) Serum IgG antibodies to C1q in hypocomplementemic urticarial vasculitis syndrome. *Arthritis Rheum*, **32**, 1119.

Wisnieski JJ, Baer AN, Christensen J, *et al.* (1995) Hypocomplementemic urticarial vasculitis syndrome. Clinical and serologic findings in 18 patients. *Medicine*, **74**, 24.

Wurzner R, Mollnes TE, Morgan BP (1997) Immunochemical Assays for Complement Components. In Johnstone AP, Turner MW (eds) *Immunochemistry 2* p 197. IRL Press, Oxford.

Yamamoto S, Kubotsu K, Kida M, *et al.* (1995) Automated homogeneous liposome-based assay system for total complement activity. *Clin Chem*, **41**, 586.

Zuraw BL, Bork K, Binkley KE, *et al.* (2012) Hereditary angioedema with normal C1 inhibitor function: consensus of an international expert panel. *Allergy Asthma Proc*, **33**(1), S145–56.

Zwirner J, Wittig A, Kremmer E, Gotze O (1998) A novel ELISA for the evaluation of the classical pathway of complement. *J Immunol Meth*, **211**, 183.

Chapter 5

Aletaha D, *et al.* (2010) 2010 Rheumatoid arthritis classification criteria: an American College of Rheumatology/European League Against Rheumatism collaborative initiative. *Arthritis Rheum*, **62**(9), 2569–81. doi: 10.1002/art.27584.

Casciola-Rosen L, Nagaraju K, Plotz P, *et al.* (2005) Enhanced autoantigen expression in regenerating muscle cells in idiopathic inflammatory myopathy. *J Exp Med*, **201**, 591–601.

Hochberg MC (1997) Updating the American College of Rheumatology revised criteria for the classification of systemic lupus erythematosus [letter]. *Arthritis Rheum*, **40**, 1725.

Myakis S, *et al.* (2006) International consensus statement on an update of the classification criteria for definite antiphospholipid syndrome (APS). *J Thromb Haemost*, **4**(2), 295–306.

Nielen MM, van Schaardenburg D, Reesink HW, *et al.* (2004) Specific autoantibodies precede the symptoms of rheumatoid arthritis: A study of serial measurements in blood donors. *Arthritis Rheum*, **50**, 380–6.

Rantapää-Dahlqvist S, de Jong BA, Berglin E, *et al.* (2003) Antibodies against cyclic citrullinated peptide and IgA rheumatoid factor predict the development of rheumatoid arthritis. *Arthritis Rheum*, **48**, 2741–9.

Stolt P, Bengtsson C, Nordmark B, *et al.* (2003) Quantification of the influence of cigarette smoking on rheumatoid arthritis: Results from a population based case-control study, using incident cases. *Ann Rheum Dis*, **62**, 835–41.

Suber TL, Casciola-Rosen L, Rosen A (2008) Mechanisms of disease: Autoantigens as clues to the pathogenesis of myositis. *Nat Clin Pract Rheumatol*, **4**(4), 201–9.

Chapter 6

Dammacco F, *et al.* (2013) Goodpasture's disease: A report of ten cases and a review of the literature. *Autoimmun Rev*, **12**(11), 1101–8.

Hellmark T, Segelmark M (2014) Diagnosis and Classification of Goodpasture's disease (Anti-GBM). *J Autoimmun*, **48–49**, 108–12.

Jennette JC, *et al.* (2013) Revised International Chapel Hill Consensus Conference Nomenclature of Vasculitides. *Arthritis Rheum*, **65**(1), 1–11.

Kallenberg CGM. (2010) Pathophysiology of ANCA-Associated Small Vessel Vasculitis. *Cur Rheumatol Rep*, **12**, 399–405.

Qin W, *et al.* (2011) Anti-phospholipase A2 receptor antibody in membranous nephropathy. *J Am Soc Nephrol*, **22**(6), 1137–43.

Mukhtyar C, *et al.* (2009) EULAR recommendations for the management of small and medium vessel vasculitis. *Ann Rheum Dis*, **68**, 310–7.

Schlumberger W (2014) Differential diagnosis of membranous nephropathy with autoantibodies to phospholipase A2 receptor 1. *Autoimmun Rev*, **13**(2), 108–13.

Chapter 7

Chorzelski TP, *et al.* (1983) IgA class endomysium antibodies in dermatitis herpetiformis and coeliac disease. *Ann NY Acad Sci*, **420**, 325–34.

Dieterich W, *et al.* (1997) Identification of tissue transglutaminase as the autoantigen of celiac disease. *Nat Med*, **3**(7), 797–801.

Chapter 9

Berg PA, Klein R (1986) Mitochondrial antigens and autoantibodies: From anti-M1 to anti- M9. *Klin Wochenschr*, **64**(19), 897–909.

Bizzaro N, Covini G, Rosina F, *et al.* (2012) Overcoming a 'probable' diagnosis in anti-mitochondrial antibody negative primary biliary cirrhosis: study of 100 sera and review of the literature. *Clin Rev Allergy Immunol*, **42**(3), 288–97.

Boberg K, Aadland E, Jahsen J, *et al.* (1998) Incidence and prevalence of primary biliary cirrhosis, primary sclerosing cholangitis and autoimmune hepatitis in a Norwegian population. *Scand J Gastroenterol*, **33**, 99–103.

Bogdanos DP, Baum H, Grasso A, *et al.* (2004) Microbial mimics are major targets of cross reactivity with human pyruvate dehydrogenase in primary biliary cirrhosis. *J Hepatol*, **40**, 31–9.

Bottazzo GF, Florin-Christensen A, Fairfax A, *et al.* (1976) Classification of smooth muscle antibodies detected by immunofluorescence. *J Clin Pathol*, **29**, 403–10.

Donaldson PT, Baragiotta A, Heneghan M, *et al.* (2006) HLA class II alleles, genotype and amino acids in primary biliary cirrhosis: A large scale study. *Hepatology*, **44**, 667–74.

Field JJ, Heathcote EJ (2003) Epidemiology of autoimmune liver disease. *J Gastroenterol Hepatol*, **18**, 1118–28.

Gregorio GV, Davies ET, Mieli-Vergani G, Vergani D (1995) Significance of extractable nuclear antigens in childhood autoimmune liver disease. *Clin Exp Immunol*, **102**, 308–13.

Gregorio GV, Portmann B, Karani J, *et al.* (2001) Autoimmune hepatitis/sclerosing cholangitis overlap syndrome in childhood: A 16-year prospective study. *Hepatology*, **33**, 544–53.

Ingelman-Sundberg M, Daly AK, Oscarson M, Nebert DW (2000) Human cytochrome P450 (CYP) genes: Recommendations for nomenclature of alleles. *Pharmacogenet Genom*, **10**, 91–3.

Liu HY, Deng AM, Zhou Y, *et al.* (2006) Analysis of HLA alleles polymorphism in Chinese patients with primary biliary cirrhosis. *Hepatobiliary Pancreat Dis Int*, **5**, 129–32.

Manns M, Gerken G, Kyriatsoulis A, Staritz M, Meyer zum Büschenfelde KH (1987) Characterisation of a new subgroup of autoimmune chronic active hepatitis by autoantibodies against a soluble liver antigen. *Lancet*, i (8528), 292–4.

Mieli-Vergani G, Vergani D (2008) Autoimmune paediatric liver disease. *World J Gastroenterol*, **14**, 3360–7.

Miyakawa H, Tanaka A, Kikuchi K, *et al.* (2001) Detection of anti-mitochondrial antibodies in immunofluorescent AMA negative patients with primary biliary cirrhosis using recombinant autoantigens. *Hepatology*, **34**(2), 243–8.

Moteki S, Leung PS, Coppel RL, *et al.* (1996) Use of a designer triple expression hybrid for three different lipoyl domains for the detection of anti-mitochondrial antibodies. *Hepatology*, **24**(1), 97–103.

Muratori P, Muratori L, Ferrari R, *et al.* (2003) Characterization and clinical impact of anti-nuclear antibodies in primary biliary cirrhosis. *Am J Gastroenterol*, **98**, 431–7.

Rizzetto M, Swana G, Doniach D (1973) Microsomal antibodies in active chronic hepatitis and other disorders. *Clin Exp Immunol*, **15**, 331–44.

Stechemesser E, Klein R, Berg PA (1993) Characterisation and clinical relevance of liver-pancreas antibodies in autoimmune hepatitis. *Hepatology*, **18**, 1–9.

Vergani D, Alvarez F, Bianchi F, *et al.* (2004) Liver autoimmune serology: A consensus statement from the committee for autoimmune serology of the International Autoimmune Hepatitis Group. *J Hepatol*, **41**, 677–83.

Chapter 10

Bataller L, Wade DF, Graus F, *et al.* (2004) Antibodies to Zic4 in paraneoplastic neurologic disorders and small-cell lung cancer. *Neurology*, **62**, 778–82.

Bernal F, Shams'ili S, Rojas I, *et al.* (2003) Anti-Tr antibodies as markers of paraneoplastic cerebellar degeneration and Hodgkin's disease. *Neurology*, **60**, 230–4.

Brain WR, Daniel PM, Greenfield JG (1951) Subacute cortical cerebellar degeneration and its relation to carcinoma. *J Neurol Neurosurg Psychiat*, **14**, 59–75.

Carvajal-González A, Leite MI, Waters P, *et al.* (2014) Glycine receptor antibodies in PERM and related syndromes: characteristics, clinical features and outcomes. *Brain*, **137**(8), 2178–92.

Chan KH, Vernino S, Lennon VA (2001) ANNA-3 anti-neuronal nuclear antibody: marker of lung cancer-related autoimmunity. *Ann Neurol*, **50**, 301–11.

Dale RC, Merheb V, Pillai S, *et al.* (2012) Antibodies to surface dopamine-2 receptor in autoimmune movement and psychiatric disorders. *Brain*, **135**(11), 3453–68.

Dalmau J, Bataller L (2006). Clinical and immunological diversity of limbic encephalitis: A model for paraneoplastic neurological disorder. *Hematol Oncol Clin North Am*, **20**, 1319–35.

Dalmau JO, Posner JB (1999) Paraneoplastic syndromes. *Arch Neurol*, **56**, 405–8.

Dalmau J, Graus F, Villarejo A, *et al.* (2004) Clinical analysis of anti-Ma2-associated encephalitis. *Brain*, **127**, 1831–44.

Dalmau J, Gleichman AJ, Hughes EG, *et al.* (2008) Anti-NMDA-receptor encephalitis: Case series and analysis of the effects of antibodies. *Lancet Neurol*, **7**, 1091–8.

European Federation of Neurological Societies/Peripheral Nerve Society (2006) Guideline on management of paraproteinemic demyelinating neuropathies. Report of a joint task force of the European Federation of Neurological Societies and the Peripheral Nerve Society. *J Peripher Nerv Syst*, **11**, 9–19.

Gallardo E, Martínez-Hernández E, Titulaer MJ, *et al.* (2014) Cortactin autoantibodies in myasthenia gravis. *Autommun Rev*, **13**(10): 1003–7.

Giometto B, Taraloto B, Graus F (1999). Autoimmunity in paraneoplastic neurological syndromes. *Brain Pathol*, **9**, 261–73.

Granerod J, *et al.* (2010) Causes of encephalitis and differences in their clinical presentations in England: a multicentre, population-based prospective study. *Lancet Infect Dis*, **10**(12), 835–44. doi: 10.1016/S1473-3099(10)70222-X.

Graus F, Cordon-Cardo C, Posner JB (1985) Neuronal antinuclear antibody in sensory neuropathy from lung cancer. *Neurology*, **35**, 538–43.

Graus F, Rowe G, Fueyo J, Darnell RB, Dalmau J (1993) The neuronal nuclear antigen recognized by the human anti-Ri autoantibody is expressed in central but not peripheral nervous system neurons. *Neurosci Lett*, **150**, 212–4.

Graus F, Dalmau J, Valldeoriola F, *et al.* (1997) Immunological characterization of a neuronal antibody (anti-Tr) associated with paraneoplastic cerebellar degeneration and Hodgkin's disease. *J Neuroimmunol*, **74**, 55–61.

Graus F, Keime-Guibert F, Rene R, *et al.* (2001) Anti-Hu-associated paraneoplastic encephalomyelitis: Analysis of 200 patients. *Brain*, **124**, 1138–48.

Graus F, Delattre JY, Antoine JC, *et al.* (2004) Recommended diagnostic criteria for paraneoplastic neurological syndromes. *J Neurol Neurosurg Psychiat*, **75**, 1135–40.

Graus F, Vincent A, Pozo-Rosich P, *et al.* (2005). Anti-glial nuclear antibody: Marker of lung cancer-related paraneoplastic neurological syndromes. *J Neuroimmunol*, **165**(1–2), 166–71.

Greene M, Lai Y, Baella N, Dalmau J, Lancaster E (2014) Antibodies to Delta/Notch-like Epidermal Growth Factor-Related Receptor in Patients With Anti-Tr, Paraneoplastic Cerebellar Degeneration, and Hodgkin Lymphoma. *JAMA Neurol*, **71**(8), 1003–8.

Grulich AE, van Leeuwen MT, Falster MO, Vajdic CM (2007) Incidence of cancers in people with HIV/AIDS compared with immunosuppressed transplant recipients: A meta-analysis. *Lancet*, **370**, 59–67.

Gultekin AH, Rosenfeld MR, Voltz R, *et al.* (2000) Paraneoplastic limbic encephalitis: Neurological symptoms, immunological findings and tumour association in 50 patients. *Brain*, **23**, 1481–94.

Hoch W, McConville J, Helms S, Newsom-Davis J, Melms A, Vincent A (2001) Auto-antibodies to the receptor tyrosine kinase MuSK in patients with myasthenia gravis without acetylcholine receptor antibodies. *Nat Med*, **7**(3), 365–8.

Höftberger R, Titulaer MJ, Sabater L, *et al.* (2013) Encephalitis and GABAB receptor antibodies: Novel findings in a new case series of 20 patients. *Neurology*, **81**(17), 1500–6.

Honnorat J, Antoine JC, Derrington E, Aguera M, Belin MF (1996) Antibodies to a subpopulation of glial cells and a 66 kDa developmental protein in patients with paraneoplastic neurological syndromes. *J Neurol Neurosurg Psychiatry*, **61**, 270–8.

Jacob S, Viegas S, Leite MI, *et al.* (2012) Presence and Pathogenic Relevance of Antibodies to Clustered Acetylcholine Receptor in Ocular and Generalized Myasthenia Gravis. *Arch Neurol*, **69**(8), 994–1001.

Juel VC, Massey JM (2007) Myasthenia gravis. *Orphanet J Rare Dis*, **2**, 44.

Karim AR, Hughes RC, Winer JB, Williams AC, Bradwell AR (2005) Paraneoplastic neurological antibodies: A laboratory experience. *Ann N Y Acad Sci*, **1050**, 274–85.

Karim AR, Hughes RG, El-Lahawi M, Bradwell AR (2007) Paraneoplastic neurological antibodies: Purkinje cell cytoplasm. In Shoenfeld Y, Gershwin E, Meroni PL (eds) *Textbook of Autoantibodies*, 2nd edition, pp. 637–43. Elsevier, New York.

Klein CJ, Lennon VA, Aston PA, *et al.* (2013) Insights from LGI1 and CASPR2 potassium channel complex autoantibody subtyping. *JAMA Neurol*, **70**(2), 229–34.

Lai M, Hughes EG, Peng X, *et al.* (2009) AMPA receptor antibodies in limbic encephalitis alter synaptic receptor location. *Ann Neurol*, **65**, 424–34.

Leite MI, Jacob S, Viegas S, *et al.* (2008) IgGl antibodies to acetylcholine receptors in 'seronegative' myasthenia gravis. *Brain*, **131**(7), 1940–52.

Lennon VA, Wingerchuk DM, Kryzer TJ, *et al.* (2004) A serum autoantibody marker of neuromyelitis optica: Distinction from multiple sclerosis. *Lancet*, **364**, 2106–12.

Meinck HM, Thompson PD (2002) Stiff man syndrome and related conditions. *Mov Disord*, **17**, 853–66.

Moll JWB., Antoine JC, Brashear HR, *et al.* (1995) Guidelines on the detection of paraneoplastic anti-neuronal-specific antibodies: Report from the Workshop to the Fourth Meeting of the International Society of Neuro-Immunology on paraneoplastic neurological disease, held October 22–23, 1994, in Rotterdam, The Netherlands. *Neurology*, **45**, 1937–41.

Pittock SJ, Lucchinetti CF, Lennon VA (2003) Anti-neuronal nuclear autoantibody type 2: Paraneoplastic accompaniments. *Ann Neurol*, **53**, 580–7.

Pittock SJ, Kryzer TJ, Lennon VA (2004) Paraneoplastic antibodies coexist and predict cancer, not neurological syndrome. *Ann Neurol*, **56**, 609–10.

Pittock SJ, Lucchinetti CF, Parisi JE, *et al.* (2005) Amphiphysin autoimmunity: Paraneoplastic accompaniments. *Ann Neurol*, **58**, 96–107.

Rees JH, (2004) Paraneoplastic syndromes: When to suspect, how to confirm, and how to manage. *J Neurol Neurosurg Psychiatry* **75** (suppl II), ii43–50.

Roberts WK, Darnell RB (2004) Neuroimmunology of the paraneoplastic neurological degenerations. *Curr Opin Immunol*, **6**, 616–22.

Rosenfeld MR, Eichen JG, Wade DF, Posner JB, Dalmau J (2001) Molecular and clinical diversity in paraneoplastic immunity to Ma proteins. *Ann Neurol*, **50**, 339–48.

Rossiñol T, Graus F (2008) Paraneoplastic neurological syndromes. In Shoenfeld Y, Cervera R, Gershwin ME (eds) *Diagnostic Criteria in Autoimmune Diseases*, pp. 421–426. Springer, New York.

Sabater L, Titulaer M, Saiz A, *et al.* (2008) SOX1 antibodies are markers of paraneoplastic Lambert–Eaton myasthenic syndrome. *Neurology*, **70**, 924–8.

Saiz A, Blanco Y, Sabater L, *et al.* (2008) Spectrum of neurological syndromes associated with glutamic acid decarboxylase antibodies: Diagnostic clues for this association. *Brain*, **131**, 2553–63.

Shams'ili S, Grefkens J, de Leeuw B, *et al.* (2003) Paraneoplastic cerebellar degeneration associated with antineuronal antibodies: Analysis of 50 patients. *Brain*, **126**, 1409–18.

Shen C, Lu Y, Zhang B, *et al.* (2013) Antibodies against low-density lipoprotein receptor-related protein 4 induce myasthenia gravis. *J Clin Invest*, **123**(12), 5190–202.

Sillevis Smitt P, Kinoshita A, De Leeuw B, *et al.* (2000) Paraneoplastic cerebellar ataxia due to autoantibodies against a glutamate receptor. *N Engl J Med*, **342**, 21–7.

Swann JB, Smyth MJ (2007) Immune surveillance of tumours. *J Clin Invest*, **117**, 1137–46.

Tan KM, Lennon VA, Klein CJ, Boeve BF, Pittock SJ (2008) Clinical spectrum of voltage-gated potassium channel autoimmunity. *Neurology*, **70**, 1883–90.

Titulaer MJ, Klooster R, Potman M, *et al.* (2009) SOX Antibodies in Small-Cell Lung Cancer and Lambert-Eaton Myasthenic Syndrome: Frequency and Relation With Survival. *J Clin Oncol*, **27**(26), 4260–7.

Titulaer MJ, McCracken L, Gabilondo I, *et al.* (2013) Treatment and prognostic factors for long-term outcome in patients with anti-NMDA receptor encephalitis: an observational cohort study. *Lancet Neurol*, **12**(2), 157–65.

Vedeler CA, Antoine JC, Giometto B, *et al.* (2006) Management of paraneoplastic neurological syndromes: Report of an EFNS Task Force. *Eur J Neurol*, **13**, 682–90.

Vernino S, Lennon VA (2000) New Purkinje cell antibody (PCA-2): Marker of lung cancer-related neurological autoimmunity. *Ann Neurol*, **47**, 297–305.

Vernino S, Hopkins S, Wang Z (2009) Autonomic ganglia, acetylcholine receptor antibodies, and autoimmune ganglionopathy. *Auton Neurosci*, **146**(1–2), 3–7.

Viegas S, Jacobson L, Waters P, *et al.* (2012) Passive and active immunization models of MuSK-Ab positive myasthenia: Electrophysiological evidence for pre and postsynaptic defects. *Exp Neurol*, **234**(2), 506–12.

Vincent A (2008) Autoimmune disorders of the neuromuscular junction. *Neurol India*, **56**, 305–13.

Voltz R, *et al.* (1999) A serologic marker of paraneoplastic limbic and brain-stem encephalitis in patients with testicular cancer. *N Engl J Med*, **340**(23), 1788–95.

Waters PJ, McKeon A, Leite MI, *et al.* (2012) Serologic diagnosis of NMO: a multicenter comparison of aquaporin-4-IgG assays. *Neurology*, **78**(9), 665–71.

Wingerchuk DM, Weinshenker BG (2014) Chapter 26—Neuromyelitis optica (Devic's syndrome). *Handb Clin Neurol*, **122**, 581–99.

Yu Z, Kryzer TJ, Griesmann K, *et al.* (2001) CRMP-5 neuronal autoantibody: Marker of lung cancer and thymoma-related autoimmunity. *Ann Neurol*, **49**, 146–54.

Zhang B, Tzartos JS, Belimezi M, *et al.* (2012) Autoantibodies to Lipoprotein-Related Protein 4 in Patients With Double-Seronegative Myasthenia Gravis. *Arch Neurol*, **69**(4), 445–51.

Chapter 12

Quillent C, Oberlin E, Braun J, *et al.* (1998) HIV-1-resistance phenotype conferred by combination of two separate inherited mutations of CCR5 gene. *Lancet*, **351**, 14–8.

Libert F, Cochaux P, Beckman G, *et al.* (1998) The deltaccr5 mutation conferring protection against HIV-1 in Caucasian populations has a single and recent origin in Northeastern Europe. *Hum Mol Genet*, **7**, 399–406.

Chapter 13

Brewerton DA, Hart FD, Nicholls A, *et al.* (1973) Ankylosing spondylitis and HL-A 27. *Lancet*, **1**, 904.

Cheng CY, Su SC, Chen CH, *et al.* (2014) HLA Associations and Clinical Implications in T-Cell Mediated Drug Hypersensitivity Reactions: An Updated Review. *J Immunol Res*, **2014**, 565320.

Fussell H, Nesbeth D, Lenhart I, *et al.* (2008) Novel detection of in vivo HLA-B27 conformations correlates with ankylosing spondylitis association. *Arthritis Rheum*, **58**(11), 3419–24.

Storb R, *et al.* (1992) Long-term follow-up of a controlled trial comparing a combination of methotrexate plus cyclosporine with cyclosporine alone for prophylaxis of graft-versus-host disease in patients administered HLA-identical marrow grafts for leukemia. *Blood*, **80**, 560–1.

Süsal C, Opelz G (2013) Current role of human leukocyte antigen matching in kidney transplantation. *Curr Opin Organ Transplant*, **18**(4), 438–44.

Terasaki PI, Marchioro TL, Starzl TE (1965) Sero-typing of human lymphocyte antigens: Preliminary trials on long-term kidney homograft survivors. In Terasaki, PI (ed.) *Histocompatibility Testing*. National Acad Sci-National Res Council, Washington, DC.

Glossary

Acetylcholine A compound found throughout the central nervous system acting as a neurotransmitter.

Acquired angioedema (AAE) is rare and due to increased consumption rather than deficient production of C1 inhibitor. Auto-antibodies to C1 inhibitor bind to the molecule in such a way as to allow it to become cleaved by other plasma proteases. These auto-antibodies may occur in association with leukaemia, lymphoma, and rarely other tumours (Type 1). They may alternatively occur in isolation or in relation to non-organ-specific autoimmune diseases such as rheumatoid arthritis and SLE (Type II).

Adaptive immunity The immunity that is acquired following sensitization with antigens.

Aetiology The cause or origin of disease.

Allergens The antigens that induce immune responses which cause allergy.

Allergy A hypersensitivity reaction initiated by immunological mechanisms.

Allotypes Allelic polymorphisms in a gene that can be determined using specific antibodies for the gene product.

Alternative pathway The complement pathway that provides a rapid, antibody-independent route for activation and amplification of complement on foreign surfaces. C3 is the key component of the alternative pathway but three other proteins, factor B (fB), factor D (fD), and properdin, are also required.

Anaphylactoid Immediate systemic reactions, with the same clinical features as anaphylaxis, but not mediated by allergen specific IgE.

Anaphylaxis occurs when there is widespread mast cell activation causing a potentially fatal reaction.

Antibodies Antigen-specific proteins that are produced by B lymphocytes in response to exposure to the antigen.

Antibody excess The state in an antibody/antigen mixture where the concentration of antibody exceeds that of antigen.

Antigen excess The state in an antibody/antigen mixture where the concentration of antigen exceeds that of antibody.

Antigens Protein molecules recognized by the immune system as foreign and against which the immune system specifically reacts.

Antisera Antibodies that are targeted against a specific antigen. Often used to identify antigens in immunological assays such as ELISA or indirect immunofluorescence (IIF).

APECED Autoimmune polyendocrinopathy, candidiasis, ectodermal dystrophy.

Apoptosis Programmed cell death.

Atopy A genetic predisposition to produce prolonged IgE antibody responses to commonly occurring allergens.

Autoantigen A self-antigen that is the target of an immune response, such as in autoimmune disease.

Autoimmune disease (autoimmunity) Breakdown of tolerance, resulting in production of antibodies and/or T cells directed against own cells and tissues.

Bence Jones proteins Monoclonal light chains found in the urine of patients with renal failure; named after the English physician Henry Bence Jones (1813–1873), who described some of their physicochemical properties in 1847.

Bullae Large blisters containing serous fluid.

Calcinosis The formation of tiny deposits of calcium in the skin.

Cationic Referring to a positively charged molecule.

Cell-mediated immunity (cellular immunity) Immune response mediated by cells such as T lymphocytes.

Cerebellar degeneration Damage to the cerebellum, with loss of muscle control and balance.

Cholangiography Imaging of the biliary tract.

Cirrhosis Irreversible change in liver tissue that results in the degeneration of functioning liver cells and their replacement with fibrous connective tissue.

Citrullinated proteins Citrullination is the post-translational modification of arginine within a protein to citrulline by enzymes called PADs (peptidylarginine deiminases) to form citrullinated proteins.

Class switch recombination The process by which a B cell upon recognition of antigen will switch the production of immunoglobulin from IgM alone to other isotypes, e.g. IgG and IgA.

Classical pathway The complement pathway that is triggered by antibody bound to particulate antigen. Many other substances including components of damaged cells, bacterial lipopolysaccharide, and nucleic acids can also trigger the classical pathway in an antibody-independent manner.

Clusters of differentiation (CD) Cell surface molecules on lymphocytes that are recognized by monoclonal antibodies to allow identification of the cell by flow cytometry.

Complement A group of blood proteins which enhance the immune response.

Complementarity determining region (CDR) A short amino acid sequence found in the variable region of an immunoglobulin.

Conjugate The term generally used to describe an immunoglobulin that has a marker attached, such as an immunofluorescent label or an enzyme. These immunoglobulins are used to label human antibodies in techniques such as IIF or ELISA.

Continuing professional development (CPD) is a process of lifelong learning, which enables you to expand and fulfil your personal and professional potential, as well as meet the present and future needs of patients and deliver health outcomes and priorities. It assures that you meet the requisite knowledge and skills levels that relate to your evolving scope of professional practice (www.IBMS.org).

CREST syndrome A limited form of scleroderma, consisting of calcinosis, Raynaud's phenomenon, oesophageal motility, sclerodactyly, and telangiectasia.

Crithidia lucillae A micro-organism with a kinetoplast that contains only double-stranded DNA. Commercial preparations of this organism are available for test purposes.

Cryofibrinogen An abnormal fibrinogen that precipitates at cold temperatures and redissolves at 37 °C.

Cryoglobulin Abnormal immunoglobulins (IgG or IgM) that precipitate when serum is cooled.

Cytokines Proteins produced by cells of the immune system that act as regulatory proteins and intercellular mediators facilitating the immune response.

Densitometry The quantitative measurement of optical density.

Dermal-epidermal junction The junction between the dermis and the epidermis (see also **hemidesmosome**).

Dermis The layer of skin between the epidermis and the sub-cutis.

Desmosome A specialized structure for cell–cell adhesion.

Encephalomyelitis Inflammation of both brain (encephalitis) and spinal cord (myelitis).

Endocytosis The process by which a cell ingests material with the formation of vesicles. Includes phagocytosis and pinocytosis.

Enteropathy A disease of the intestinal tract.

Entopy Localized mucosal allergic disease in the absence of circulating allergen specific IgE.

Epidermis The outermost layer of the skin.

Epiphenomenon A secondary symptom that appears during the course of a disease, secondary to the existing disease symptoms.

Epitope The region on an antigen that is recognizable by the immune system.

Erythema Reddening of the skin.

Fixative A compound (such as ethanol or formaldehyde) that preserves or stabilizes tissues and cells for microscopic study.

Fluorochrome A fluorescent chemical that emits a specific colour when illuminated by light.

Gastritis Inflammation of the stomach lining.

Genotyping The process of defining the genotype of an individual using laboratory techniques such as DNA sequencing and PCR. This is useful in determining if an individual has disease-associated genes.

L-Glutamate The main excitatory neurotransmitter in the central nervous system. It acts via voltage-gated ion channels (ionotropic) or G-protein coupled (metabotropic) receptors.

Graft versus host disease (GVHD) A T cell response by donor cells driven by HLA mismatch with the recipient, such that donor cells recognize the recipient as foreign antigen and cause an immune response, which may be life threatening.

Grand Round A conference in which clinicians/experts present the case studies of individual patients, or new topics in the field of medicine, and use this as an educational tool for other staff members.

Granulocytes White blood cells filled with granules containing enzymes which enable digestion of micro-organisms and production of inflammatory responses. Includes neutrophils, eosinophils, and basophils.

Granuloma A mass of immune cells (lymphocytes, macrophages) that accumulates at sites of inflammation, injury, or infection.

Graves' disease Autoimmune hyperthyroidism.

Haematemesis Vomiting blood.

Haematuria Blood in urine.

Haemolytic uraemic syndrome (HUS) A syndrome consisting of the triad of thrombocytopenia, Coombs negative microangiopathic haemolytic anaemia, and acute renal failure; deficiency of or mutations in factor H and factor I can lead to a susceptibility to HUS.

Haemoptysis Coughing up blood.

Hapten A complex of a small molecule with a carrier, usually protein.

Hemidesmosome Stud-like structures on the inner layer of keratinocytes in the epidermis that allow cell adhesion to the extracellular matrix.

Hepatitis Inflammation of the hepatocytes in the liver.

Hereditary angioedema (HAE) Genetic mutations resulting in the absence of C1 esterase inhibitor in serum are found in approximately 85% of patients (type I). The remaining 15% of patients have normal or elevated serum concentrations, but the protein produced by one allele is dysfunctional (type II). In either case, this clinically results in angioedema.

Heterophile An antibody against an antigen from one species that also reacts against antigens from other species. Often seen in indirect immunofluorescence.

Human leukocyte antigen (HLA) A genetically determined series of markers (antigens) present on human white blood cells (leukocytes) and on tissues that are important in histocompatibility.

Humoral immunity Immune response mediated by B cells and antibodies.

Hypergammaglobulinaemia An increase of gammaglobulins in serum.

Hypersensitivity The reaction that causes reproducible signs or symptoms, following exposure to a defined stimulus, in a susceptible individual.

Hyperthyroidism Excessive production of thyroid hormones caused by overactivity of the thyroid gland.

Hypoparathyroidism Underactivity of the parathyroid, the gland that controls calcium levels in both blood and bone.

Hypothyroidism A reduction in the production of thyroid hormones caused by underactivity of the thyroid gland.

Idiopathic Of an unknown cause.

Immune complexes Antigen and antibody complexes which can be soluble or insoluble. This depends on the size of the complex and the presence of complement.

Immune paresis Suppression of normal immunoglobulin production by a malignant bone marrow plasma cell clone.

Immunodeficiency Defects in the immune system resulting in gaps in the body's defence against pathogens.

Immunofixation Process in which a specific antibody is used to 'fix' antigens within a gel after electrophoresis by means of the formation of antibody–antigen complexes. After removing unfixed molecules by washing and then staining the fixed complexes, the presence or absence of specific molecules in the original sample can be demonstrated.

Immunological memory The ability of the immune system to 'recall' a previous encounter with an antigen resulting in a stronger immunological response.

Immunosuppression A suppression of the immune system with a reduction in number, reactivity, expansion, or differentiation of T and/or B lymphocytes.

Infectious mononucleosis Also known as glandular fever. An acute disease characterized by fever and swollen lymph nodes and an abnormal increase of mononuclear leucocytes or monocytes.

Inflammation A characteristic physiological response of tissues to injury. The signs of inflammation are heat, redness, swelling, and pain.

Innate immunity The natural immunity that exists prior to sensitization from an antigen. It is often non-specific.

Lambert–Eaton myasthenic syndrome (LEMS) Muscle weakness, fatigue, difficulty swallowing, and autonomic symptoms.

Lectin pathway The complement pathway that provides a second antibody-independent means of activation of complement on bacterial and other micro-organism surfaces. It is highly analogous to the classical pathway and shares C2, C3, and C4 with it.

Limbic encephalitis Inflammation of the brain leading to memory loss, drowsiness, confusion, disorientation, and seizures.

Lipodystrophy The progressive loss of fat. Lipodystrophy may be congenital or acquired, and can affect all of the body (generalized lipodystrophy) or just parts of the body (partial lipodystrophy).

Lupus anticoagulant An auto-antibody which interferes with blood coagulation, as well as *in vitro* tests of clotting function, causing elevation in the partial thromboplastin time.

Lymphocytes A type of white blood cell of which there are three subtypes: B cells, which give rise to humoral immunity; T cells, which give rise to cellular immunity; and natural killer cells.

Macrocytic anaemia An anaemia in which the red blood cells are larger in volume than normal (raised mean corpuscular volume [MCV]).

Macrophages Phagocytic cells found in the tissues that ingest, kill, and digest bacteria, foreign cells, and tissue debris. These cells also play a role in antigen presentation in the immune system.

Major histocompatibility complex (MHC) A group of genes that code for cell-surface histocompatibility antigens and are the principal determinants of tissue type and transplant compatibility.

Membrane attack complex (MAC) A large transmembrane pore formed from the terminal complement components which can cause lysis of the target cell by allowing free diffusion of molecules in and out of the cell.

Membrane attack pathway The membrane attack pathway involves the non-covalent association of complement C5b with the four terminal complement components to form an amphipathic membrane-inserted complex, the membrane attack complex (MAC).

Membranoproliferative glomerulonephritis (MPGN) A disorder of the kidney caused by immune complex deposition in the glomerular basement membrane. Complement activation results in inflammation of the glomeruli, causing disrupted kidney function and can progress to chronic renal failure.

Microcytic anaemia An anaemia in which the red blood cells are smaller in volume than normal (reduced mean corpuscular volume [MCV]).

Mitosis Division of a somatic cell to form two genetically identical daughter cells.

Monoclonal antibodies Antibodies produced from a single clone of cells, consisting of identical molecules.

Monoclonal gammopathy (MG) Disease characterized by the finding of monoclonal immunoglobulin in the serum and/or urine.

Monoclonal gammopathy of undetermined significance (MGUS) Monoclonal gammopathy in which the monoclonal quantification and clinical features do not meet the diagnostic criteria for any specific disease.

Mononuclear cells White blood cells with only one nucleus. Includes monocytes and lymphocytes.

Multidisciplinary team meetings (MDTs) Whereby different groups of professionals (i.e. doctors, nurses, and scientists) meet to discuss individual patients, using the knowledge from each discipline to work towards effective diagnosis and treatments.

Multisystem disease A disease affecting more than one component of the body. An example is rheumatoid arthritis which can affect the joints, lungs, kidneys and blood vessels.

Myasthenia gravis Weakness and rapid fatigue of voluntary muscles.

Myeloma Disease associated with a malignant monoclonal proliferation of bone marrow plasma cells, characterized by lytic bone lesions, plasma cell accumulation in the bone marrow and the presence of monoclonal immunoglobulin in the serum and/or urine.

Necrosis Unprogrammed cell death.

Negative selection T cell recognition of self-antigen in the thymus resulting in deletion by apoptosis.

Neoantigen A newly acquired and expressed antigen; often present after a cell is infected by an oncogenic virus.

Neuromyotonia Abnormal nerve impulses from peripheral motor neurons causing twitching, stiffness, cramps, and slowed movement.

Neuropathy Disorder of peripheral nervous system involving motor, sensory, and/or autonomic nerves.

Neutrophils Phagocytic white blood cells that ingest and destroy bacteria as part of the innate immune response. These cells rapidly accumulate, in large numbers, at sites of infection and inflammation.

Oesophageal dysmotility Involvement of the oesophagus in scleroderma.

Opsoclonus-myoclonus (OM) Rapid, irregular eye movements (opsoclonus) coupled with quick, involuntary muscle jerks (myoclonus).

Opsonization The binding of complement and antibodies to the surface of a pathogen or foreign substance to aid phagocytosis.

Oral allergy syndrome (OAS) Mild oral symptoms, usually mouth tingling or itching. Patients usually have hay fever and the reaction is caused by cross-reactive PR-10 components in pollen and plant derived foods.

Overflow proteinuria Proteinuria caused by glomerular filtration of levels of protein which exceed the reabsorption capacity of the renal tubules.

Paraprotein An abnormal (usually monoclonal) protein seen in a monoclonal gammopathy such as MGUS or myeloma.

Pathogenesis The origination and development of a disease.

Pathogenic Causing disease.

Plasmoblast A precursor cell of the plasmocyte, which constitutes 1% of the nucleated white blood cells. Not commonly seen in the peripheral blood of normal people, but can be seen in chronic infections, granulomatous and allergic diseases, and plasma cell myeloma.

Polymorphism Variations in a gene locus at a frequency greater than 1% (adj. **polymorphic**).

Positive selection The survival of a T cell through the TCR binding to MHC with weak affinity, ensuring T cells can recognize self and are non-reactive.

Prodrome An early symptom of disease.

Protein electrophoresis The separation of the protein molecules within a solution (usually serum, urine, or CSF) as a result of their differing motilities within an electric field.

Proteinuria The presence of protein in the urine. Proteins filtered through the kidney glomeruli should be actively reabsorbed in the tubules and so proteinuria should normally be absent or minimal.

Pruritis Itch.

Raynaud's phenomenon Spasm of the tiny artery vessels supplying the blood to the extremities during periods of low ambient temperature.

Scalded skin syndrome Staphylococcal infection of the skin, leading to a generalized red blistering rash also known as bullous impetigo.

Scanning densitometry (densitometry) The determination of the density of stain along a protein electrophoresis strip by means of light absorption. If the stain density is linear in relation to the amount of protein present, the densitometric scan can be used to determine the amount of protein in a given area, e.g. within a monoclonal band.

Sclerodactyly Localized thickening and tightness of the skin of the fingers or toes.

Sensitivity The ability of an assay to correctly identify disease. The number of false negatives.

Seroconversion The detection of antibodies in response to an antigen (infectious organism). In HIV infection, the conversion from an antibody-negative to an antibody-positive state can take from one week to several months.

Somatic hypermutation The introduction of mutations into the variable region of an antibody, to increase the antibody affinity.

Specificity Lack of interference from other elements other than the analyte being measured. The number of false positives.

Stiff person syndrome (SPS) Progressive, severe muscle stiffness or rigidity, mainly in spine and legs.

Sub-cutis The deepest/innermost layer of the skin.

Synovial membrane The thin membrane that lines the inside of a joint. Its function is to lubricate the joint and produce synovial fluid.

Telangiectasias Dilated capillaries that form tiny red areas, frequently on the face.

Thrombosis The formation of a blood clot (thrombus) within the blood vessels.

Thyrotoxicosis The condition resulting from an excess of thyroid hormones.

Vasculitis Inflammation of the blood vessels.

Viraemia The presence of virus in plasma.

Abbreviations

AAE	Acquired angioedema
ACE	Angiotensin converting enzyme
AChR	Acetylcholine receptor antibody
ACTH	Adenocorticotrophic hormone
ADCC	Antibody-dependent cell-mediated cytotoxicity
AGA	Anti-ganglioside antibodies
AIDS	Acquired immune deficiency syndrome
AIRE	Autoimmune regulator gene
ALBIA	Addressable laser bead immunoassay
ALTM	All laboratories trimmed mean
AMPAR	α-Amino-3-hydroxy-5-methyl-4-isoxazole propionic acid receptor
ANNA1	Anti-neuronal nuclear antibody type 1 (Hu is an alternative name)
ANNA2	Anti-neuronal nuclear antibody type 2 (Ri is an alternative name)
APC	Antigen-presenting cell
APECED	Autoimmune polyendocrinopathy, candidiasis, ectodermal dystrophy
APS	Autoimmune polyglandular syndrome (*also* anti-phospholipid syndrome)
AQP4	Aquaporin 4 antibody (NMO is an alternative name)
ATP	Adenosine triphosphate
CCD	Cross-reactive carbohydrate determinants
CCR3	C-C Chemokine receptor type 3
CD	Cluster of differentiation
CDC	Complement dependent cytotoxicity
CDR	Complementarity determining region
CGD	Chronic granulomatous disease
CLR	Collagen-like region
CML	Chronic myeloid leukaemia
CNS	Central nervous system
CPD	Continuing professional development
CRD	Component-resolved diagnosis
CRMP-5	Collapsin response-mediator brain proteins
CRP	C-reactive protein
CSF	Cerebrospinal fluid
CTLA	Cytotoxic T-lymphocyte antigen
CV-2	Alternative name for CRMP-5 antibody
CZE	Capillary zone electrophoresis
DAF	Decay-accelerating factor
DBPCC	Double-blind placebo-controlled challenge
DNP	Deoxyribonucleoprotein
DSA	Donor-Specific Antibody
DTT	Dithiothreitol
EAACI	European Academy of Allergy and Clinical Immunology
ECP	Eosinophil cationic protein
EGTA	Ethylene glycol tetra-acetic acid
ELISA	Enzyme-linked immunosorbent assay
EFI	European Federation of Immunogenetics
EQA	External quality assessment
ENA	Extractable nuclear antigens
ESR	Erythrocyte sedimentation rate
EUROEQAS	European External Quality Assessment Service
FBC	Full blood count
FcεRI	High affinity IgE receptor
FCXM	Flow cytometric crossmatching
FPIA	Fluorescent polarization immunoassay
FTT	Failure to thrive
G6PD	Glucose-6-phosphate dehydrogenase
GAD	Glutamic acid decarboxylase
GINA	Global Initiative for Asthma
GVHD	Graft versus host disease
H&I	Histocompatibility and Immunogenetics
HAE	Hereditary angioedema
HbA_1c	Glycosylated haemoglobin
HCV	Hepatitis C virus
HIDS	Hyper IgD syndrome
HIV	Human immunodeficiency virus
HLA	Human leukocyte antigen
HUVS	Hypocomplementaemic urticarial vasculitis
IA-2	Insulinoma-like antigen-2
ICA	Islet cell antibody
IgA	Immunoglobulin A
IgD	Immunoglobulin D
IgE	Immunoglobulin E
IgG	Immunoglobulin G
IgM	Immunoglobulin M
IIF	Indirect immunofluorescence
IL	Interleukin
IFCC	International Federation of Clinical Chemistry

IQC	Internal quality control
IUIS	International Union of Immunological Societies
JDF	Juvenile Diabetes Foundation
kU/L	Kilo units per litre
kUA/L	Kilo allergen specific units per litre
LADA	Latent autoimmune diabetes of adults
LEMS	Lambert–Eaton myasthaenic syndrome
LFT	Liver function test
LTP	Lipid transfer protein
MAC	Membrane attack complex
MAG	Myelin-associated glycoprotein antibodies
MASP	MBL-associated serine protease
MBL	Mannan-binding lectin
MCP	Membrane cofactor protein
MCTD	Mixed connective tissue disease
MCV	Mean cell volume
MDT	Multidisciplinary team
MG	Myasthenia gravis
mGluR1	Anti-metabotropic glutamate receptor 1
MGUS	Monoclonal gammopathy of undetermined significance
MHC	Major histocompatibility complex
MICA	MHC class 1-related gene A
MKD	Mevalonate kinase deficiency
MPGN	Membranoproliferative glomerulonephritis
MPO	Myeloperoxidase
MRBIS	Mean running bias index score
MRI	Magnetic resonance imaging
MRVIS	Mean running variance index score
MS	Multiple sclerosis
MuSK	Muscle-specific kinase
NHSBT	NHS Blood and Transplant
NICE	National Institute of Health and Care Excellence
NIDG	UK Neuroimmunology Discussion Group
NK	Natural killer (cells)
NKAS	National Kidney Allocation Scheme
NMDAR	N-methyl D-aspartate receptor
NMJ	Neuromuscular juction
NMO	Neuromyelitis optica
NMT	Neuromyotonia
NSAID	Nonsteroidal anti-inflammatory drug
OAS	Oral allergy syndrome
OM	Opsoclonus–myoclonus
OMRVIS	Overall mean running variance index score
PAD	Peptidylarginine deiminase
PCA-1	Purkinje cell cytoplasmic antibody type 1 (Yo is an alternative name)
PCA-2	Purkinje cell cytoplasmic antibody type 2
PCA-Tr	Purkinje cell cytoplasmic antibody type Tr (Tr is an alternative name)
PCD	Paraneoplastic cerebellar degeneration
PCNA	Proliferating cell nuclear antigen
PCR	Polymerase chain reaction
PEG	Polyethylene glycol
PEM	Paraneoplastic encephalomyelitis
PLE	Paraneoplastic limbic encephalitis
PNA	Paraneoplastic neurological antibody
PNH	Peripheral nerve hyperexcitability
PNS	Paraneoplastic neurological syndrome
POM	Paraneoplastic opsoclonus–myoclonus
PR-10	Family 10 of pathogenesis related proteins
RAST	Radioallergosorbent test
RF	Rheumatoid factor
RNP	Ribonucleoproteins
RSV	Respiratory syncitial virus
SCLC	Small-cell lung cancer
SDBIS	Standard deviation of the bias index score
SEP	Serum electrophoresis
SFLC	Serum κ and λ free light chains
sIgE	Allergen-specific immunoglobulin E
SIT	Specific immunotherapy
SLE	Systemic lupus erythematosus
SPS	Stiff person syndrome
T_3	Tri-iodothyronine
T_4	Thyroxine
TCC	Terminal complement complex
TCR	T cell receptors
TNF	Tumour necrosis factor
TPO	Thyroid peroxidase
TSH	Thyroid-stimulating hormone
TSHRAB	TSH receptor antibody
tTG	Tissue transglutaminase
U&E	Urea and electrolytes (test)
UKNEQAS	United Kingdom National External Quality Assessment Service
UEP	Urine electrophoresis
VGCC	Voltage-gated calcium channel antibody
VGKC	Voltage-gated potassium channel antibody
WAO	World Allergy Organization
WHO	World Health Organization

Hints and tips for discussion questions

Chapter 1

1.1

- Good knowledge of more than one discipline.
- Ability to interpret results from different disciplines, as results from one discipline should be considered together with those from the other disciplines for meaningful interpretation and diagnosis.
- Biomedical scientists usually specialize in one discipline but they need, at least, to have a basic understanding and to be aware of the scope of the other disciplines.
- Greater opportunity for career progression, as trained in more than one discipline.

1.2

- An internationally recognized benchmark of quality and excellence.
- Biomedical Scientists can register as a chartered scientist if they have achieved the level of qualification required, show evidence of continual profession development, and have the minimum level of work experience required.
- Demonstration of practising science at the full professional level.

Chapter 2

2.1

- Immunoglobulin molecule subunits are called domains and are named according to their location in the immunoglobulin molecule, e.g. constant region heavy chain domain 1 is CH1. Within each domain the polypeptide chain is folded into beta-pleated sheets held by intrachain disulphide bonds.

2.2

- a) CH2
- b) CH3
- c) VH.

2.3

- IgG: Complement activation + +, IgG Fc receptor II & III binding + + + +, placental transfer + +, produced to peptide antigens.
- IgG2: Complement activation +, IgG Fc receptor II & III binding +, placental transfer +, produced to polysaccharide antigens.
- IgG3: Complement activation + + +, IgG Fc receptor II & III binding + + +, placental transfer + +, produced to peptide antigens.
- IgG4: Complement activation 0, IgG Fc receptor II & III binding +, placental transfer +, produced to peptide antigens.

2.4

- As a fixed amount of antibody is combined with increasing amounts of antigen, the immune complex which is formed becomes larger. When antigen exceeds available antibody, the large complexes break apart leaving small or single antibody immune complexes which generate a small optical signal similar to that generated by low concentrations of antigen. This is described by the Heidelberger–Kendall curve.

Chapter 3

3.1

- Natural extracts should contain the relevant allergenic components.
- Extraction processes may destroy the allergenicity of the final product.
- There can be problems with reproducibility of reagents and variability between commercial suppliers.
- Recombinant technology allows the production of single proteins with defined allergenic epitopes.
- Recombinant allergens can be used as diagnostic tools to supplement natural extracts or as single reagents.
- Testing with recombinant allergens can lead to component resolved diagnosis.
- Reagents which are based on recombinant allergens may not cover the complete repertoire of allergenic epitopes.

3.2

- Internal quality control using sera and/or commercial preparations of known sIgE concentrations in the assay.
- Assay verification undertaken by monitoring Levy–Jennings plots and by applying Westgard rules.
- Impractical to undertake internal quality control for every allergen. Therefore, choose most appropriate and test at relevant sIgE concentrations.
- Undertake external quality assessment, e.g. UKNEQAS scheme.
- Compare performance with peer group because of potential variability in allergen preparations.
- Enrol in web-based educational programmes.

3.3

- Most common approach is in assessing basophil activation.
- Applicable in situations where specific IgE tests are unavailable or have poor diagnostic sensitivity or specificity, e.g. drug allergy.
- May be useful when skin/challenge testing cannot be undertaken.

- May provide diagnostic evidence when sIgE results are equivocal as the method may more accurately reflect the in vivo pathophysiological pathway.

Chapter 4

4.1

- Opsonization.
- Mediates an inflammatory response.
- Activates endothelium.
- Recruits and activates phagocytes.
- Lysis of target cells by membrane attack complex.

4.2

- C1 esterase inhibitor.
- Autosomal dominant inheritance.
- Symptoms: episodes of angioedema which can affect any part of the body; intra-abdominal swellings can lead to obstruction; airway swellings can lead to death by asphyxiation.
- Treatments: tranexamic acid (which inhibits some of the proteases which cleave C1 inhibitor); androgenic steroids danazol or stanozolol (which increase transcription of many genes, including the normally functioning copy of C1 inhibitor); C1 esterase inhibitor concentrate (a blood product); bradykinin inhibitors.

4.3

- Activation is different: antibody–antigen pathways for the classical pathway and components of bacterial cell walls for the lectin pathway.
- The initial proteins are different. However, there is homology between them with C1q, C1r, and C1s being structurally similar to MBL, MASP1, and MASP2.
- Subsequently the pathways converge, with cleavage of C4 and C2 leading on to the production of C3 convertase, C5 convertase, and formation of the membrane attack complex.

Chapter 5

5.1

- Malar rash
- Discoid rash
- Photosensitivity
- Oral ulcers
- Nonerosive arthritis
- Involving > 2 peripheral joints
- Pleuritis or pericarditis
- Renal disorder
- Persistent proteinuria or cellular casts
- Neurological disorder
- Seizures or psychosis in the absence of drugs or known metabolic disorders
- Haematologic disorder
- Haemolytic anaemia or leukopenia or lymphopenia or thrombocytopenia
- Immunologic disorder
- Antibodies to dsDNA or Sm or positive finding of antiphospholipid antibodies (anti-cardiolipin, lupus anticoagulant, or a false positive syphilis test)
- Positive anti-nuclear antibodies.

Four out of the eleven criteria need to be present for the diagnosis to be made.

5.2

Method	Advantages	Disadvantages
Indirect immunofluorescence	Good screening test to eliminate negative sera. Low cost. Semi-quantitative (titration).	Antibody specificity not identified. Will detect other non-clinically relevant auto-antibodies. Requires experienced staff to read accurately.
ELISA/FPIA/bead immunoassay	Antibody specificity identified. Automatable tests. Quantitative measurement.	
Western blot	Antibody specificity identified.	Qualitative test. Not useful for monitoring.
Dot blot	Antibody specificity identified.	Qualitative test. Not useful for monitoring.

5.3

- Proliferation of cells within the synovial membrane.
- Migration of immune cells to site of inflammation.
- Release of pro-inflammatory cytokines and chemokines within the fluid of the joint.
- Auto-antibodies in the circulation of patients with RA including rheumatoid factor and antibodies to citrullinated proteins.
- The presence of cryoglobulins.
- Increase of proteins associated with an acute phase response such as fibrinogen and C-reactive protein.
- Increased complement breakdown products (C3d or C4d).
- Presence of circulating immune complexes.

Chapter 6

6.1

Method	Advantages	Disadvantages
Indirect immunofluorescence	Good screening test to eliminate negative sera. Low cost.	Antibody specificity not identified. Will detect other auto-antibodies, e.g. ANA. Requires experienced staff to read accurately. Semi-quantitative (titration)..
ELISA/FPIA/bead immunoassay	Antibody specificity identified. Automatable tests. Quantitative measurement.	
Western blot	Antibody specificity identified.	Qualitative test. Not useful for monitoring.
Dot blot	Antibody specificity identified.	Qualitative test. Not useful for monitoring.

6.2

General:

- Weight loss.
- Night sweats.
- Fatigue.
- Arthritis.

Specific:

- Changes in blood biochemistry indicating decreasing kidney function: increased urea, increased creatinine.
- Haemoptysis (blood in sputum).
- Haematuria (blood in urine).
- Kidney biopsy showing damage to glomeruli with crescent formation. Immunochemistry shows no immunoglobulin or complement present (in ANCA associated diseases), or liner IgG staining of the glomerular basement membrane sometimes accompanied by associated complement deposition (anti-GBM disease).
- X-ray showing infiltrates (granulomas).

6.3

- Antibody titres in many patients show a direct relationship to disease activity.
- They are capable of binding to primed neutrophils and initiate a respiratory burst, which leads to degranulation and the release of proteolytic enzymes, which are capable of causing damage to surrounding tissues.
- The antibodies may also bind directly to endothelial cells and thus render them to damage by cell mediated or complement mediated cytotoxicity.

6.4

- There are two methods: ELISA (recombinant PLA2R) and indirect immunofluorescence (HEK298 cell lines expressing PLA2R).
- PLA2R antibodies are important to determine whether membranous nephropathy is due to a primary or secondary cause.

6.5

- Untreated mortality is up to 90% in ANCA associated vasculitis. With conventional treatment there is only a 10% 1-year mortality. The recommended therapies are potent immunosuppressants, in the form of steroids and steroid sparing agents, or plasma exchange, depending on the severity at presentation. The regimes are induction and remission, with more potent therapies used for induction.

Chapter 7

7.1

- Firstly, the patient needs to be genetically susceptible to the disease. Also within this sphere are endogenous factors such as hormone balance.
- Secondly, the patient requires some form of trigger to break tolerance. Often this trigger is unknown but infections are commonly thought to be involved (sometimes called 'molecular mimicry').
- Finally, the patient requires an element of bad luck, as even identical twins brought up in the same environment do not always both get the disease.

7.2

- Auto-antibodies may be detected in some members of the normal, healthy population.
- Also note that the transient appearance of auto-antibodies, particularly during and after a viral infection, is a common occurrence.
- Most patients do not go on to develop autoimmune disease, although some do.

- Where this balance is not restored the patient may go on to develop autoimmune disease.
- Those with persistent antibody on retesting are more likely to develop the associated autoimmune disease in the future.

7.3

- Hypothyroidism: Hashimoto's thyroiditis, atrophic thyroiditis, post partum thyroiditis, sub-clinical hypothyroidism, focal thyroiditis, juvenile lymphocytic thyroiditis.
- Hyperthyroidism: Graves' disease.

7.4

- IgA responses predominate and are the more important in diagnosis; however, IgA deficiency is about ten times more common in patients with coeliac disease than in the general population. If a patient is IgA deficient, then IgA tests for coeliac disease will be negative.

7.5

- The destruction of parietal cells in the stomach leads to a lack of intrinsic factor, which is necessary for efficient vitamin B_{12} absorption.
- Intrinsic factor auto-antibodies can further impair the absorption of vitamin B_{12}, either by preventing B_{12} binding to intrinsic factor or by interfering with the binding of intrinsic factor to receptors in the ileum.

Chapter 8

8.1

- The immunology laboratory can undertake serology testing for basement membrane antibodies and intercellular antibodies and rule out associated disorders such as dermatitis herpetiformis.

8.2

- Pemphigus and pemphigoid are both treated with steroids and steroid sparing immune suppression: whereas pemphigoid may be treated with topical treatment, pemphigus is nearly always treated with systemic therapies.

Chapter 9

9.1

- All the variables that constitute the assay; the serum screening dilution1/10, in line with the international consensus document as the antibody may be present in very low concentration; the use of appropriate control sera; choice and dilution of FITC conjugate (must do chequerboard titration to ensure optimum performance); optimization of microscope optics and light source; competence of the observers (there should be two experienced observers); use of an antigen-specific based assay to confirm microscopic findings; and participation in external quality assurance scheme.

9.2

- Result suggests AMA negative PBC or is IIF not sufficiently sensitive? Use an anti-M2 specific ELISA or immunoblot. Better still use a recombinant ELISA with three target M2 antigens to increase sensitivity. If these are negative then sample is probably anti-M2 negative. However there are ANAs associated with PBC, rim, MND, and centromere. Test the sample on HEp-2 cells or one of the derivative cell lines to look for these auto-antibodies. Ultimately the liver biopsy will confirm or deny presence of PBC.

9.3

- A high titre anti-M2 will mask the presence of other auto-antibodies of lower titre. The use of HEp-2 cells may reveal ANA but F-actin SMA will probably be lost in the M2 fluorescence of the HEp-2 cytoplasm. Anti-LKM 1 and anti-LC 1are unlikely in PBC/AIH overlap and again would be lost in the anti-M2 pattern. Use alternative techniques: ELISA and/or immunoblot for liver disease related auto-antibodies. The blots are easy to use and provide all the potential auto-antigen targets (more efficient than using four separate ELISAs).
- Also the blots contain an SLA antigen which is not detectable in IIF even in the absence of anti-M2. In this scenario anti-SLA was detected along with the expected anti-M2 on immunoblot. This is not an infrequent pair of auto-antibodies to find in PBC/AIH overlap.

Chapter 10

10.1

- Infiltration of immune mediators in the affected areas of the brain and antibodies from patients with PNS can be shown to bind to the brain tissue.

10.2

- Neuronal antigens expressed in the tumour cause immune response against tumour and brain cell (neuron) antigens.

10.3

- A diagnosis of paraneoplastic neurological syndrome is confirmed if the classical neurological syndrome and a well-characterized PNA are present together.

10.4

- Irreversible neurological damage. The objective is usually to stabilize the syndrome and improve quality of life; death can occur from tumour burden or associated severe neurological problems.

Chapter 11

11.1

- They enable B cells to class switch, i.e. make IgG (without T cells' help would only make IgM).
- Activate macrophage killing of pathogens.

- CD4⁺ T cells help CD8⁺ T cells to kill cells infected with virus.

11.2

- XLA and B-SCID.
- Set up a lymphocyte panel including HLA-DR.
- XLA would have normal T cells, i.e. normal CD4/CD8 ratio and normal activation.
- SCID would have no T cells (MFE or Omenn's: T cells would be very activated).

11.3

- Lymphadenopathy/hepatosplenomegaly, autoimmune cytopenias.
- Defect in apoptosis.
- Look for the presence of increased numbers of double negative TCR αβ T cells.

11.4

- SCID
- XLA
- CGD
- (SCID) SCID, non random X inactivation of the T cells
- (XLA) Normal BTK in all B cells, 50:50 normal/abnormal BTK in the monocytes
- (CGD) 2 populations of neutrophils one with normal and one with abnormal oxidative burst.

Chapter 12

12.1

- HIV infection is usually determined using an ELISA which combines the testing of p24 antigen and anti-HIV antibodies, together with other HIV-1 antigens, such as gp160, gp41. Some HIV tests differentiate between HIV-1 and HIV-2 although confirmation is usually by Western blot or line probe assays—reactivity to gp120 and gp41 indicative of HIV-1 infection while samples positive for HIV-2 would react with gp105 and gp36, but not with gp120 and gp41. In developing countries, point of care or rapid screening tests may be offered.

12.2

- Yes. As noted under question 12.1, most ELISAs differentiate between HIV-1 and HIV-2, although confirmation of HIV-1 or HIV-2 infection is usually by Western blot.

12.3

- The term seroconversion refers to the development of antibodies following infection or immunization, i.e. the change from an antibody negative to antibody positive state. In HIV-1 infection, however, individuals are said to have 'seroconverted' following a 'seroconvertion illness', which may precede the development of antibodies and may be marked by a significant viraemia.

12.4

- During seroconversion illness patients may experience flu-like symptoms, myalgia, pyrexia, and lymphadenopathy. Occasionally patients present with a mobilliform rash.

12.5

- Long term non-progressors or elite controllers (those who maintain a viral loads of < 50 copies/ml) are individuals who have been infected with HIV virus but have sustained low-level viraemia and normal CD4 counts in the absence of antiretroviral therapy.

12.6

- Disease progression and/or therapy efficacy can be determined by monitoring CD4 counts and HIV viral load. In treatment naïve patients, approximately one third will present with a CD4 count of < 200 cells/μl—these patients, even after commencing antiretroviral therapy, will have a significantly higher risk of disease progression or death than those starting with higher CD4 counts. Patients presenting with low CD4 counts may have contracted the disease a long time ago and the CD4 count may be a reflection of the progressive damage to the immune system over time. Predictions may be made about possible disease progression from initial CD4 count and viral load.

12.7

- Treatment failure may occur for a number of reasons: development of resistant strains, suboptimal absorption, or may be due to patient non-compliance.

12.8

- If mutations are not detected following genotypic resistance testing, a failure in antiretroviral therapy may be due to non-compliance or poor absorption—therapeutic drug monitoring may be useful in this circumstance.

12.9

- The failure to produce an effective HIV-1 vaccine is in part down to the high mutation rate of the HIV-1 virus, and the inability of the immune system to produce a broad spectrum of cross-neutralizing antibodies capable of recognizing a range of target envelope antigens.

Chapter 13

13.1

- See Figures 13.1 and 13.2.

13.2

- MHC class I and II both present peptides that interact with the TCR. Class I is a closed binding groove with more restricted peptide length than class II. MHC I uses CD8 as a co-receptor, whereas MHC II uses CD4.

13.3

- HLA alleles are named as:

HLA–Gene-*-two digit allele group: three digit protein group: two digit synonym: two digit non coding variance: expression digit, e.g. HLA-A*02:101:01:02N

13.4

- HLA molecular typing may either be by PCR-SSP, PCR-SSOP, or sequence based typing. Both SSP and SSOP require that the allele is already known, since sequence-specific probes are generated. With sequence based typing new alleles can be identified and characterized, since a whole HLA sequence will be generated.

13.5

- HLA antibodies may be detected by ELISA or LUMINEX technologies.

13.6

- Kidneys are allocated based on need and probability of greatest benefit. Included in this are age, cold ischaemia time, and HLA match.

Tier	Patients
A	000 mismatched paediatric patients–highly sensitized* or HLA-DR homozygous
B	000 mismatched paediatric patients–others (all except those in Tier A)
C	000 mismatched adult patients–highly sensitized* or HLA-DR homozygous
D	• 000 mismatched adult patients–others (all except those in Tier C) • Favourably matched paediatric patients (100, 010, 110 mismatches)
E	All other eligible patients

- Usually one kidney is retained locally and the other offered nationally unless the donor is under 5 or over 50 years old, in which case both are retained locally.

13.7

- Crossmatching may be 'real' or virtual. Virtual cross matching uses known donor specific antibody status in the recipient and compares this with the HLA antigens of the donor. Live cross matching may be by complement dependent cytotoxicity (CDC) assay, flow cross match, or solid phase assay.

13.8

- The ability of the T cell adaptive immune system to see antigens is dependent on the MHC binding of a peptide and then presenting this to T cells. Certain HLA types will preferentially bind and present certain antigens. In extreme cases individuals will only develop a disorder if they have the specific HLA haplotype that allows the presentation of immune pathogenic peptides. Coeliac disease is a good example where only certain DQ2/8 heterodimers allow presentation of deamidated gladin peptides which cause disease.

Index

A

Q

R

S

T

U